Serono Symposia USA
Norwell, Massachusetts

Springer
New York
Berlin
Heidelberg
Barcelona
Hong Kong
London
Milan
Paris
Singapore
Tokyo

PROCEEDINGS IN THE SERONO SYMPOSIA USA SERIES

ART AND THE HUMAN BLASTOCYST
Edited by David K. Gardner and Michelle Lane

QUALITY OF THE BODY CELL MASS: Body Composition in the Third Millennium
Edited by Richard N. Pierson, Jr.

OVULATION: Evolving Scientific and Clinical Concepts
Edited by Eli Y. Adashi

THE TESTIS: From Stem Cell to Sperm Function
Edited by Erwin Goldberg

BIOLOGY OF MENOPAUSE
Edited by Francis L. Bellino

THERAPEUTIC OUTCOME OF ENDOCRINE DISORDERS:
Efficacy, Innovation and Quality of Life
Edited by Brian Stabler and Barry B. Bercu

EMBRYO IMPLANTATION: Molecular, Cellular and Clinical Aspects
Edited by Daniel D. Carson

SEX-STEROID INTERACTIONS WITH GROWTH HORMONE
Edited by Johannes D. Veldhuis and Andrea Giustina

MALE STERILITY AND MOTILITY DISORDERS:
Etiological Factors and Treatment. A Serono Symposia S.A. Publication
Edited by Samir Hamamah, Roger Mieusset, François Olivennes, and René Frydman

NUTRITIONAL ASPECTS OF OSTEOPOROSIS. A Serono Symposia S.A. Publication
Edited by Peter Burckhardt, Bess Dawson-Hughes, and Robert P. Heaney

GERM CELL DEVELOPMENT, DIVISION, DISRUPTION AND DEATH
Edited by Barry R. Zirkin

CELL DEATH IN REPRODUCTIVE PHYSIOLOGY
Edited by Jonathan L. Tilly, Jerome F. Strauss III, and Martin Tenniswood

INHIBIN, ACTIVIN AND FOLLISTATIN: Regulatory Functions
in System and Cell Biology. A Serono Symposia S.A. Publication
Edited by Toshihiro Aono, Hiromu Sugino, and Wylie W. Vale

PERIMENOPAUSE
Edited by Rogerio A. Lobo

GROWTH FACTORS AND WOUND HEALING: Basic Science and
Potential Clinical Applications
Edited by Thomas R. Ziegler, Glenn F. Pierce, and David N. Herndon

POLYCYSTIC OVARY SYNDROME
Edited by R. Jeffrey Chang

IDEA TO PRODUCT: The Process
Edited by Nancy J. Alexander and Anne Colston Wentz

Continued after Index

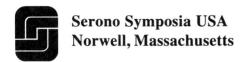

Serono Symposia USA
Norwell, Massachusetts

David K. Gardner   Michelle Lane
Editors

ART and the Human Blastocyst

With 41 Figures

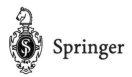

Springer

David K. Gardner, D.Phil.
Michelle Lane, Ph.D.
Colorado Center for Reproductive Medicine
Englewood, CO 80110
USA

Proceedings of the International Symposium on ART and the Human Blastocyst, sponsored by Serono Symposia USA, Inc., held March 30 to April 2, 2000, in Dana Point, California.

For information on previous volumes, contact Serono Symposia USA, Inc.

Library of Congress Cataloging-in-Publication Data
ART and the human blastocyst / edited by David K. Gardner, Michelle Lane.
   p. cm.
   Proceedings of the Serono symposia.
   Includes bibliographical references and index.
   ISBN 0-387-95245-4 (alk. paper)
   1. Ovum implantation—Congresses. 2. Human reproductive technology—Congresses.
3. Blastocyst—Congresses. I. Gardner, David K. II. Lane, Michelle.
RG133.5 .A76 2001
618.1'7806—dc21   00-067927

Printed on acid-free paper.

© 2001 Springer-Verlag New York, Inc.
All rights reserved. This work may not be translated or copied in whole or in part without the written permission of the publisher (Springer-Verlag New York, Inc., 175 Fifth Avenue, New York, NY 10010, USA), except for brief excerpts in connection with reviews or scholarly analysis. Use in connection with any form of information storage and retrieval, electronic adaptation, computer software, or by similar or dissimilar methodology now known or hereafter developed is forbidden.
The use of general descriptive names, trade names, trademarks, etc., in this publication, even if the former are not especially identified, is not to be taken as a sign that such names, as understood by the Trade Marks and Merchandise Marks Act, may accordingly be used freely by anyone.
While the advice and information in this book are believed to be true and accurate at the date of going to press, neither the authors, nor the editors, nor the publisher, nor Serono Symposia USA, Inc., can accept any legal responsibility for any errors or omissions that may be made. The publisher makes no warranty, express or implied, with respect to the material contained herein.
Authorization to photocopy items for internal or personal use, or the internal or personal use of specific clients, is granted by Springer-Verlag New York, Inc., provided that the appropriate fee is paid directly to Copyright Clearance Center, 222 Rosewood Drive, Danvers, MA 01923, USA (Telephone: (508) 750-8400), stating the ISBN number, the volume title, and the first and last page numbers of each article copied. The copyright owner's consent does not include copying for general distribution, promotion, new works, or resale. In these cases, specific written permission must first be obtained from the publisher.

Production coordinated by Chernow Editorial Services, Inc., and managed by Francine McNeill; manufacturing supervised by Erica Bresler.
Typeset by KP Company, Brooklyn, NY.
Printed and bound by Edwards Brothers, Inc., Ann Arbor, MI.
Printed in the United States of America.

9 8 7 6 5 4 3 2 1

ISBN 0-387-95245-4   SPIN 10793875

Springer-Verlag New York Berlin Heidelberg
A member of BertelsmannSpringer Science+Business Media GmbH

SYMPOSIUM ON ART AND THE HUMAN BLASTOCYST

Scientific Committee

    David K. Gardner, D.Phil., Chair
    Michelle Lane, Ph.D.
    Thomas B. Pool, Ph.D.
    William B. Schoolcraft, M.D.

Organizing Secretary

    Cindy J. Bell, Pharm.D., Executive Director
    Serono Symposia USA, Inc.
    100 Longwater Circle
    Norwell, Massachusetts

Preface

The field of human artificial reproductive technology (ART) is continually advancing and has witnessed significant changes since the inception of Louise Brown in 1978. Though Louise Brown herself was conceived after the transfer of a blastocyst, there remain significant confusion and debate regarding the stage at which the human embryo conceived in the laboratory should be replaced in the mother. Developments in culture media formulations, leading to the introduction of sequential media, have brought the role of the blastocyst in human ART back into the spotlight. It was due to this resurgence of interest in the niche of extended culture in human infertility treatment that the symposium on "ART and the Human Blastocyst" was held.

The proceedings of this meeting within this volume bring to the forefront the main issues raised with the transfer of embryos at the blastocyst stage. It is evident from the chapters that follow that ART needs to be perceived as a continuum of procedures, each one dependent on the preceding one, and all equally as important as each other. That is to say, the development of a competent embryo is ultimately dependent on the quality of the gametes from which it was derived. With regard to the oocyte, this then places the emphasis on the physician to use a stimulation protocol that both produces quality oocytes and does not impair endometrial function. Maintenance of gamete and embryo quality is the laboratory's role. It is beyond the ability of the laboratory to increase the viability of the conceptus. It is evident that culture media used in a laboratory are but one part of the culture system. Differences in results between laboratories, therefore, may not reflect on the culture media, but they may be due to other aspects of laboratory procedures and other factors impacting media performance (which in turn reflects on laboratory quality assurance). This should always be borne in mind when results from one group do not agree with those of another. Blastocyst culture and transfer are not a panacea for other problems within the IVF clinic. The culmination of the treatment cycle is the embryo transfer procedure and luteal phase support, both critical in determining the final outcome, and both as diverse in their clinical application between clinics, and therefore a large source of variation in results.

Although the final role of the blastocyst in human ART awaits further clinical studies, the one niche it has already claimed is in the reduction of high-order multiple gestations. For many patients blastocyst culture and transfer will facilitate the successful move to a single embryo transfer.

This symposium and subsequent proceedings could not have been possible without the tireless work of Cindy Bell and the staff of Serono Symposia USA. Our gratitude also goes to Thomas Pool and William Schoolcraft for their assistance with the program. The success of the symposium itself was due to the quality presentations and manuscripts provided by leaders in the field of human ART and mammalian embryology. We are indebted to them for taking the time to participate in this project.

DAVID K. GARDNER
MICHELLE LANE

Contents

Preface vii
Contributors xiii

Part I. Gamete Quality and Pregnancy Outcome

1. The Impact of High-Order Multiple Pregnancies 3
   JOHN A. SCHNORR AND HOWARD W. JONES, JR.

2. Patient Stimulation and Effect on Outcomes 21
   DAVID R. MELDRUM

3. New Developments in Imaging and Hormonal
   Stimulation of the Ovaries 29
   ROGER A. PIERSON

4. Paternal Effects on Fertilization, Embryo
   Development, and Pregnancy Outcome 38
   DENNY SAKKAS, GIANCARLO MANICARDI, DAVIDE BIZZARO,
   ODETTE MOFFATT, AND MATHEW TOMLINSON

Part II. Physiology of the Embryo

5. The Cell Biology of Preimplantation Development 51
   RICHARD J. TASCA

6. Metabolism of the Early Embryo:
   Energy Production and Utilization 61
   HENRY J. LEESE, ISABELLE DONNAY, DONALD A. MACMILLAN,
   AND FRANCHESCA D. HOUGHTON

7. Blastomere Homeostasis 69
   MICHELLE LANE AND DAVID K. GARDNER

8. Cell Junctions and Cell Interactions in Animal and
   Human Blastocyst Development 91
   TOM P. FLEMING, M. REZA GHASSEMIFAR, JUDITH ECKERT,
   ASPASIA DESTOUNI, FAY THOMAS, JANE E. COLLINS,
   AND BHAVWANTI SHETH

Part III.   Blastocyst Development in Culture

9. Blastocyst Development in Culture:
   The Role of Macromolecules 105
   THOMAS B. POOL

10. Culture Systems and Blastocyst Development 118
    DAVID K. GARDNER, MICHELLE LANE, AND WILLIAM B. SCHOOLCRAFT

11. Apoptosis in the Human Blastocyst: Role of Survival Factors 144
    KATE HARDY AND SOPHIE SPANOS

12. Predictors of Viability of the Human Blastocyst 155
    NATALIE A. CEKLENIAK, KATHARINE V. JACKSON,
    AND CATHERINE RACOWSKY

Part IV.   Blastocyst Transfer and Fate

13. Which Patients Should Have Blastocyst Transfer? 167
    KEVIN DOODY

14. Embryo Transfer and Luteal Phase Support 184
    WILLIAM B. SCHOOLCRAFT

15. Cryopreservation of Blastocysts 188
    YVES MENEZO, DENNY SAKKAS, AND ANNA VEIGA

Part V. Implantation

16. Embryo–Maternal Dialogue in the Apposition
    and Adhesion Phases of Human Implantation 199
    CARLOS SIMÓN, JOSE LOUIS DE PABLO, JULIO C. MARTIN,
    MARCOS MESEGUER, ARANCHA GALÁN, AND ANTONIO PELLICER

17. Biomarkers and the Assessment of Uterine Receptivity 210
    BRUCE A. LESSEY

18. Endometrial Pinopodes: Relevance for
    Human Blastocyst Implantation 227
    URSULA BENTIN-LEY AND GEORGE NIKAS

19. The Future: Toward Single Embryo Transfer 236
    LARS HAMBERGER, PETER SVALANDER, AND MATTS WIKLAND

20. The Niche of the Blastocyst in Human ART 241
    JESSE HADE AND ALAN H. DECHERNEY

Author Index 247

Subject Index 249

Contributors

URSULA BENTIN-LEY, The Fertility Unit, Department of Obstetrics and Gynecology, Herlev Hospital, University of Copenhagen, Herlev, Denmark.

DAVIDE BIZZARO, Department of Animal Biology, University of Modena, Modena, Italy.

NATALIE A. CEKLENIAK, Department of Obstetrics, Gynecology and Reproductive Biology, Brigham and Women's Hospital, Harvard Medical School, Boston, Massachusetts, USA.

JANE E. COLLINS, Division of Cell and Molecular Medicine, School of Medicine, University of Southampton, Southampton, UK.

ALAN H. DECHERNEY, Department of Obstetrics and Gynecology, School of Medicine, University of California at Los Angeles, Los Angeles, California, USA.

JOSE LOUIS DE PABLO, Instituto Valenciano de Infertilidad Foundation (FIVIER), Valencia, Spain.

ASPASIA DESTOUNI, Division of Cell Sciences, School of Biological Sciences, University of Southampton, Southampton, UK.

ISABELLE DONNAY, Veterinary Unit, Catholic University of Louvain, Louvain-la-Neuve, Belgium.

KEVIN DOODY, Center for Assisted Reproduction, Bedford, Texas, USA.

JUDITH ECKERT, Division of Cell Sciences, School of Biological Sciences, University of Southampton, Southampton, UK.

TOM P. FLEMING, Division of Cell Sciences, School of Biological Sciences, University of Southampton, Southampton, UK.

ARANCHA GALÁN, Instituto Valenciano de Infertilidad Foundation (FIVIER), Valencia, Spain.

DAVID K. GARDNER, Colorado Center for Reproductive Medicine, Englewood, Colorado, USA.

M. REZA GHASSEMIFAR, Division of Cell Sciences, School of Biological Sciences, University of Southampton, Southampton, UK.

JESSE HADE, Department of Obstetrics and Gynecology, School of Medicine, University of California at Los Angeles, Los Angeles, California, USA.

LARS HAMBERGER, Department of Obstetrics and Gynecology, University of Gothenburg, Gothenburg, Sweden.

KATE HARDY, Department of Reproductive Science and Medicine, Division of Pediatrics, Obstetrics and Gynecology, Imperial College School of Medicine, Hammersmith Hospital, London, UK.

FRANCHESCA D. HOUGHTON, Department of Biology, University of York, York, UK.

KATHARINE V. JACKSON, Department of Obstetrics, Gynecology and Reproductive Biology, Brigham and Women's Hospital, Harvard Medical School, Boston, Massachusetts, USA.

HOWARD W. JONES, JR., Division of Reproductive Endocrinology and Infertility, Jones Institute for Reproductive Medicine, Norfolk, Virginia, USA.

MICHELLE LANE, Colorado Center for Reproductive Medicine, Englewood, Colorado, USA.

HENRY J. LEESE, Department of Biology, University of York, York, UK.

BRUCE A. LESSEY, Department of Obstetrics and Gynecology, Division of

Reproductive Endocrinology and Infertility, University of North Carolina at Chapel Hill, Chapel Hill, North Carolina, USA.

DONALD A. MACMILLAN, Department of Biology, University of York, York, UK.

GIANCARLO MANICARDI, Department of Animal Biology, University of Modena, Modena, Italy.

JULIO C. MARTIN, Instituto Valenciano de Infertilidad Foundation (FIVIER), Valencia, Spain.

DAVID R. MELDRUM, Reproductive Partners Medical Group, Redondo Beach, California, USA.

YVES MENEZO, Laboratoire Marcel Merieux, Bron, France.

MARCOS MESEGUER, Instituto Valenciano de Infertilidad Foundation (FIVIER), Valencia, Spain.

ODETTE MOFFATT, Assisted Conception Unit, Birmingham Women's Hospital, Edgbaston, Birmingham, UK.

GEORGE NIKAS, Department of Obstetrics and Gynecology, Huddinge Hospital, Karolinska Institute, Stockholm, Sweden.

ANTONIO PELLICER, Department of Pediatrics, Obstetrics and Gynecology, Valencia University, and Instituto Valenciano de Infertilidad Foundation (FIVIER), Valencia, Spain.

ROGER A. PIERSON, Department of Obstetrics, Gynecology and Reproductive Sciences, College of Medicine, University of Saskatchewan, Saskatoon, Saskatchewan, Canada.

THOMAS B. POOL, Fertility Center of San Antonio, San Antonio, Texas, USA.

CATHERINE RACOWSKY, Department of Obstetrics, Gynecology and Reproductive Biology, Brigham and Women's Hospital, Harvard Medical School, Boston, Massachusetts, USA.

DENNY SAKKAS, Assisted Conception Unit, Birmingham Women's Hospital, Edgbaston, Birmingham, UK.

JOHN A. SCHNORR, Division of Reproductive Endocrinology and Infertility, Jones Institute for Reproductive Medicine, Norfolk, Virginia, USA.

WILLIAM B. SCHOOLCRAFT, Colorado Center for Reproductive Medicine, Englewood, Colorado, USA.

BHAVWANTI SHETH, Division of Cell Sciences, School of Biological Sciences, University of Southampton, Southampton, UK.

CARLOS SIMÓN, Department of Pediatrics, Obstetrics and Gynecology, Valencia University, and Instituto Valenciano de Infertilidad Foundation (FIVIER), Valencia, Spain.

SOPHIE SPANOS, Department of Reproductive Science and Medicine, Division of Pediatrics, Obstetrics and Gynecology, Imperial College School of Medicine, Hammersmith Hospital, London, UK.

PETER SVALANDER, Vitrolife AB, Gothenburg, Sweden.

RICHARD J. TASCA, National Institute of Child Health and Human Development, National Institutes of Health, Bethesda, Maryland, USA.

FAY THOMAS, Division of Cell Sciences, School of Biological Sciences, University of Southampton, Southampton, UK.

MATHEW TOMLINSON, Assisted Conception Unit, Birmingham Women's Hospital, Edgbaston, Birmingham, UK.

ANNA VEIGA, Department of Obstetrics and Gynecology, Institute Universitari Dexeus, Barcelona, Spain.

MATTS WIKLAND, Fertility Center, Carlanderska Hospital, Gothenburg, Sweden.

Part I

Gamete Quality and Pregnancy Outcome

1
The Impact of High-Order Multiple Pregnancies

JOHN A. SCHNORR AND HOWARD W. JONES, JR.

Introduction

Between 1980 and 1997 the number and rate of twin, triplet, and higher-order multiple births has climbed at an unprecedented pace within the United States. The number of live births in twin deliveries rose 52% between 1980 and 1997, and the number of live births in triplet and higher-order multiple pregnancies increased an astounding 404%. In sharp contract, single births during the same time period rose 6%. The last several years has witnessed an even more remarkable aspect to the trend in multiple pregnancies in that there was nearly a 1,000% increase in the incidence of multiple gestation among women 45–49 years of age between 1980 and 1997 (1). These extraordinary increases in the incidence of multiple pregnancy is a public health concern due to the considerable medical, social, and financial consequences of multiple gestation.

Trends in Twin, Triplet, and High-Order Multiple Births

The most recent statistics available from the U.S. Department of Health and Human Services (published September 14, 1999) demonstrates an alarming trend in twin, triplet, and high-order multiple births. The number of infants born between 1980 and 1997 in multiple deliveries rose at a remarkable pace. Twin births since 1980 have risen 52% from 68,339 to 104,137 births. The number of triplet and higher-order gestations has quadrupled, climbing from 1,337 to 6,737 births. Within the category of triplet and higher-order multiple births, triplet births have increased 142%, quadruplet pregnancies increased 123%, and quintuplet and higher-order births increased 98% between 1989 and 1997 (Fig. 1.1) (1).

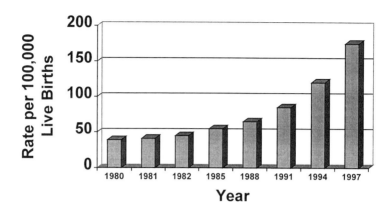

FIGURE 1.1. Triplets and other higher-order multiples on the rise.

Broken down by age group, twinning rates for all groups rose between 1980 and 1997, but the increases were most pronounced among women 30 years of age and older. During the same time interval, twin births rose by 12% for teenage mothers, 41% for women in their thirties, 63% for women 40–44 years of age, and nearly 1,000% among women 45–49 years of age. In 1990 there were only 39 twin deliveries for women between the age of 45 and 49, but there were 444 twin deliveries in 1997.

There appears to be significant geographic variation in the incidence of multiple births because twin and triplet birth rates within the United States for the 50 states and the District of Columbia for 1995–1997 ranged widely. The twin birth rate for Massachusetts and Connecticut was 32.6 per 1,000 births, which is at least 25% higher than the rate for the entire United States and 75% higher than that for Hawaii. Triplet and higher-order birth rates for Nebraska (323.6 per 100,000 births) and New Jersey (306.6 per 100,000 birth) were twice the U.S. level of 151.2 births per 100,000 births. Among the factors that may be influencing the variation in state twin and higher-order birth rates are state differences in maternal age, distributions, and access to fertility clinics that are concentrated mostly in the Northeast, where twin and triplet birth rates tend to be higher (2,3).

A dramatic increase in low birth weight infants is associated with this dramatic increase in the multiple pregnancy rates. Between 1980 and 1997 twins were noted to have an eightfold increase, and triplet and higher-order multiple pregnancies a 33-fold increase, in the incidence of being born at a weight less than 1,500 g, which is typically classified as very low birth weight (VLBW). More than half of all twins and nearly all triplet and higher-order multiple births, compared with only 6% of single gestations, are born in the low birth weight (LBW) group at less than 2,500 g.

The ultimate price of multiple pregnancies is perhaps reflected in the infant mortality rate. Multiple births born to women at any age are high-risk births. Twins are four times, triplets 10 times, quadruplets 13 times, and quintuplets 30 times more likely than singletons to die within the first month of life (1,4).

The significant increase in multiple births appears to coincide with two overlapping and related trends. The first is the older age at childbearing, which within spontaneous conceptions older women are more likely to have a multiple birth. Second, there is an increase in the availability and use of fertility-enhancing therapies that typically result in a high percentage of multiple pregnancies. It has been estimated that approximately one third of the increase in multiple births since the early 1980s has been attributed to a shift in maternal age distribution, whereas the remaining two thirds is likely the result of fertility-enhancing therapies (5–8). If these estimates are reliable, the fertility-enhancing therapies translate into more than 225,000 multiple births over the 1980–1997 study period (1).

The Cost of the Problem

Multiple pregnancies represent a health risk to both the mother and fetus, which subsequently places immense financial and psychosocial pressures upon the family and surrounding community. The maternal increased health risk starts early in gestation with an increase in the risk of miscarriage and vanishing twin syndrome. Anemia is also frequently reported in multiple gestations due to the increase in blood volume compared with red cell mass, which lowers the hemoglobin concentration.

In the second and third trimester, preterm labor and delivery (before 37 weeks gestation) occur with increasing frequency as the number of fetuses in utero increases. This poses significant risks to the mother due to the need for hospitalization and intravenous tocolytic therapy thereby placing the mother at risk for major cardiovascular events such as pulmonary edema (9,10).

The incidence of pregnancy-induced hypertension, preeclampsia, and eclampsia are all increased in multiple pregnancies. Primigravida women with a twin pregnancy have a fivefold greater risk of severe pre-eclampsia than it does with a singleton pregnancy. Multigravida with a multiple gestation are at 10-fold greater risk relative to that of a singleton pregnancy (11).

Other maternal risks associated with a multifetal gestation include hydramnios, antepartum hemorrhage, and antepartum fetal death. Intrapartum risks include an increased risk for an operative delivery and significantly increased likelihood of cesarean delivery (4). Postpartum complications can include postpartum hemorrhage and significant psychosocial stressors associated with the demand of two or more babies.

The fetus is also at significant increased risk in a multiple gestation. Reports from Australia, the United Kingdom, and the United States of America have demonstrated that multiple pregnancy was associated with a significant increase in perinatal mortality. It was estimated that the perinatal mortality rate of twins is up to 10-fold that of singleton gestations; however, if a broader definition is used to include late abortion and late neonatal death, the risk is further doubled (1,4).

Preterm delivery (before 37 completed weeks gestation) is the greatest threat to fetuses in multiple gestations. The median duration of pregnancy decreases as the number of fetuses in utero increases as illustrated in Figure 1.2. The average number of weeks completed by singleton gestation is 39 weeks. Twin gestations average 35 weeks, triplet gestations 33 weeks, and quadruplet gestations 29 completed weeks (12). The overall incidence of preterm delivery in a twin gestation approaches 50% which is 12 times higher than that seen in singleton pregnancies. Most neonatal deaths in multiple premature births are associated with gestations of less than 32 weeks and birth weights of under 1,500 g.

Fetuses of multiple gestations are also at increased risk for intrauterine growth restriction. Up to two thirds of twin infants show clinical and objective signs of intrauterine growth restriction. There can also be disparity in the growth rates between twins and other gestations in utero. This is most prominent in twin–twin transfusion syndrome that occurs in approximately 15% of monochorionic twin pregnancies and in these situations the perinatal mortality rate for both twins is high.

Major congenital anomalies are twice as common in multiple pregnancies compared with singletons. Abnormalities found exclusively in multiple pregnancy are conjoined twins and acardia. Neural tube defects, bowel atresia, and cardiac anomalies have also been associated with increased incidence in multiple gestations.

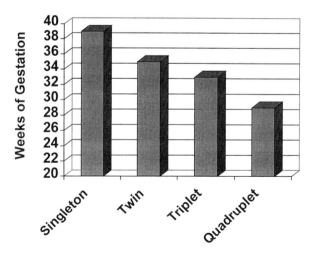

FIGURE 1.2. Average length of gestation in relation to number of fetuses.

Intrapartum complications of a multiple pregnancy are also significantly increased above that of a singleton pregnancy. The intrapartum complications can include malpresentation, cord prolapse, cord entanglement, and fetal distress. Locking or collision of twins is possible, however extremely rare.

The financial costs associated with multifetal pregnancy include the costs associated with prenatal care, maternal hospitalization, and most significantly with the mean number of days a neonate spends in the neonatal intensive care unit (NICU). The amount of time a neonate spends within the intensive care unit is directly related to his or her gestational age at delivery. The mean NICU length of stay based upon gestational age which ranges from more than 80 days of hospitalization at 25 weeks of delivery to 28 days at 32 weeks of delivery and less than 5 days with term deliveries (Fig. 1.3) (13). The cost per day hospitalized in the NICU can vary widely; however, it is estimated that each day costs approximately $1,000 per infant in the NICU. This results in a neonatal cost alone in excess of $80,000 for each infant delivered at 25 weeks and $28,000 for infants delivered at 32 weeks.

High-order multiple births are associated both with increased maternal and perinatal mortality and morbidity; rather, they also stretch the mother, family, and community resources because of the many complications associated with their pregnancy, birth, and future development. One study of 20 consecutive triplet pregnancies in a Boston hospital revealed that the average maternal hospitalization was 16.7 days costing $20,067. The average neonatal stay was 13.6 days per live born with an average cost of $36,885, resulting in a total cost per triplet pregnancy of more than $64,000. This is a significant increase in cost above that associated with a singleton gestation that is typically less than $9,000 (14).

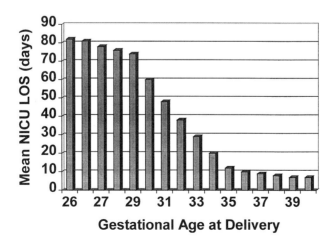

FIGURE 1.3. Mean NICU length of stay based on gestational age.

The Cause of Increased Multiple Gestations

The increase in the incidence of twin, triplet, and higher-order gestation has been associated with two overlapping trends within the United States. The first trend is the older age at childbearing, which physiologically increases the likelihood of a multiple birth within a spontaneous conception cycle. It has been estimated that approximately one third of the increase in multiple births since the 1980s has been attributed to the shift in maternal age distribution; however, the remainder of the increase is due to the use of assisted reproductive technologies.

Assisted reproductive technologies can be divided into two categories: artificial ovulation induction alone with the use of clomiphene citrate, and/or injectable gonadotropins, which results in the development of multiple mature follicles and a possibility for high-order multiple pregnancies. Unlike the other forms of assisted reproductive technology, physicians do not have as much control over the number of fertilized embryos available for implantation.

It is difficult to ascertain the impact of artificial ovulation induction alone with regards to the multiple pregnancy rates. Levene et al. (15) studied 156 consecutive triplet and higher order multiple pregnancies. Of the 156 pregnancies, 144 were triplet gestations and 12 were quadruplet and quintuplet gestations. Table 1.1 details the method of conception in the 156 pregnancies. Forty-seven of the 144 (32%) triplet pregnancies were spontaneous pregnancies, and none of the quadruplet and quintuplet pregnancies were spontaneous. Forty-four out of the 144 (30%) triplet pregnancies were a consequence of ovarian stimulation alone, and 8 out of the 12 (66%) quadruplet and quintuplet pregnancies were from ovarian stimulation. In vitro fertilization and gamete intrafallopian transfer (GIFT) accounted for 53 of the triplet pregnancies or 36% and four or 33% of the quadruplet and quintuplet pregnancies (15).

The significant impact of the sole use of fertility-enhancing drugs alone was further identified in a study by Derom et al., who studied 458 twin and 78 triplet pregnancies resulting from assisted reproductive technologies. An

TABLE 1.1. Method of conception in 156 triplet and higher multiple pregnancies.

Method of conception	Triplets	Quads and quins
Natural conception	47	0
Ovarian stimulation	44	8
IVF-ET	36	1
GIFT	14	3
Total	144	12

Source: Data from Levene et al. (15).

analysis revealed that the majority of multiple pregnancies were from ovulation induction alone and did not result from advance technologies such as in vitro fertilization (IVF), GIFT, or ZIFT. In 77% (351 out of 458) of the twin pregnancies and 72% (56 out of 78) of the triplet pregnancies, artificial induction of ovulation alone was the only treatment (16).

IVF allows more control over the multiple pregnancy rates by allowing the patient and physician to determine the optimum number of embryos to transfer. It is often a difficult decision for the physician and patient due to the heavy focus on maximizing a woman's chance of becoming pregnant. One common practice at maximizing the chance of pregnancy is to transfer multiple embryos into the uterine cavity. As expected, this also results in a dramatic increase in the multiple pregnancy rate.

In 1999 Schieve et al. (17) examined the association between the number of embryos transferred in IVF and the live birth and multiple birth rate in 35,554 IVF transfer procedures performed within the United States. As an increasing number of embryos are transferred, the pregnancy rate increases until three embryos or more are transferred (Fig. 1.4). Three or more embryos transferred generally results in a plateauing of the pregnancy rate; however, the multiple pregnancy rate continues to increase with each additional embryo transferred. The only exceptions are women aged 35–39 years and 40–44 years, which demonstrate a continued increase in pregnancy rates before the plateau occurs at four embryos transferred in a 35–39 age group and five embryos in the 40–44 age group (17).

A similar study by Templeton et al. analyzed 44,236 cycles within the United Kingdom to study the factors associated with an increased risk of multiple births. Their study also noted no significant statistical difference between the pregnancy rate with the transfer of two or three embryos in those patients with greater than four fertilized embryos (Fig. 1.5); however, the multiple pregnancy rate in women aged 30–35 years increased from 28.6% with the transfer of two embryos to 39.4% with the transfer of three embryos, which is a statistically significant change. This study was unable to examine elective transfer of high number of embryos due to the United Kingdom limits of number of embryos transferred to three (18).

Actual Versus Theoretical Pregnancy and Multiple Pregnancy Rates

Physicians are commonly confronted with pressure from patients and competing programs to transfer more embryos in an effort to increase pregnancy rates. The result of these pressures is illustrated through the use of simple calculations to determine the estimated pregnancy rate and estimated rate of multiple gestations based upon the number of embryos transferred. In this theoretical example, an implantation rate of 14% for all fresh transfers is

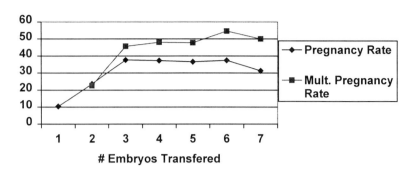

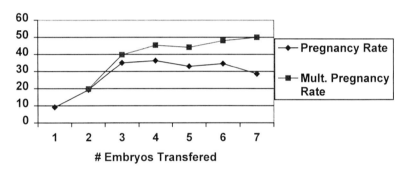

FIGURE 1.4. Pregnancy and multiple pregnancy rates based upon the number of embryos transferred in IVF-ET cycles (17).

utilized based upon our average fresh-cycle implantation rate at the Jones Institute for Reproductive Medicine between October 1987 and June 1999. The transfer of one embryo would accordingly yield a pregnancy rate of 14% with 100% of those pregnancies being singleton gestations. With the transfer of two embryos, the theoretical pregnancy rate increases to 26.04%, with 92.47% of those pregnancies being singleton and 7.53% being twin gestation. The transfer for three embryos results in a pregnancy rate of 36.39%, 85% of which are singleton, 13.89% are twins, and 0.75% triplets. The transfer of four embryos results in a pregnancy rate of 45.3%, of which 78.63% are singletons, 19.2% are twins, 2.8% are triplets, and quadruplets account for 0.08% (Table 1.2).

The actual results are quite different. The transfer of one mature embryo in 46 cycles resulted in four pregnancies or pregnancy rate per transfer of 9% (Table 1.3). The transfer of two mature embryos in 96 cycles resulted in 19 pregnancies

Age 34 thru 39

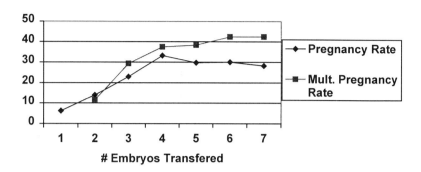

Age 40 thru 44

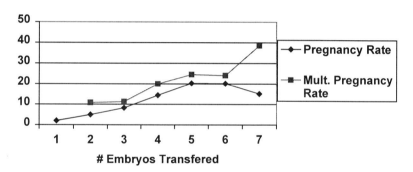

FIGURE 1.4. *Continued.*

with a resulting pregnancy rate of 20%. Of those pregnancies, four or 21% were twins. The transfer of three mature embryos resulted in 152 pregnancies from 436 transfers or a pregnancy rate of 35%, of which 23% were twins, 8% triplets, and 0.6% quadruplets. The transfer of four mature embryos resulted in 393 pregnancies of 989 transfers with a pregnancy rate of 40%, 21% of which are twins, 9% triplets, and the quadruplet rate was 2%. The transfer of five mature embryos in 384 cycles resulted in 158 pregnancies, or a pregnancy rate of 41%. This resulted in 22% of pregnancies being twin gestations, one triplet, one quadruplet, and one quintuplet gestation. The transfer of six embryos occurred in 89 cycles with 27 pregnancies or pregnancy rate of 30%. Of those pregnancies, 7% were twins and 7% were triplets.

There is considerable difference between the theoretical and actual pregnancy and multiple pregnancy rates. The increased frequency of multiple pregnancies relative to the predicted frequency based upon a fixed implantation rate suggests that there are "extraembryo" factors that significantly affect each embryo within a given cycle. These extraembryo factors could

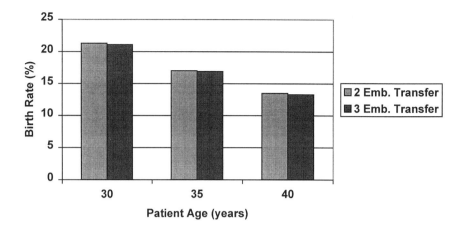
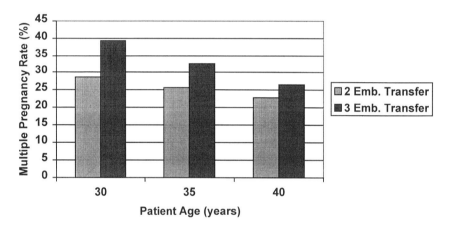

FIGURE 1.5. Pregnancy and multiple pregnancy rates per embryo transferred in patients with more than 4 fertilized eggs in the United Kingdom (18).

include specific endometrial factors, embryo transfer techniques, and embryo culture conditions.

Attempted Solutions to the High-Order Multiple Pregnancies

A significant portion of the multiple pregnancy rates (about two thirds, according to a British study [15]) are due to reproductive technologies.

For ovulation induction, multiple pregnancies are avoidable by monitoring the degree of ovarian stimulation through a combination of serum estradiol levels and the identification of the number of follicles developing by

TABLE 1.2. Theoretical fresh pregnancy rate and multiple pregnancy rate assuming an implantation rate of 14%.

No. transferred	Pregnancy rate	Singleton	Twin	Triplet	Quadruplet
1	14.0%	100%			
2	26.04%	92.5%	7.5%		
3	36.39%	85.4%	13.9%	0.8%	
4	45.30%	78.6%	19.2%	2%	0.1%

ultrasound imaging. Several options are available when too many follicles are developing. The cycle can be halted and the injection of hCG, which stimulates ovulation, can be withheld. Other options include converting the cycle into IVF, which will allow the retrieval of eggs and the controlled placement of a limited number of embryos into the uterine cavity. A portion of the follicles can also be aspirated and discarded before giving hCG, thereby limiting the number of available eggs. An editorial by Hershlag reviewed various options for this problem (19).

It is of significance that no official or unofficial body has offered any regulations or guidelines to avoid high-order multiple pregnancies due to ovulation induction.

It seems that a third to perhaps as many as one half, of the problem of high-order multiple pregnancies can be attributed to IVF and its variants.

There has been a considerable international effort to solve this problem. This has taken the form of the issuance of guidelines or regulations by unofficial or official bodies, indicating a maximum number of preembryos considered allowable to transfer.

Under the aegis of the International Federation of Fertility Societies (IFFS), a compilation of these guidelines, regulations, or the absence of either, was made for 38 nations (20). Although this compilation concerned multiple aspects of assisted reproductive technologies, only the compilation in relation to the number of preembryos to transfer is pertinent to this discussion. The survey of sovereign political entities (i.e., nations or states) fell into three

TABLE 1.3. Actual fresh pregnancy and multiple pregnancy rate at the Jones Institute between October 1987 and June 1999.

No. transferred	Pregnancy rate	Singleton	Twin	Triplet	Quadruplet and higher
1	9.0%	100%			
2	20.0%	79%	21%		
3	35.0%	68.4%	23%	8%	0.6%
4	40.0%	68%	21%	9%	2%
5	41%	76.2%	22%	0.6%	1.2%
6	30%	86%	7%	7%	

categories: (1) those with legislation, (2) those with voluntary guidelines, and (3) those with neither. Among the 23 entities with legislation (Table 1.4), there are nine entities that limit the number of embryos to be transferred, with that number varying from two to a maximum of four. Regulations are often rather specific, and allow no exceptions. The penalties for violation are not trivial. For instance, a clinic's license to practice might be withdrawn (United Kingdom), there could be a fine or imprisonment (Germany), and imprisonment and a fine of at least FS1 million (Switzerland), loss of license, probably imprisonment (South Australia, Australia), and loss of license (Sweden). It is interesting enough that 14 of the nations operating with legislation do not indicate a limit to the number to be transferred.

Four of the 10-guideline countries specifically limit the number to transfer, although in the nature of the thing, there is no enforcement mechanism. One country (the United States) when surveyed, even though it was not specific in the number to be transferred, nevertheless burdened the individual programs with transferring no more than will result in a 2% or less triplet rate among all pregnancies. Since the survey, the United States has issued guidelines through the practice committee of the American Society for Reproductive Medicine specifying exact numbers that are acceptable to transfer.

Six of the 10 guidelines countries in the IFFS today do not have any specifications with the number to transfer.

None of the sovereign states operating without legislation or guidelines has a limit on the number of embryos to be transferred, as might be expected. Nevertheless, it is interesting that the respondents of all seven countries indicated that it was customary in their countries to transfer two or three, although it was stated in the case of one country (Canada) that up to six were transferred in certain circumstances.

Effectiveness of Surveillance

It seems clear that the voluntary guideline system in the United States has not solved the problem of multiple gestations. There are at least four aspects to an explanation of the failure.

First, there is the intense desire of the patient to become pregnant. When informed of the risks of multiples, many patients are prepared to accept the risks. There is need for more education of the patient public. This would include materials and their dissemination.

Second, there is need for backbone in the medical profession. Even though we are in an era of patient participation in therapy, it is inescapable that the physician should accept at least equal responsibility for preventing untoward results. The physician is unfortunately many times prepared to be a risk taker for competitive reasons, of which more will be said shortly. As a minimum, the physician must be sure that the informed consent signed by the patient is clear and detailed as to the multiple pregnancy risk.

TABLE 1.4. ART: The number to transfer.

Country	Legislation	Guidelines	Neither	Transfer limit	Unlimited
Argentina		+			+
Australia (West)	+				+
Australia (South)	+			3	
Australia (Victoria)	+				+
Australia (Remainder)		+		2(3)	
Austria	+				+
Belgium			+		+ (2–4+)
Brazil	+			4	
Canada			+		+ (2–4+)
Czech Republic		+		4	
Denmark	+			2–3	
Egypt		+			+
Finland		+			+ (2–3)
France	+				+
Germany	+			3	
Greece			+		+ (6)
Hong Kong			+		+ (2–3)
Hungary	+			3–4	
India			+		+ (4–5)
Ireland		+			+ (3)
Israel	+				+
Italy		+		3–4	
Japan		+		3–4	
Jordan		+			+
Korea		+			+
Mexico	+				+
The Netherlands	+				+ (2–3)
Norway	+				+
Poland		+		2–3	
Portugal			+		+ (3–5)
Saudi Arabia	+			4(3)	
Singapore	+			3	
South Africa	+				+
Spain	+				+
Sweden	+			2–3	
Switzerland	+			*	
Taiwan	+				+
Turkey	+				+
United Kingdom	+			3	
United States		+			+**

Source: Reproduced with permission from Jones and Cohen (30).
Note: Number in parentheses indicates customary number transferred.
*The number of human oocytes that may be developed up to embryo stage outside the woman's body is restricted to the number that can be immediately replaced in the uterus.
**Transfer no more embryos than would lead to a more than 2% triplet rate.

Third, there is the unfortunate aspect of competition among assisted reproductive technology programs to achieve a high pregnancy rate. The high pregnancy rate is considered desirable to assure the prosperity of any program in question. Patients generally lack adequate medical sophistication to interpret a program's specific pregnancy rates. As they now exist, program-specific pregnancy rates do not give consideration to the multiple variables involved in achieving a specific pregnancy rate. Thus, specific pregnancy rates are misleading. Furthermore, in clinic-specific reporting, as it now exists, no consideration is given to the prevalence of fetal reduction in the calculation of multiple pregnancy rates.

If these observations are correct it would be in the best interest of the patient to take whatever steps are necessary to eliminate clinic-specific reporting as it now exists. The American Society of Reproductive Medicine (ASRM) bears a heavy responsibility in this regard.

Fourth, scientific advances have inadvertently contributed to the problem. If any given program has adjusted the number to transfer to eliminate undesirable multiples, then any improvement in the implantation rate will pari passu reintroduce undesirable multiples.

The elimination of multiples due to scientific advance is difficult, to say the least. The best to be hoped for is a very prompt adjustment of the number transferred when improvement in implantation rates is perceived.

Patients need to be warned of the down side of scientific advance; indeed, some paragraph about this might be appropriate to include in informed consent forms.

Surveillance in Millennium 2000 (USA)

It seems inescapable that voluntary guidelines as they now exist have failed to control the multiple pregnancy problems in IVF in the United States (Fig. 1.6). There are several considerations. There would probably be general agreement that avoidance of Federal regulations is a most desirable aim. Furthermore, there seems to be a constitutional requirement that such regulation be assigned to states; therefore, any Federal action would likely take the form of a recommendation to the states of a model law, which would have to be adopted state by state. The attempt at surveillance of embryological laboratories, which is now in progress, is an example of the compliance with this constitutional requirement.

Is There a Workable Voluntary Way?

The Voluntary Licensing Authority (VLA) of Great Britain might be considered as an example. As a result of the study by Dame Warnock in the United Kingdom, there was a recommendation for a licensing authority. In view of the anticipated delay in action by the Parliament, the Royal College of

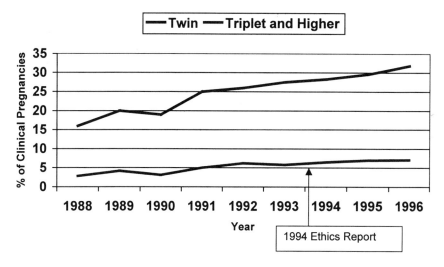

FIGURE 1.6. Multiple pregnancy rate per clinical pregnancy in the United States (21–29).

Obstetricians and Gynecologists established a voluntary licensing authority, the basis of which was the inspection according to announced guidelines of the various programs and the issuance of a license to that program as having fulfilled the requirements previously set forth by the College. In the event of violation of any of the requirements, the licensing authority was permitted to withdraw the license. This seemed to work well. There was no official governmental imposition, and the patient had the opportunity to be sure that the program in which they were being treated had indeed been licensed by the Authority. This gave considerable patient assurance.

It is true that the VLA has now become official under the name of the Human Embryology and Fertilization Authority (HEFA) and it continues to operate by issuing licenses and the withdrawal of them for violations, but there is reason to argue that the authority was as effective on a voluntary basis as it is when it is official.

Serious consideration should be given in the United States for attempting to establish what amounts to a voluntary licensing authority molded to the American system.

An attempt was made to do that previously by the then–American Fertility Society and the American College of Obstetricians and Gynecologists (ACOG) in the establishment of the National Advisory Board on Ethics in Reproduction (NABER), but NABER did not seize the opportunity to pursue this goal and rather concerned itself with reevaluating the ethical aspects of matters that had been considered by the ethics committee of the American Fertility Society and indeed update some of these requirements. This was unfortunate and it might be that a new start needs to be made. The ASRM and ACOG bear heavy responsibility in this regard and it is to be devoutly hoped that this conference would somehow or other call the necessity to the attention of ASRM and ACOG for them to take action to attempt to establish a national body that would be willing to undertake the duties of voluntary licensing that might very well work to overcome the problem of multiple pregnancies without governmental interference.

Summary

The number of twin, triplet, and higher-order multiple births has climbed at an unprecedented pace since 1980. Between 1980 and 1997, the number of twin births increased 52%, and the number of triplet and higher-order multiple deliveries has soared 404%. These multiple pregnancies place the mother and fetus at increased risk for adverse outcomes including preterm delivery, low birth rate, congenital malformations, and long-term morbidity. Twins are five times as likely, and triplets and higher-order infants 13 times as likely as singleton infants to die within the first year of life.

The vast majority of these multiple pregnancies are due to patients being treated at infertility clinics. Ovulation induction alone accounts for 66–75% of triplet and higher-order multiple pregnancies due largely to the inability of physicians to control the number of eggs that fertilize and are available for implantation (15,16). These high-order multiple pregnancies, however, can be predicted based upon high serum estradiol concentrations and the number of follicles present with ultrasound monitoring. Multiple options are available that include cancellation of the cycle, follicular aspiration, and/or conversion to IVF.

IVF also contributes to the multiple pregnancy rate and newer options including blastocyst culture, and transfer has been developed over the past several years. Additional options include limiting the number of embryos transferred and the use of cryopreservation for excess embryos.

The soaring multiple pregnancy rate is iatrogenic in origin and a public health concern due to the increased health risk to the mother and child along with multiple psychosocial difficulties. This condition, most importantly, is preventable!

References

1. Martin JA, Park MM. Trends in twin and triplet births: 1980–97. National Vital Statistics Report. Hyattsville, Maryland: National Center for Health Statistics, 1999;47:24.
2. Assisted reproductive technology success rates: 1996. National Summary and Fertility Clinic Reports. Atlanta, GA: Centers for Disease Control and Prevention, 1998.
3. Ventura SJ, Martin JA, Curtin SC, Mathews TJ. Births: Final data for 1997. National Vital Statistics Reports. Hyattsville, Maryland: National Center for Health Statistics, 1999;47:18.
4. Doyle P. The outcome of multiple pregnancy. Hum Reprod 1996;11(Suppl. 4):110–17; discussion 118–20.

5. Jewell SE, Yip R. Increasing trends in plural births in the United States. Obstet Gynecol 1995;85:229–32.
6. Martin JA, MacDorman MF, Mathews TJ. Triplet births: Trends and outcomes, 1971–94. Hyattsville, Maryland: National Center for Health Statistics, 1997.
7. Wilcox LS, Kiely JL, Melvin CL, Martin MC. Assisted reproductive technologies: estimates of their contribution to multiple births and newborn hospital days in the United States. Fertil Steril 1996;65:361–66.
8. Kiely JL, Kleinman JC, Kiely M. Triplets and higher-order multiple births. Time trends and infant mortality. Am J Dis Child 1992;146:862–68.
9. Suidan JS. Cardiopulmonary complications of selective beta 2 adrenergic tocolytic therapy. Middle East J Anesthesiol 1989;10:247–59.
10. Makhseed M, Al-Sharhan M, Egbase P, Al-Essa M, Grudzinskas JG. Maternal and perinatal outcomes of multiple pregnancy following IVF-ET. Int J Gynaecol Obstet 1998;61:155–63.
11. MacGillivray I. Management of twin pregnancies. In: MacGillivray I, Thompson B, Campbell DM, eds. Twinning and twins. Chichester, UK: John Wiley & Sons, Ltd., 1988:111–39.
12. Caspi E, Ronen J, Schreyer P, Goldberg MD. The outcome of pregnancy after gonadotrophin therapy. Br J Obstet Gynaecol 1976;83:967–73.
13. Ross MG, Downey CA, Bemis-Heys R, Nguyen M, Jacques DL, Stanziano G. Prediction by maternal risk factors of neonatal intensive care admissions: evaluation of >59,000 women in national managed care programs. Am J Obstet Gynecol 1999;181:835–42.
14. Chelmow D, Penzias AS, Kaufman G, Cetrulo C. Costs of triplet pregnancy. Am J Obstet Gynecol 1995;172:677–82.
15. Levene MI, Wild J, Steer P. Higher multiple births and the modern management of infertility in Britain. The British Association of Perinatal Medicine. Br J Obstet Gynaecol 1992;99:607–13.
16. Derom C, Derom R, Vlietinck R, Maes H, Van den Berghe H. Iatrogenic multiple pregnancies in East Flanders, Belgium. Fertil Steril 1993;60:493–96.
17. Schieve LA, Peterson HB, Meikle SF, et al. Live-birth rates and multiple-birth risk using in vitro fertilization. JAMA 1999;282:1832–38.
18. Templeton A, Morris JK. Reducing the risk of multiple births by transfer of two embryos after in vitro fertilization [see comments pp. 624–25]. N Engl J Med 1998;339:573–77.
19. Hershlag A. Multifetal prophylaxis—a reality? [editorial; comment]. Fertil Steril 1999;72:973–74.
20. International Federation of Fertility Societies International Conference. IFFS Surveillance 98. Fertil Steril 1999;71:1S–34S.
21. Assisted reproductive technology in the United States: 1996 results generated from the American Society for Reproductive Medicine/Society for Assisted Reproductive Technology Registry. Fertil Steril 1999;71:798–807.
22. In vitro fertilization-embryo transfer in the United States: 1988 results from the IVF-ET Registry. Medical Research International. Society for Assisted Reproductive Technology. American Fertility Society. Fertil Steril 1990;53:13–20.
23. In vitro fertilization-embryo transfer (IVF-ET) in the United States: 1989 results from the IVF-ET Registry. Medical Research International, Society for Assisted Reproductive Technology, The American Fertility Society. Fertil Steril 1991;55:14–22; discussion 22–23.

24. In vitro fertilization-embryo transfer (IVF-ET) in the United States: 1990 results from the IVF-ET Registry. Medical Research International. Society for Assisted Reproductive Technology (SART), The American Fertility Society [published erratum appears in Fertil Steril 1993 Jan;59(1):250]. Fertil Steril 1992;57:15–24.
25. Assisted reproductive technology in the United States and Canada: 1991 results from the Society for Assisted Reproductive Technology generated from the American Fertility Society Registry. Fertil Steril 1993;59:956–62.
26. Assisted reproductive technology in the United States and Canada: 1992 results generated from the American Fertility Society/Society for Assisted Reproductive Technology Registry. Fertil Steril 1994;62:1121–28.
27. Assisted reproductive technology in the United States and Canada: 1993 results generated from the American Society for Reproductive Medicine/Society for Assisted Reproductive Technology Registry. Fertil Steril 1995;64:13–21.
28. Assisted reproductive technology in the United States and Canada: 1994 results generated from the American Society for Reproductive Medicine/Society for Assisted Reproductive Technology Registry. Fertil Steril 1996;66:697–705.
29. Assisted reproductive technology in the United States and Canada: 1995 results generated from the American Society for Reproductive Medicine/Society for Assisted Reproductive Technology Registry. Fertil Steril 1998;69:389–98.
30. Jones HW Jr., Cohen J, eds. ART—the number to transfer. Fertil Steril 1999;71: 12s–13s.

2

Patient Stimulation and Effect on Outcomes

DAVID R. MELDRUM

Routine Use of Gonadotropin-Releasing Hormone (GnRH) Agonists

Benefits of GnRH Agonists for Assisted Reproductive Technology

Use of GnRH agonists has become routine for preparation of the ovaries for oocyte retrieval because of reduced cancellations and more oocytes and embryos (1), and a twofold increase of pregnancy (2). The lower cancellation rate is predominately by preventing premature luteinizing hormone (LH) surges, as well as because of fewer poor responses (3). Improved response is probably due to suppression of intraovarian androgens (4). A concomitant of the augmented response is a higher incidence of ovarian hyperstimulation syndrome (OHSS) (5), particularly in women with polycystic ovaries (PCO). The higher rate of pregnancy may be by suppressing LH and ovarian androgens (4), as well as by having more embryos from which to select for transfer. More extra embryos also result in a higher pregnancy rate with frozen embryo replacement.

GnRH Agonist Regimens

The best overall results have been with the long or downregulation protocol. One controlled study found a significantly higher pregnancy rate with midluteal initiation of suppression (6), which also largely avoids the prolonged agonist effect and cyst formation accompanying an early follicular phase start of therapy (7). Better ovarian responses are observed with a mid- to late-luteal initiation compared with an early luteal initiation of the GnRH agonist (8).

The short or flare protocol produces fewer oocytes and is associated with more variable results (9,10). The lower stimulation with flare protocols probably is due to stimulation of ovarian androgens during the early stage of follicle recruitment (11). The timing of hCG administration also appears to be critical, with even a 1-day delay being associated with a dramatic fall in the pregnancy rate (12). On the other hand, the flare protocol is briefer and requires less exogenous gonadotropin.

Use of Oral Contraceptive Pretreatment

Oral contraceptive (O.C.) pretreatment is increasingly being utilized to aid in scheduling, to avoid ovarian cyst formation, and to augment the ovarian response. The first hint that O.C. pretreatment does not reduce response was the finding by Gonen et al. (13) that response to a clomiphene citrate/human menopausal gonadotropin stimulation was modestly improved following O.C. administration. It is of interest that no LH surges were noted, indicating that prior O.C. suppression of the pituitary together with the suppressive effect of factor(s) released by the hyperstimulated ovary (gonadotropin surge inhibiting factors) together effectively prevent premature pituitary LH release. One study has documented a marked decrease of the incidence of follicular cysts and a significant increase of ovarian response (14). O.C. pretreatment allows scheduling of the oocyte retrieval by varying the duration of O.C. therapy, whereas accomplishing this same goal by extending the duration of GnRH agonist desensitization results in significant menopausal side effects (i.e., headache, difficulties with recent memory) (15). O.C. therapy could also improve the outcome with the short or flare protocol by suppressing ovarian androgens (16).

GnRH Agonist Regimens for Poor Responders

Poor response can be due to excessive suppression due to dose or potency of the particular agonist used. In one study response was noted to be improved with a "minidose" of agonist (17), but that lower dose was comparable to standard doses of other agonists such as leuprolide acetate (LA) because it is so much more potent (18). The most common dose of LA is 1.0 mg, which decreases to 0.5 mg when stimulation is begun. This dose may be cut in half when poor response is observed or anticipated. It was suggested based on an uncontrolled study that response is improved by stopping the agonist when stimulation is begun (19), but two previous (20,21) and one subsequent controlled studies (22) showed no improved response and, in fact, a slightly higher response in the control groups. These findings again suggest that suppression of ovarian androgens augments the ovarian response.

Use of a miniflare LA regimen following O.C. pretreatment has been reported to improve follicular response in poor responders (23), with good pregnancy outcome. O.C. pretreatment and the very small LA dose may limit any LH and androgen response to the agonist.

The Role of LH in Ovarian Stimulation Using GnRH Agonists

It has been controversial whether addition of LH to the stimulation regimen can improve the response of some women to FSH stimulation because of varying doses and potencies of different agonists. There are clearly improved outcomes (fertilization) with hMG versus pure FSH with some agonist regimens that are more effective in suppressing endogenous LH (24,25). Because the O.C./GnRH-a combination further suppresses LH, there has been concern that stimulation may be blunted; clinically, this has been observed, and reversed by adding a small amount of hMG to the stimulation. It has also been found in one retrospective analysis that the full dose of LA was associated with a significant improvement of the rate of blastocyst implantation with addition of hMG to pure FSH for ovarian stimulation (26). This may become somewhat clearer when a study is completed of the addition of recombinant LH to pure FSH (27). Using low dose lupron, preliminary results suggested that additional LH was deleterious in women who have an LH concentration more than 1.5 mIU/ml. Because about two thirds of the women had LH over this threshold, addition of hMG to low-dose LA appears unnecessary and may be harmful. There were trends toward better implantation in the one third of women who have LH levels below the chosen threshold. The full dose of LH would be expected to result in marked suppression of LH in the majority of women (4), which suggests that addition of LH could be beneficial. On the other hand, one retrospective study found improved oocyte quality and pregnancy outcome with pure FSH with full dose LA (28). Prospective randomized studies are necessary to determine whether added LH is beneficial or deleterious at various agonist doses with and without O.C. pretreatment. Although the regimen chosen may predict the optimal gonadotropin stimulation to a certain degree, it may be necessary to measure LH in the individual woman to determine the degree of suppression.

Management of Excessive Ovarian Response with GnRH Agonist

Management of hyperresponders is benefited by a 3–4-week pretreatment with O.C. overlapping with a full dose of LH (29). If the response is still excessive the agonist can be continued while the gonadotropin stimulation is stopped ("coasting"). This has resulted in a reduced incidence of OHSS with similar success rates to patients not coasted (30–33).

GnRH Antagonists for ART

Advantages of Using GnRH Antagonists

Since GnRH antagonists suppress LH within hours (34), they can be started late in follicular development to prevent excessive LH release and a premature LH surge. This dramatically shortens the duration of drug administration, avoids the agonist phase, which can cause ovarian cyst formation, and avoids the menopausal symptoms caused by GnRH agonist suppression of the ovary before the estrogen response to stimulation.

GnRH Antagonist Regimens

GnRH antagonists have been given as a single large dose (35) or smaller daily doses (36). The single dose approach has mainly been using cetrorelix. Small series of cycles have been reported with satisfactory results. To detect any differences in outcomes compared with GnRH agonists requires large randomized studies. This has been carried out with ganirelix using daily doses. First, the optimum daily dose was determined from a dose-ranging study (36) using pure recombinant FSH for stimulation. Below the optimum 250-µg dose, LH suppression was insufficient and lower implantation rates were noted. At doses exceeding 250 µg, LH levels were very low and the implantation rate dropped dramatically suggesting either that embryo quality was reduced with insufficient LH exposure to the oocytes and/or that the GnRH antagonist itself may have a direct effect inhibiting implantation. The former mechanism is suggested from a study in monkeys receiving Antide, a potent GnRH antagonist, that shows better blastocyst development and cryosurvival by adding recombinant LH to the stimulation (37). The latter mechanism is suggested by the observation that frozen embryos from the high-dose ganirelix cycles had a satisfactory rate of implantation after thawing (38).

A randomized multicenter study has been done (39) comparing full dose LA with 250 µg of ganirelix begun on Day 6 of FSH stimulation. There were two fewer embryos with ganirelix compared with LA (11 vs. 13). This may indicate that LA augments ovarian response by suppressing ovarian androgens because response was greater despite a similar daily dose of FSH and lower levels of endogenous gonadotropins in the LA group prior to stimulation. The ongoing pregnancy rate was slightly lower with ganirelix (31.3 vs. 35.3%). Although this was not statistically significant, these preliminary results suggest a slight decrease of implantation in GnRH antagonist cycles.

Future GnRH Antagonist Protocols

Because suppression of ovarian androgens may play an important role in ovarian response during GnRH agonist cycles, pretreatment with O.C. would be expected to augment the stimulation response by suppressing ovarian androgens. Use of O.C. will also add back the flexibility that is otherwise lost with GnRH antagonist cycles by allowing scheduling of retrieval by varying the length of time on the O.C. One would predict that the best time to start stimulation after O.C. would be Day 4 or 5, when gonadotropins and estradiol are beginning to rise. Because this may vary with different O.C. preparations, we strongly advise using one for which the recovery phase has been thoroughly evaluated (40). If stimulation is started too soon, response may be blunted due to lack of recovery of endogenous gonadotropins (41). The speed of recovery also appears to be influenced by age, with slower recovery in women over age 35 (42). We therefore recommend waiting until the fifth day after O.C. in older women and in poor responders.

Initiation of the ganirelix was arbitrarily fixed at Day 6. This might be too early in slow responders and could increase the dose of exogenous gonadotropin. In rapid responders, LH levels may not be suppressed early enough. It is possible that individualizing the start of antagonist by diameter of the leading follicle or estradiol level may improve the overall outcomes.

It is remarkable that the results with ganirelix at the first pass at a standard fixed research protocol were so close to the reference treatment with which the investigators had more than 10 years of experience. It is likely that these and other refinements will yield an antagonist regimen with outcomes indistinguishable from GnRH agonists, with a shorter duration of therapy and fewer side effects.

References

1. Meldrum, DR. GnRH agonists as adjuncts for in vitro fertilization. Obstet Gynecol Surv 1989;44:314–18.
2. Hughes EG, Fedorkow DM, Daya S, Sagle MA, Van de Koppel P, Collins JA. The routine use of gonadotropin-releasing hormone agonists prior to in vitro fertilization and gamete intrafallopian transfer: a meta-analysis of randomized controlled trials. Fertil Steril 1992;58:888–96.
3. Serafini P, Stone B, Kerin J, Batzofin J, Quinn P, Marrs RP. An alternate approach to controlled ovarian hyperstimulation in "poor responders": pretreatment with a gonadotropin-releasing hormone analog. Fertil Steril 1988;49:90–95.
4. Cedars MI, Surey E, Hamilton F, Lapolt P, Meldrum DR. Leuprolide acetate lowers circulating bioactive luteinizing hormone and testosterone concentrations during ovarian stimulation for oocyte retrieval. Fertil Steril 1990;53:627–31.
5. Smitz J, Camus M, Devroey P, Erard P, Wisanto A, Van Steirtegham AC. Incidence of severe ovarian hyperstimulation syndrome after GnRH agonist/HMG superovulation for in-vitro fertilization. Hum Reprod 1990;5:933–37.
6. Urbancsek J, Witthaus E. Midluteal buserelin is superior to early follicular phase buserelin in combined gonadotropin-releasing hormone analog and gonadotropin stimulation in in vitro fertilization. Fertil Steril 1996;65:966–71.
7. Meldrum DR, Wisot A, Hamilton F, Gutlay AL, Huynh D, Kempton W. Timing of initiation and dose schedule of leuprolide influence the time course of ovarian suppression. Fertil Steril 1988;50:400–2.
8. Pellicer A, Simon C, Miro F, et al. Ovarian response and outcome of in-vitro fertilization in patients treated with gonadotropin-releasing hormone analogues in different phases of the menstrual cycle. Hum Reprod 1989;4:285–89.
9. Tan S-L, Kingsland C, Campbell S, et al. The long protocol of administration of gonadotropin-releasing hormone agonist is superior to the short protocol for ovarian stimulation for in vitro fertilization. Fertil Steril 1992;57:810–14.
10. San Roman GA, Surrey ES, Judd HL, Kerin JF. A prospective randomized comparison

of luteal phase versus concurrent follicular phase initiation of gonadotropin-releasing hormone agonist for in vitro fertilization. Fertil Steril 1992;58:744–49.
11. Filicori M, Flamigni C, Cognigni GE, et al. Different gonadotropin and leuprorelin ovulation induction regimens markedly affect follicular fluid hormone levels and folliculogenesis. Fertil Steril 1996;65:387–93.
12. Clark L, Stanger J, Brinsmead M. Prolonged follicle stimulation decreases pregnancy rates after in vitro fertilization. Fertil Steril 1991;55:1192–94.
13. Gonen Y, Jacobson W, Casper RF. Gonadotropin suppression with oral contraceptives before in vitro fertilization. Fertil Steril 1990;53:282–87.
14. Biljan MM, Mahutte NG, Dean N, Hemmings R, Bissonnette F, Tan S-L. Effects of pretreatment with an oral contraceptive on the time required to achieve pituitary suppression with gonadotropin-releasing hormone analogues and on subsequent implantation and pregnancy rates. Fertil Steril 1998;70:1063–69.
15. Varney NR, Syrop G, Kubu CS, Struchen M, Hahn S, Franzen K. Neuropsychologic dysfunction in women following leuprolide acetate induction of hypoestrogenism. J Assist Reprod Genetics 1993;10:53–57.
16. Andersen CY, Ziebe S. Serum levels of free androstenedione, testosteone and oestradiol are lower in the follicular phase of conceptual than of non-conceptual cycles after ovarian stimulation with a gonadotropin-releasing hormone agonist protocol. Hum Reprod 1992;7:1365–70.
17. Feldberg D, Farhi J, Ashkenazi J, Dicker D, Shalev J, Ben-Rafael Z. Minidose gonadotropin-releasing hormone agonist is the treatment of choice in poor responders with high follicle-stimulating hormone levels. Fertil Steril 1994;62:343–46.
18. Vale WW, Rivier C, Perrin M, Smith M, Rivier J. Pharmacology of gonadotropin-releasing hormone: a model regulatory peptide. In: Martin JB, Reichlin S, eds. Neurosecretion and brain peptides. New York: Raven Press; 1981:609–25.
19. Faber BM, Mayer J, Cox B. Cessation of gonadotropin-releasing hormone agonist therapy combined with high dose gonadotropin stimulation yields favorable pregnancy results in low responders. Fertil Steril 1998;69:826–30.
20. Pantos K, Meimeth-Damianaki T, Vaxevanoglou T, Kapetanakis E. Prospective study of a modified gonadotropin-releasing hormone agonist long protocol in an in vitro fertilization program. Fertil Steril 1994;61:709–13.
21. Smith J, Van Den Abbeel E, Bollen N, et al. The effect of gonadotropin-releasing hormone (GnRH) agonist in the follicular phase on in-vitro fertilization outcome in normo-ovulatory women. Hum Reprod 1992;7:1098–102.
22. Dirnfeld M, Fruchter O, Yshai D, Lissak A, Ahdut A, Abramovici K. Cessation of gonadotropin-releasing hormone analogue (GnRH-a) upon down-regulation versus conventional long GnRH-a protocol in poor responders undergoing in vitro fertilization. Fertil Steril 1999;72:406–11.
23. Schoolcraft W, Schlenker T, Gee M, Stevens J, Wagley L. Improved controlled ovarian hyperstimulation in poor responder in vitro fertilization patients with a microdose follicle-stimulating hormone flare, growth hormone protocol. Fertil Steril 1997;67:93–97.
24. Westergaard LG, Erb K, Laursen S, Rasmussen PE, Rex S. The effect of human menopausal gonadotropin and highly purified, urine-derived follicle stimulating hormone on the outcome of in-vitro fertilization in down-regulated normogonadotrophic women. Hum Reprod 1996;11:1209–13.

25. Soderstrom-Anttila V, Foudila T, Hovatta O. A randomized comparative study of highly purified follicle stimulating hormone and human menopausal gonadotrophin for ovarian hyperstimulation in an oocyte donation programme. Hum Reprod 1996;11: 1864–70.
26. Schoolcraft WB, Gardner DK, Lane M, Schlenker T, Hamilton F, Meldrum DR. Blastocyst culture and transfer: analysis of results and parameters affecting outcome in two in vitro fertilization programs. Fertil Steril 1999;72:604–9.
27. Weathersbee P, Kelly E, Nebiolo L, Ferrande L. Open, multicenter, prospective randomized study comparing r-hFSH therapy alone versus combination therapy (r-hFSH + r-hLH) in patients desensitized with low dose luteal GnRH agonist protocol: preliminary results. Sydney: IVF World Congress; 1999.
28. Mercan R, Mayer JF, Walker D, et al. Improved oocyte quality is obtained with follicle stimulating hormone alone than with follicle stimulating hormone/human menopausal gonadotropin combination. Hum Reprod 1997;12:1886–89.
29. Damario MA, Barmat L, Liu H-C, Davis OK, Rosenwaks Z. Dual suppression with oral contraceptives and gonadotropin releasing-hormone agonists improves in-vitro fertilization outcome in high responders. Hum Reprod 1997;12:2359–65.
30. Benadiva CA, Davis O, Kligman I, Moomjy M, Liu H-C, Rosenwaks Z. Withholding gonadotropin administration is an effective alternative for the prevention of ovarian hyperstimulation syndrome. Fertil Steril 1997;67:724–27.
31. Tortoriello DV, McGovern PG, Colon JM, Skurnick JH, Lipetz K, Santoro N. "Coasting" does not adversely affect cycle outcome in a subset of highly responsive in vitro fertilization patients. Fertil Steril 1998;69:454–60.
32. Waldenstrom U, Kahn J, Marsk L, Nilsson S. High pregnancy rates and successful prevention of severe ovarian hyperstimulation syndrome by "prolonged coasting" of very hyperstimulated patients: a multicenter study. Hum Reprod 1999;14:294–97.
33. Fluker MR, Hooper WM, Yuzpe AA. Withholding gonadotropins ("coasting") to minimize the risk of ovarian hyperstimulation during superovulation and in vitro fertilization-embryo transfer cycles. Fertil Steril 1999;71:294–301.
34. Mortola JF, Sathanandan M, Pavlou S, et al. Suppression of bioactive and immunoreactive follicle-stimulating hormone and luteinizing hormone levels by a potent gonadotropin-releasing hormone antagonist: pharmacodynamic studies. Fertil Steril 1989;51:957–62.
35. Olivennes F, Fanchin R, Bouchard P, Taleb J, Selva J, Frydman R. Scheduled administration of a gonadotrophin-releasing hormone antagonist (cetrorelix) on day 8 of in-vitro fertilization cycles: a pilot study. Hum Reprod 1995;10:1382–86.
36. The ganirelix dose-finding study group. A double-blind, randomized, dose-finding study to assess the efficacy of the gonadotropin-releasing hormone antagonist ganirelix (Org 37462) to prevent premature luteinizing hormone surges in women undergoing ovarian stimulation with recombinant follicle stimulating hormone (Puregon). Hum Reprod 1998;13:3023–31.
37. Weston AM, Zelinski-Wooton MB, Hutchison JS, Stouffer RL, Wolf DP. Developmental potential of embryos produced by in-vitro fertilization from gonadotrophin-releasing hormone antagonist-treated macaques stimulated with recombinant follicle-stimulating hormone alone or in combination with luteinizing hormone. Hum Reprod 1996;11:608–13.
38. Kol S, Lightman A, Hillensjo T, et al. High doses of gonadotrophin-releasing hormone

antagonist in in-vitro fertilization cycles do not adversely affect the outcome of subsequent freeze-thaw cycles. Hum Reprod 1999;14:2242–44.
39. North American Ganirelix Study Group. Results of a prospective, randomized, multicenter study to assess the efficacy and safety of a gonadotropin releasing hormone (GnRH) antagonist - Org 37462 (Ganirelix Acetate) treatment in women undergoing controlled ovarian hyperstimulation (COH) Annual Meeting, American Society of Reproductive Medicine, Toronto, Canada, Sept. 25–30, 1999.
40. Van Heusden AM, Fauser BCJM. Activity of the pituitary-ovarian axis in the pill-free interval during use of low-dose combined oral contraceptives. Contraception 1999;59:237–43.
41. Benadiva CA, Ben-Rafael Z, Blasco L, Tureck R, Mastroianni, L, Flickinger GL. Ovarian response to human menopausal gonadotropin following suppression with oral contraceptive. Fertil Steril 1988;50:516–18.
42. Fitzgerald C, Elstein M, Spona J. Effect of age on the response of the hypothalamo-pituitary-ovarian axis to a combined oral contraceptive. Fertil Steril 1999;71:1079–84.

3

New Developments in Imaging and Hormonal Stimulation of the Ovaries

ROGER A. PIERSON

In the frontispiece of William Harvey's book on the generation of animals published in Latin (1651) there is a wonderful engraving of the god Zeus liberating living beings from an egg (1). On the egg Zeus holds in his hands is inscribed *ex ovo omnia* (all things come from eggs). As I wondered about my contribution to this volume on the blastocyst, I finally developed the corollary *ex folliculi ovo*. Although I cannot claim perfection in the Latin declination of that statement, the sentiment is that all eggs come from follicles. We believe that good eggs are more capable of fertilization and make good embryos and that good embryos survive our culture methods and become good blastocysts.

Introduction

We have traditionally been limited to gross anatomy and classical histology techniques to study the ovary. Although we have learned a great deal from these methods they are not compatible with studying ovarian function in living creatures. Radioimmunoassay techniques became available in the 1960s and we have used them to infer ovarian function by determining the levels of the reproductively active hormones in the systemic circulation. We began to appreciate the dynamic changes in the ovarian follicle population with the development of real-time ultrasonography in the early 1980s. The standard of practice in ovarian stimulation regimens used to obtain oocytes for the assisted reproductive technologies in which we are all so interested is now a combination of serum assay for estradiol-17β and ultrasonography to determine the number and diameter(s) of follicles responding to the gonadotropins that we administer.

Ovarian Imaging

Ovarian follicular development and ovulation have been the focus of research in our laboratory for the past several years. We have been using high-resolution transvaginal ultrasonographic imaging to study the ovary and all of the changes in the follicles, both physiologically dominant and subordinate in situ. Transvaginal imaging has brought all of the process of human reproduction within our "visual" field. We can finally see what is actually going on within the body. The beauty of the transvaginal imaging technique lies in our ability to follow changes in individual follicles as they progress through their life cycles. All of us tend to see ultrasonography of the ovary as a group of black dots (the fluid-filled antra of follicles) on the viewing screen of a somewhat mystical machine. It is really much more than meets our eyes. With color Doppler ultrasonography, we are able to visualize the arterioles and veins that comprise the vascular supply of individual follicles. We may use this information to evaluate differences in tissues as minute as those of the stratum granulosum and theca interna.

We also know from our study of the acoustic physics of image making with ultrasonography that there is much more information contained within the images that we see than we are able to detect with our naked eyes. In many instances we are able to visualize structures as small as the oocyte-cumulus complex within the follicle. There is exquisite detail available in the images that we are simply unable to appreciate; however, we have been able to develop computer-assisted algorithms that enable us to take advantage of the image data and display it in a manner that we may easily interpret (2). We believe that blending the technological advances of imaging and image analysis with the fine art of ovarian stimulation based in a firm foundation of knowledge of ovarian physiology with allow us to harvest more oocytes of higher quality. This in turn will allow the development of more quality embryos and play a role in the development of more and better blastocysts.

Ultrasonographic Image Analysis

The image analysis techniques that we have developed in our laboratory are variants of three relatively simply ideas (2). The simplest method of analyzing the pixels that comprise the ultrasonographic image in a quantitative manner is to select a small circular area of interest in the image. The computer can be used to report the precise grey-scale value of each of the pixels within the selected spot easily and present a mean numeric value and a measure of central tendency. This simple technique may be used to compare the pixel values in various portions of the image or among images generated at different time points. In our interest here are portions of the follicle wall from different follicles developed during ovarian stimulation. Sequential images may also be evaluated to detect changes in the follicles that may be characteristic of impending ovulation and ovulatory failure and atresia.

Linear and time-series analyses are implemented by drawing a line across a specified section of the image of the follicle and viewing a graph of the numerical pixel values along the line. The graph depicts the amplitude of the echoes located along the line. To perform a time-series analysis, the linear pixel intensity graphs drawn across each individually identified follicle on each day are concatenated into a composite image. The composite is then subjected to a shading algorithm that allows detailed analysis of the surface contours of the follicular walls and follicular fluid as a follicle grows from the time that it is first identified (approximately 10 mm) to the day of ovulation or ovulatory failure. The three dimensions in this type of graphic display are follicle diameter, numerical pixel value, and time. Visual assessment of the surface features representing various portions of the follicles provide important clues regarding the physiologic status at different time points during follicle development or regression. Physiologically important time periods may be identified with this technique, and specific images may be selected for more detailed analysis.

The most promising technique for evaluating the physiologic status of individual follicles involves overlaying a computer-generated grid onto a selected area of the two-dimensional image of a follicle and generating a three-dimensional framework representing processed pixel intensities. Placing a computer-generated opaque "film" over the wire framework representing numerical pixel values comprising the ultrasound image yields a three-dimensional contoured surface. This type of analysis is designed to highlight detail or enhance perception of either surface features (texture) or the portion of the image comprised of echo intensities of particular interest (proportional area). If desired, color may be applied to this construction to further enhance the perception of fine detail. In contrast to the time-series analyses, the X and Y coordinates represent distance in two dimensions on the image (i.e., length and width) and Z represents numerical pixel value. This technique allows discriminatory examination of the surfaces and rapid visual assessment of ultrasonographic attributes associated with follicle health (state of viability of atresia).

The techniques we have developed have undergone extensive testing in in vitro and in vivo animal model systems. The imaging system has been instrumental in the development of our ability to ascertain the viability of individual follicles of different diameters and to assess their probability of ovulation and their individual contribution to the systemic estradiol concentrations (2–4). We have been able to substantiate that the image analysis techniques may be used to distinguish between follicles that are dominant and those destined for atresia in human follicles as small as 10 mm (Pierson, unpublished). The task that remains is to implement these techniques in ovarian stimulation protocols to assess the ovarian response to the drugs and protocols used so that we may collect several physiologically healthy oocytes capable of being fertilized in our culture systems.

Folliculogenesis Revisited

In natural menstrual cycles, there are follicles of many diameters in the ovaries at all times. As reproductive endocrinologists interested in obtaining oocytes for use in our assisted reproductive technologies, we are typically most interested in the late follicular phase of the cycle when we may follow the development of the follicle physiologically selected to ovulate. We are usually able to identify the preovulatory follicle on the basis of its greater diameter approximately 7 days following the onset of menstruation. It then grows at an approximate rate of 2 mm per day (5–10). The dominant preovulatory follicle produces most of the estradiol present in the circulation, and the increase seen in the estradiol curve follows the development of the dominant follicle (8,11).

The dominant follicle also has a much more extensive and permeable vascular network than does the nonselected follicles in the ovary, which are committed to atresia and is ultrasonographically different than subordinate follicles (12). The take-home lesson is that dominant follicles (i.e., those that are biologically selected to produce oocytes) are different from those that are not destined for ovulation, and that the natural process with which physiologic dominance of the follicle is manifest is exactly what we wish to duplicate with our ovarian stimulation schemes. Although we know that all follicles contain oocytes (*ex folliculi ova*), this seemingly obvious difference between preovulatory and atretic follicles is the basis for our work to try to distinguish those follicles destined for oocyte production from those not so fated. In concept, physiologic selection of a dominant follicle is the mechanism that we must overcome to cause the development of more than one dominant follicle for oocyte collection.

Hormonal Control of the Ovaries

All of us in the business of assisted reproductive technologies use many different exogenous hormones and techniques to stimulate the ovaries for oocyte collection. We also use many different exogenous compounds with estrogenic and progestational effects to suppress ovarian function when we are interested in contraception. Although these two uses for exogenous reproductively active hormones may at first seem diametrically opposed, they are really just opposite sides of the same coin. They are based on different ideas about how to coax the ovaries into forgetting how to select a dominant follicle, go against the natural order and give us many competent follicles from which to choose or to try to remove the physiologic selection mechanism from the list of things that the body must "do." Various combinations of both ovarian suppression and stimulation in our attempts to have many follicles develop for oocyte retrievel.

Oral Contraceptives

Oral contraceptives work by having a woman ingest various combinations of ethinyl estradiol and various progestins. The most common progestins are norgestimate, levonorgestral, or desogestral. Although progestin pills do exist, the estrogen and progestin combination pills are used most commonly. The exogenous hormones suppress ovarian function, in part, by providing the hormones that the body needs to maintain female characteristics and suppressing the hypothalamus and pituitary in its ability to produce follicle stimulating hormone (FSH) and luteinizing hormone (LH). As long as the pills are taken as indicated, ovarian follicular development is effectively curtailed. When the pills are stopped and the hormonal suppression removed, FSH levels immediately rebound, follicular growth is reinitiated, estradiol production from the follicles resumes, and the steps leading toward physiologic selection of a dominant follicle are reinstated. It is not uncommon to see follicles develop to ostensible preovulatory size during the "pill free" interval in oral contraceptive cycles, and ovulation of these follicles has been documented (13). Computer-assisted analysis of ultrasonographic images of follicles developing during oral contraceptive regimens has revealed substantial variability in the apparent quality of the follicles, depending on the progestin used.

Ovarian Superstimulation

In assisted reproductive technologies, we work to overcome the physiologic selection mechanism that nature has designed to limit our natural fecundity and cause the development of as many oocytes capable of being fertilized as possible. We collect the oocytes with transvaginal ultrasound-directed ovarian puncture and deliver them to our embryologists.

Clomiphene Citrate

The simplest method used for ovarian stimulation is an oral medication, clomiphene citrate. Clomiphene citrate is a weak estrogen agonist that works by binding to estrogen receptors in the hypothalamus and pituitary, and stimulating the endogenous production of FSH, which will cause the development of one or more dominant preovulatory follicles. When we look at the follicles that clomiphene assists in their development, however, the image analysis pictures that we see are indicative of follicles with thin, apparently atretic walls and intrafollicular fluid that is quantitatively different from that of follicles analyzed during natural mentstrual cycles (Pierson, unpublished).

Exogenous Gonadotropins

Most ovarian superstimulation is done by administering exogenous gonadotropins derived of either biological (human menopausal gonadotropin) or recombinant sources. We use many techniques to accomplish this single goal.

We know that there is a wide range of values reported for the diameter of a preovulatory follicle during both natural menstrual cycles and for ovulation induction cycles. This wide variance precludes simple assessment of diameter as an index for the prediction of ovulation (8,14–16). Diameter of the follicle, however, appears to be more accurate as an impeding ovulation index than does assessment of circulation FSH, LH, or estradiol (17). For all practical purposes, this means that we are actually guessing about the time that is optimal for the collection of oocytes for IVF.

There are cycles where gonadotropins are administered after ovarian suppression and cycle synchronization with oral contraceptives or where the gonadotropins are initiated at specific times of natural unstimulated cycles. We administer the gonadotropins at constant levels throughout the stimulation cycle, "step-up" cycles where the levels of gonadotropin start out low and are increased through the stimulation cycle, and "step-down" cycles where the initial doses of gonasdotropins are high and are then decreased throughout the stimulation cycle. We use GnRH agonists to downregulate and suppress the endogenous FSH and LH while we take over control of the amount and type of exogenous gonadotropin that the body "sees" in long agonist protocols and in short agonist protocols. The agonists also ensure precise control over the timing of the final phases of follicular maturation by allowing us to suppress the endogenous LH surge completely and provide our own version by the administration of exogenous hCG or recombinant LH. We also use many variants and combinations of each of the protocols. It is interesting that we really do not have any idea what any of the compounds that we use actually do to oocytes. Their function is simply to grow follicles that give us oocytes to fertilize.

In a long series of studies that is only beginning to be published, we have followed the development of individual follicles during ovarian stimulation and ovulation-induction cycles (Newstead, Hess, and Pierson, Pierson et al. unpublished). In brief, we learned that not all follicles that attain preovulatory diameter are capable of responding to the ovulation-inducing bolus injection of human chorionic gonadotropin (hCG). Women in our ovulation induction cycles had quite varied responses to our therapies. Only approximately 20% of women ovulated all of the follicles that developed to preovulatory diameter in their ovaries. Approximately 15% failed to ovulate completely. The remaining majority ovulated one or more, but not all of their preovulatory diameter follicles. We have learned from this series of studies that follicular development in women undergoing ovarian stimulation are extremely variable, as is the ovulatory response in women undergoing ovulation induction. If we are able to take the leap of faith that in ovulation-induction cycles follicles that ovulate are somehow better then those that do not, then one of the lessons here appears to be that more oocytes does not necessarily mean better oocytes.

When we examine the image attributes of physiologically selected small follicles in natural cycles (<6 mm) they include higher amplitude walls and smooth echotexture of follicular fluid compared with subordinate follicles of the cohort. Time series analyses applied to follicles stimulated by exogenous gonadotropins show marked differences between ovulatory and atretic follicles (2). Follicles that eventually ovulated, or provided superior grades of oocytes, exhibited walls that are thicker and of quantitatively lower peak pixel values throughout their development than did the walls of follicles that were atretic or from which lower-grade oocytes were recovered. In addition, follicles that ovulate typically had smooth, even textures in the areas corresponding to follicular fluid, whereas images of follicles that do not ovulate exhibit rough surfaces in the fluid areas and higher (brighter) walls. The associations among computer-assisted analyses, intrafollicular hormone levels and histologic appearances were to be very high (2–4). The implications for timing oocyte retrievel from small follicles for in vitro maturation are profound. If acoustic markers for follicle and/or oocyte competence are able to be determined we may eventually time our oocyte-retrievel procedures based on the quality of the follicles as opposed to waiting for some arbitrary time depending on systemic estradiol levels. This may be especially valuable as the techniques for in vitro maturation become more developed.

An important observation during these studies was that when the circulating estradiol data were partitioned according to complete ovulatory response, partial ovulatory response, or ovulatory failure there were no statistically significant differences seen. That is, even though the women were producing similar numbers of follicles, we could not predict their ovulatory responses by examining circulating estradiol levels.

Mathematical Modeling

One of the newest methods of investigating ovarian function, especially under ovarian stimulation conditions, is mathematical modeling of follicular development (18). Our working hypothesis has been that imaging attributes derived from ultrasonography or magnetic resonance imaging (MRI) may be integrated into a comprehensive model of ovarian folliculogenesis, which includes a mathematical description of growth of ovarian follicles in a competitive environment under the influence of estradiol and other hormones, such as FSH and LH (16,19). We integrate image attributes from our ultrasonographic images into the mathematical model to allow inference of hormone levels from noninvasive image data and obviate the need for routine hormonal analyses. We are close to being able to assess the per follicle estradiol contribution to the concentration of estradiol in the systemic circulation. In the model's simplest form, the growth of every follicle is governed by a first order nonlinear differential equation where the follicle's maturity is measured by the intrafollicular estradiol content, circulating estradiol level, and imaging characteristics determined by ultrasonography. This allows us to create a visual picture of the ovarian stimulation cycle and examine the mathematical curves for physiologically important events. Using this technique, we have been able to determine ovarian stimulation cycles with a high probability of ovulation and conception from those with low probabilities of ovulation. Work to predict high-percentage collection of good oocytes in IVF cycles is ongoing.

Conclusions

The point here is not to discuss the merits of the various protocols that are used; rather, it is to point out that the goal of each of the protocols are the same. It is to overwhelm the natural selection mechanism, cause the synchronous development of many follicles, and obtain many oocytes capable of being fertilized. It seems like such a simple goal; however, over the past three decades the most consistent finding in the substantial literature on ovarian stimulation is that there is an extreme variability in the ovarian response to exogenous gonadotropins. In fact, it was the only consistent feature of the literature that we found. Obtaining high-quality oocytes is one of the most important rate-limiting steps in the success of our assisted reproductive technology programs. The work in our laboratory is focused on using imaging technology and its image analysis variants to help provide kinder, gentler ovarian stimulations based on fundamental knowledge of the patterns and rhythms underlying follicular development, and which will result in the consistent production of oocytes with the highest probability for fertilization, embryonic development to the blastocyst stage in culture.

Acknowledgments. Original research in the Women's Health Imaging Research Laboratory is supported by the Medical Research Council of Canada. The contributions of John Deptuch, Angela Hess, Jennifer Hilton, Nadia Jilwah, Jill Newstead, Lissa Ogieglo, Dr. Gord Sarty, and Dr. Gregg Adams are gratefully acknowledged.

References

1. Needham J, Hughes A. A history of embryology. New York: Abelard-Schuman, 1959:139.
2. Pierson RA, Adams GP. Computer-assisted image analysis, diagnostic ultrasonography and ovulation induction: strange bedfellows. Theriogenology 1995;43:105–12.
3. Singh J, Pierson RA, Adams GP. Ultrasound image attributes of bovine ovarian follicles: endocrine and functional correlates. J Reprod Fertil 1998;112:19–29.
4. Tom JW, Pierson RA, Adams GP. Quantitative echotextural analysis of bovine ovarian follicles. Theriogenology 1998;50:339–46.
5. Hodgen GD. The dominant ovarian follicle. Fertil Steril 1982;38:281–300.

3. New Developments in Imaging and Hormonal Stimulation of the Ovaries 37

6. Guraya SS. Biology of ovarian follicles in mammals. New York: Springer-Verlag, 1985:320.
7. Baird DT. A model for follicular selection and ovulation: lessons from superovulation. J Steroid Biochem 1987;27:15–23.
8. Bomsel-Helmreich O. Ultrasound and the preovulatory human follicle. Oxford Rev Reprod Biol 1985;7:1–72.
9. Leerentveld RA, VanGent I, DerStoep M, Wladimiroff JW. Ultrasonographic assessment of Graafian follicle growth under monofollicular and multifollicular conditions in clomiphene citrate stimulated cycles. Fertil Steril 1985;40:461–65.
10. Gougeon A. Dynamics of follicular growth in the human: a model from preliminary results. Hum Reprod 1986;1:81–87.
11. Hackelöer BJ, Fleming R, Robinson HP, Adam AH, Coutts JRT. Correlation of ultrasonic and endocrinologic assessment of human follicular development. Am J Obstet Gynecol 1979;135:122–29.
12. Martinuk SD, Chizen DR, Pierson RA. Ultrasonographic morphology of the human preovulatory follicle wall prior to ovulation. Clin Anat 1992;5:1–14.
13. Pierson RA. The scientific basis for improving contraceptive regimens. Processings of the Society of Obstetricians and Gynecologists of Canada Annual Conference, International Symposium on the Scientific Basis for Improving Oral Contraceptive Regimens 1999:30–42. June 25, 1999. Ottawa, Ontario.
14. Queenan JT, O'Brien GD, Bains LM, Simpson J, Collins WP, Campbell S. Ultrasound scanning of ovaries to detect ovulation in women. Fertil Steril 1980;34:99–105.
15. Lenz S. Ultrasonic study of follicular maturation, ovulation and development of corpus luteum during normal menstrual cycles. Acta Obstet Gynecol Scand 1985;64:15–19.
16. Hanna MD, Chizen DR, Pierson RA. Characteristics of follicular evacuation during human ovulation. J Ultrasound Obstet Gynaecol 1994;4:488–93.
17. Pierson RA, Chizen DR, Olatunbosun OA. Ultrasonographic Assessment of Ovulation Induction. In: Jaffe R, Pierson RA, Abramowicz JS, eds. Imaging in Infertility and Reproductive Endocrinology. Lippincott, Philadelphia USA 1994:155–66.
18. Bryce RL, Shuter B, Sinosich MJ, Stiel JN, Picker RH, Saunders DM. The value of ultrasound, gonadotropin, and estradiol measurements for precise ovulation prediction. Fertil Steril 1982;37:42–45.
19. Sarty GE, Pierson RA. Analysis of ovarian follicular response to superstimulation in a three dimensional parametric space. Fertil Steril 1998;70(Suppl. 3):S183.

4

Paternal Effects on Fertilization, Embryo Development, and Pregnancy Outcome

DENNY SAKKAS, GIANCARLO MANICARDI, DAVIDE BIZZARO,
ODETTE MOFFATT, AND MATHEW TOMLINSON

It has long been recognized that oocyte factors can drastically influence fertilization, embryo development and pregnancy outcome in the human. The role that the spermatozoon plays, however, has not been thought to be as important. Much of this was probably related to the idea that the paternal influence was an "all or nothing" event: If the semen parameters of a male were poor (i.e., low sperm concentration, motility, and morphology), then they would not ensue in fertilization. If poor sperm were not even able to create an embryo, then that was believed to be the end of the story. It is now becoming more evident that some of the intrinsic properties of spermatozoa may influence the ensuing embryo, including anomalies in the sperm nucleus (1), the organelles (2) and even the elaborate cytoskeleton of the sperm (3).

Effects of Radiation on Male Germ Cells

The majority of the evidence highlighting paternal influences has come from animal studies, in particular the rodent. Indeed, many of these studies have concentrated on the role of radiation or toxic chemicals and have shown that germ cell DNA damage can lead to spontaneous abortions, malformations, and increased incidence of cancer (4–7). Models are more difficult to obtain in the human than they are in the rodent, but a number of studies have tried to determine the role of radiation on the male germ cell. One example is a series of studies that have investigated the transgenerational effects of paternal preconceptional irradiation in the offspring of male radiation workers at the Sellafield nuclear reprocessing plant in the United Kingdom. An increased risk has been shown in the children born to male radiation workers by investigating the sex ratio and adverse health outcomes of their children (e.g., stillbirth, infant death, and cancer) (8–10). The true influence of paternal effects in the human, however, is still in dispute (11–12).

As stated earlier the data from animal models is more conclusive than that so far reported in the human. One interesting series of studies has been conducted by the group of Robaire during the late 1980s and early 1990s. They have performed a series of studies indicating that damage to rat spermatozoal nuclear DNA may be linked to an increase in early embryo death. They reported that treatment of male rats with cyclophosphamide had little effect on the male reproductive system, but caused single strand DNA breaks in the cauda epididymal spermatozoa and altered the decondensation potential of spermatozoa (13–14). It is more disturbing that similar treatment protocols using cyclophosphamide were already known to produce an increase in postimplantation loss and malformations (15–17) and that these were shown to be transmissible to the next generation (18).

In the human there are real concerns that offspring born from defective male gametes may be at risk. Which scenarios would lead to defective male gametes being used to create offspring in the human? As stated earlier males may produce offspring after being exposed to certain toxins or agents that would cause damage to their gametes. These agents would not influence their semen parameters to the extent that they could not reproduce normally, but their gametes would carry certain anomalies most likely in the nuclear DNA. Another form of transferring faulty male gametes has now become more predominant in that many males with poor semen parameters are assisted in reproduction with techniques such as in vitro fertilization (IVF) and, more so, with intracytoplasmic sperm injection (ICSI).

Males with Abnormal Semen Parameters

A large body of evidence has accumulated showing that men with poor sperm parameters can have problems in their spermatozoa at the nuclear (19), organelle (20,21), and cytoskeletal (22) levels. In this chapter we will concentrate on the role that anomalies in the sperm nuclear DNA may give rise to once they enter into an oocyte during fertilization and what may ensue in the developing embryo and offspring.

The presence of spermatozoa in the human ejaculate that have damaged nuclear DNA has been confirmed by a number of studies (19,23–27). In addition to the previous studies it has been shown that men with poor semen parameters possess anomalies in the composition of their sperm nuclei, displaying higher levels of loosely packaged chromatin and damaged DNA (28–34) (Fig. 4.1). As a result the males that possess spermatozoa with damaged nuclear DNA are those more likely to have semen parameters that would require assisted reproduction. In the majority of cases these males will ultimately be treated with ICSI. In treating infertile men the statistical chances

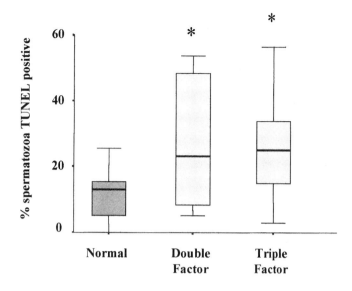

FIGURE 4.1. The percentage of spermatozoa possessing nuclear DNA damage, as assessed by the TUNEL assay, in males with normal sperm parameters (> 20 million sperm per ml, > 50% motility, and >15% normal forms) compared with a combination of two anomalies in sperm concentration, motility, and morphology (Double Factor) and a combination of all three anomalies (Triple Factor). The results are expressed in a box plot. *Denotes significantly greater ($p < 0.01$) when compared with normals.

are therefore higher that, during the ICSI procedure, spermatozoa possessing defective nuclear DNA would be selected and used. By performing techniques (e.g., ICSI) we remove many of the barriers set in place to select the best sperm for fertilization. We have therefore become less discriminating with the quality of paternal nuclear material we introduce into the egg because the onus on sperm selection is left purely on the ICSI operator.

The Effect of an Abnormal Sperm Nucleus on Fertilization

We have previously shown that sperm from men with high levels of nuclear DNA damage and anomalies in their chromatin packaging are more likely to exhibit anomalies in decondensation after ICSI (35). We observed that after ICSI patients who had a high percentage of DNA-damaged sperm and high levels of abnormal chromatin were more likely to have unfertilized oocytes containing sperm that had remained condensed. A number of studies have shown an association between increased DNA fragmentation and decreased fertilization rates (30,36). Lopes et al. (31) investigated the relationship between the outcome of ICSI and the percentage of spermatozoa possessing nuclear DNA damage, as assessed by the TUNEL assay, and found a significant negative association between the percentage of sperm with DNA fragmentation and the ICSI fertilization rate. Indeed, they found that men who had more than 25% of their sperm possessing DNA damage were more likely to experience fertilization rates of less than 20% after ICSI.

Esterhuizen et al. (33) reported that poor chromatin packaging, as assessed using Chromomycin A_3, was related to poor IVF rates. The Chromomycin A_3 fluorochrome is a useful tool for assessing the packaging quality of the chromatin in sperm and allows an indirect visualization of protamine deficiency (24,37). In a study conducted by Twigg et al. (38) it was found that although sperm exposed to hydrogen peroxide, NADPH, or activated leucocytes showed increased amounts of DNA strand breakage, their rate of decondensation and pronuclear formation, when microinjected into hamster oocytes, was the same as untreated control sperm. They went on to state that the ability of genetically damaged spermatozoa to achieve normal fertilization had implications for assisted conception therapy.

The Effect of an Abnormal Sperm Nucleus on Embryo Development

A number of authors have suggested that semen quality and embryo development may be related (39–41). In one study, Filatov et al. (42) found that disordered sperm chromatin packing was related to a decline in rates of embryo cleavage. The majority of the previous studies, which have indicated a paternal effect, have been based on using routine IVF insemination procedures, where cleavage rates and embryo quality may be influenced by the timing of fertilization. In addition, they only examined preimplantation embryo development for 2 or 3 days. Extended culture to the blastocyst stage may give us a broader insight as to the paternal effects on embryo development. Indeed, Janny and Menezo (43) reported that frozen sperm and abnormal sperm both gave rise to embryos with a significantly lower cleavage rate and potential to form blastocysts.

In a previous study we examined the development of supernumerary embryos after ICSI and IVF to the blastocyst stage (44). Embryos were cultured to the blastocyst stage using the Vero cell coculture system (45). It is of interest that the development of blastocysts after ICSI was found to be significantly less than that after routine IVF. Furthermore, in the same study, when we compared the IVF and ICSI embryos at the Day 2 stage, the overall morphology and cell number of the IVF embryos did not greatly exceed that of the ICSI embryos. The differences between IVF and ICSI embryos manifested themselves between the Day 2 stage and the time of blastocyst formation. We proposed that the inability to develop after Day 2 might have been linked to a postembryonic genome activation event when the influence of the paternal genome is more likely to have consequence. In human embryos, embryonic genome activation has been shown to occur between the four- to eight-cell stage (46). Sperm that had the ability to fertilize may not necessarily be able to contribute to further embryonic development. A number of other reports have shown that ICSI embryos have a lower capability to develop to the blastocyst stage (47,48).

It is of note that it would be expected that the resulting poor rate of blastocyst development would also manifest itself as a decreased pregnancy rate in ICSI patients. This does not appear to be the case. In addition, when comparing ICSI-generated embryos to IVF the question of whether the ICSI technique itself may influence embryo development comes into play, as Blake et al. (49) have shown that even the sperm deposition site during ICSI can effect embryo quality.

The Assessment of Sperm Nuclear DNA Damage and Fertility

We have investigated whether a relationship exists between sperm nuclear DNA damage and pregnancy rates after IVF and ICSI. We examined the percentage of sperm that had endogenous DNA damage, using the in situ nick translation technique (26), in the raw semen sample and after separation using density gradient centrifugation with PureSperm (Nidacon, Gothenburg, Sweden). The sperm separated using PureSperm is that used for performing either the insemination when doing IVF or ICSI. In addition, using PureSperm significantly reduces the percentage of sperm possessing nuclear DNA damage (50). When we examined the outcomes for IVF and ICSI patients who achieved pregnancy, we found that of the parameters tested the level of DNA damage in their prepared samples was significantly different, whereas other sperm parameters did not differ significantly (Table 4.1). Although this data is preliminary, it indicates that the persistence of high levels of DNA-damaged sperm, even after preparation by density gradient centrifugation, could jeopardize IVF and ICSI outcome.

Further evidence of a relationship between sperm nuclear DNA integrity and fertility has been reported in two studies that have shown the sperm chromatin structure assay (SCSA) could be used as a prognostic factor for human fertility (51,52). The SCSA measures the susceptibility of sperm nuclear DNA to heat or acid-induced denaturation in situ. In the Evenson study (51) they found that men who had an SCSA value of greater or equal to 30% had difficulties in achieving pregnancy. This was considered a threshold level not compatible with good fertility. In addition, using selected cut-off values, the SCSA data predicted 7 of 18 miscarriages (39%). The Spano study (52) reported that if an individual had a high fraction of sperm with abnormal chromatin he was a good candidate not to conceive. The probability of fathering a child sharply declined when the fraction of cells with abnormal chromatin was more than 20% and was negligible when a value of 40% was

TABLE 4.1. A comparison of pregnant and non-pregnant patients after treatment by IVF or ICSI in relation to various sperm parameters.

Parameter	Not pregnant	Pregnant	p
No. of cycles	76	36	
Sperm concentration (million per ml)	62.9 ± 5.5	67.1 ± 7.3	0.5
% motile sperm (forward progression)	50.5 ± 2.2	52.9 ± 3.2	0.6
% sperm with normal forms	12.9 ± 0.8	13.3 ± 1.1	0.6
Mean % of DNA damaged sperm after preparation	4.8 ± 0.7	3.1 ± 0.5	0.03
No. of oocytes collected	12.6 ± 1.4	14.0 ± 1.2	0.2
Fertilization rate (%)	58.3 ± 3.3	62.4 ± 2.8	0.8
No. of embryos transferred	2.2 ± 0.1	2.2 ± 0.1	0.5

Statistical analysis was performed using the Mann-Whitney test. Values given are means ± SEM.

obtained. These studies showed that the SCSA, which is an indicator of abnormal nuclear chromatin organization, was highly indicative of male subfertility, regardless of the concentration, motility, and morphology of spermatozoa from an individual patient.

Conclusions

The influence that DNA-damaged human spermatozoa can have on the outcome of normal or assisted conception is not clear. Many of the studies reported in the human are not definitive in their conclusions and are rarely drawn from experimental models. The main question that needs to be considered is "what are the consequences once a defective male gamete has fertilized an oocyte?" Once fertilized, the oocyte may have the capability to repair the damaged DNA of sperm. Matsuda and Tobari (53) showed that newly fertilized eggs were capable of repairing some of the deliberately damaged DNA of mouse spermatozoa irradiated with UV or treated with alkylating agents; however, although there may be in-built mechanisms to guard against the incorporation of damaged DNA, the results from the studies of Robaire and colleagues are highly indicative that these systems may not be foolproof. Our data (44) indicate that some effects of a defective male gamete may be seen in postembryonic genome activation. The implementation of blastocyst culture in human IVF programs may help us answer this question.

A number of scenarios may therefore be envisaged if defective paternal DNA enters into an egg (Fig. 4.2) (54). During fertilization the oocyte may: (1) reject the sperm and fail to be fertilized, (2) it could repair the DNA and complete fertilization, or (3) attempt to repair the DNA and complete fertilization after

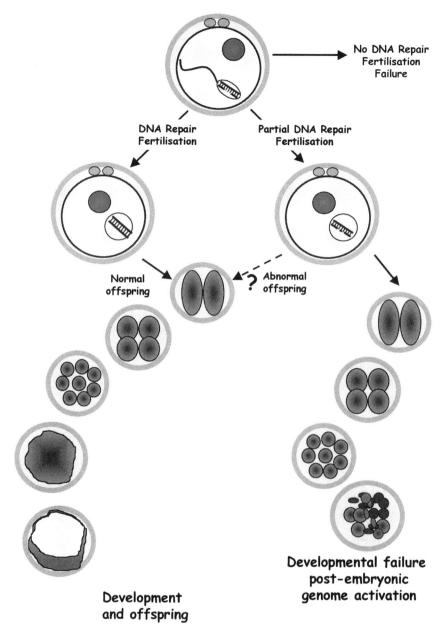

FIGURE 4.2. Consequences of fertilization by sperm with nuclear DNA damage. During fertilization the oocyte may: (1) reject the sperm and fail to be fertilized, (2) repair the DNA and complete fertilization, or (3) attempt to repair the DNA and complete fertilization after only partially completing the repair process. Partial repair of damaged sperm DNA could then lead to a failure in embryo development or possibly to the development of offspring. Reproduced with kind permission from Sakkas et al. (50).

only partially completing the repair process. Either of the first two events should not have any deleterious effects. If an embryo develops from the third scenario it may develop normally with no further consequences, falter in its development once the embryonic genome is activated, or develop and implant carrying a defective paternal genome. The consequences of this final possibility may not be seen until various stages: during the pregnancy, at birth, during the lifetime of the offspring, or even not until the second generation.

The paternal effects on fertilization, embryo development, and pregnancy outcome has not been adequately examined in the human. The exposure of males to environmental and work-related factors that may reduce their sperm quality and the treatment of males who display abnormal sperm characteristics (e.g., nuclear DNA damage) using assisted reproductive techniques such as ICSI both increase the chances of generating offspring from abnormal male gametes. A greater understanding of the male gamete, its abnormalities and the influences it has once it enters the oocyte, is therefore required.

References

1. Sakkas D, Urner F, Bizzaro D, Manicardi G, Bianchi PG, Shoukir Y, et al. Sperm nuclear DNA damage and altered chromatin structure: effect on fertilization and embryo development. Hum Reprod 1998;13(Suppl. 4):11–19.
2. Shoubridge EA. Transmission of mammalian mitochondrial DNA. In: Gagnon C, ed. The male gamete: from basic science to clinical applications. Vienna, IL: Cache River Press, 1999:283–90.
3. Hewitson L, Simerly C, Sutovsky P, Dominko T, Takahashi D, Schatten G. The fate of sperm components within the egg during fertilization: implications for infertility. In: Gagnon C, ed. The male gamete: from basic science to clinical applications. Vienna, IL: Cache River Press, 1999:273–82.
4. Jacobs P, Hassold T, Harvey J, May K. The origin of sex chromosome aneuploidy. Prog Clin Biol Res 1989;311:135–51.
5. Dellarco VL. Genetic anomalies in mammalian germ cells and their significance for human reproductive and developmental risk. Environ Health Perspect 1993;101 (Suppl. 2):5–11.
6. Luke GA, Riches AC, Bryant PE. Genomic instability in haematopoietic cells of F1 generation mice of irradiated male parents. Mutagenesis 1997;12:147–52.
7. Lord BI, Woolford LB, Wang L, Stones VA, McDonald D, Lorimore SA, et al. Tumour induction by methyl-nitroso-urea following preconceptional paternal contamination with plutonium-239. Br J Cancer 1998;78:301–11.
8. Dickinson HO, Parker L, Binks K, Wakeford R, Smith J. The sex ratio of children in relation to paternal preconceptional radiation dose: a study in Cumbria, northern England. J Epidemiol Community Health 1996;50:645–52.
9. Parker L, Craft AW, Smith J, Dickinson H, Wakeford R, Binks K, et al. Geographical distribution of preconceptional radiation doses to fathers employed at the Sellafield nuclear installation, West Cumbria. Br Med J 1993;307:966–71.
10. Parker L, Pearce MS, Dickinson HO, Aitkin M, Craft AW. Stillbirths among offspring of male radiation workers at Sellafield nuclear reprocessing plant. Lancet 1999;354:1407–14.

11. Doll R, Evans HJ, Darby SC. Paternal exposure not to blame. Nature 1994;367: 678–80.
12. Inskip H. Stillbirth and paternal preconceptional radiation exposure. Lancet 1999;354:1400–1.
13. Qiu J, Hales BF, Robaire B. Damage to rat spermatozoal DNA after chronic cyclophosphamide exposure. Biol Reprod 1995;53:1465–73.
14. Qiu J, Hales BF, Robaire B. Effects of chronic low-dose cyclophosphamide exposure on the nuclei of rat spermatozoa. Biol Reprod 1995;52:33–40.
15. Trasler JM, Hales BF, Robaire B. A time-course study of chronic paternal cyclophosphamide treatment in rats: effects on pregnancy outcome and the male reproductive and hematologic systems. Biol Reprod 1987;37:317–26.
16. Trasler JM, Hales BF, Robaire B. Chronic low dose cyclophosphamide treatment of adult male rats: effect on fertility, pregnancy outcome and progeny. Biol Reprod 1986;34:275–83.
17. Trasler JM, Hales BF, Robaire B. Paternal cyclophosphamide treatment of rats causes fetal loss and malformations without affecting male fertility. Nature 1985;316: 144–46.
18. Hales BF, Crosman K, Robaire B. Increased postimplantation loss and malformations among the F2 progeny of male rats chronically treated with cyclophosphamide. Teratology 1992;45:671–78.
19. Evenson DP, Darzynkiewicz Z, Melamed MR. Relation of mammalian sperm chromatin heterogeneity to fertility. Science 1980;210:1131–33.
20. Cummins JM. Mitochondrial DNA: implications for the genetics of human male fertility. In: Barratt CL, De Jonge CJ, Mortimer D, Parinaud J, eds. Genetics of human male infertility. Paris: Editions EDK, 1997:287–307.
21. Cummins JM, Jequier AM, Kan R. Molecular biology of human male infertility: links with aging, mitochondrial genetics, and oxidative stress? Mol Reprod Dev 1994;37: 345–62.
22. Simerly C, Wu GJ, Zoran S, Ord T, Rawlins R, Jones J, et al. The paternal inheritance of the centrosome, the cell's microtubule-organizing center, in humans, and the implications for infertility. Nat Med 1995;1:47–52.
23. Evenson DP. Flow cytometry of acridine orange stained sperm is a rapid and practical method for monitoring occupational exposure to genotoxicants. Prog Clin Biol Res 1986;207:121–32.
24. Bianchi PG, Manicardi GC, Bizzaro D, Bianchi U, Sakkas D. Effect of deoxyribonucleic acid protamination on fluorochrome staining and in situ nick-translation of murine and human mature spermatozoa. Biol Reprod 1993;49:1083–88.
25. Gorczyca W, Traganos F, Jesionowska H, Darzynkiewicz Z. Presence of DNA strand breaks and increased sensitivity of DNA in situ to denaturation in abnormal human sperm cells: analogy to apoptosis of somatic cells. Exp Cell Res 1993;207:202–5.
26. Manicardi GC, Bianchi PG, Pantano S, Azzoni P, Bizzaro D, Bianchi U, et al. Presence of endogenous nicks in DNA of ejaculated human spermatozoa and its relationship to chromomycin A3 accessibility. Biol Reprod 1995;52:864–67.
27. Sailer BL, Jost LK, Evenson DP. Mammalian sperm DNA susceptibility to in situ denaturation associated with the presence of DNA strand breaks as measured by the terminal deoxynucleotidyl transferase assay. J Androl 1995;16:80–87.
28. Foresta C, Indino M, Mioni R, Scanelli G, Scandellari C. Evidence of sperm nuclear chromatin heterogeneity in ex-cryptorchid subjects. Andrologia 1987;19:148–52.

29. Bianchi PG, Manicardi GC, Urner F, Campana A, Sakkas D. Chromatin packaging and morphology in ejaculated human spermatozoa: evidence of hidden anomalies in normal spermatozoa. Mol Hum Reprod 1996;2:139–44.
30. Sun JG, Jurisicova A, Casper RF. Detection of deoxyribonucleic acid fragmentation in human sperm: correlation with fertilization in vitro. Biol Reprod 1997;56:602–7.
31. Lopes S, Sun JG, Jurisicova A, Meriano J, Casper RF. Sperm deoxyribonucleic acid fragmentation is increased in poor-quality semen samples and correlates with failed fertilization in intracytoplasmic sperm injection. Fertil Steril 1998;69:528–32.
32. Host E, Lindenberg S, Kahn JA, Christensen F. DNA strand breaks in human sperm cells: a comparison between men with normal and oligozoospermic sperm samples. Acta Obstet Gynecol Scand 1999;78:336–39.
33. Esterhuizen AD, Franken DR, Lourens JG, Prinsloo E, van Rooyen LH. Sperm chromatin packaging as an indicator of in-vitro fertilization rates. Hum Reprod 2000;15:657–61.
34. Irvine DS, Twigg JP, Gordon EL, Fulton N, Milne PA, Aitken RJ. DNA integrity in human spermatozoa: relationships with semen quality. J Androl 2000;21:33–44.
35. Sakkas D, Urner F, Bianchi PG, Bizzaro D, Wagner I, Jaquenoud N, et al. Sperm chromatin anomalies can influence decondensation after intracytoplasmic sperm injection. Hum Reprod 1996;11:837–43.
36. Hoshi K, Katayose H, Yanagida K, Kimura Y, Sato A. The relationship between acridine orange fluorescence of sperm nuclei and the fertilizing ability of human sperm. Fertil Steril 1996;66:634–39.
37. Bizzaro D, Manicardi GC, Bianchi PG, Bianchi U, Mariethoz E, Sakkas D. In-situ competition between protamine and fluorochromes for sperm DNA. Mol Hum Reprod 1998;4:127–32.
38. Twigg JP, Irvine DS, Aitken RJ. Oxidative damage to DNA in human spermatozoa does not preclude pronucleus formation at intracytoplasmic sperm injection. Hum Reprod 1998;13:1864–71.
39. Ron-el R, Nachum H, Herman A, Golan A, Caspi E, Soffer Y. Delayed fertilization and poor embryonic development associated with impaired semen quality. Fertil Steril 1991;55:338–44.
40. Chan SY, Tucker MJ, Leung CK, Leong MK. Association between human in vitro fertilization rate and pregnancy outcome: a possible involvement of spermatozoal quality in subsequent embryonic viability. Asia Oceania J Obstet Gynaecol 1993;19:357–73.
41. Parinaud J, Mieusset R, Vieitez G, Labal B, Richoilley G. Influence of sperm parameters on embryo quality. Fertil Steril 1993;60:888–92.
42. Filatov MV, Semenova EV, Vorob'eva OA, Leont'eva OA, Drobchenko EA. Relationship between abnormal sperm chromatin packing and IVF results. Mol Hum Reprod 1999;5:825–30.
43. Janny L, Menezo YJ. Evidence for a strong paternal effect on human preimplantation embryo development and blastocyst formation. Mol Reprod Dev 1994;38:36–42.
44. Shoukir Y, Chardonnens D, Campana A, Sakkas D. Blastocyst development from supernumerary embryos after intracytoplasmic sperm injection: a paternal influence? Hum Reprod 1998;13:1632–37.
45. Sakkas D, Jaquenoud N, Leppens G, Campana A. Comparison of results after in vitro fertilized human embryos are cultured in routine medium and in coculture on Vero cells: a randomized study. Fertil Steril 1994;61:521–25.

46. Braude P, Bolton V, Moore S. Human gene expression first occurs between the four- and eight-cell stages of preimplantation development. Nature 1988;332:459–61.
47. Jones GM, Trounson AO, Lolatgis N, Wood C. Factors affecting the success of human blastocyst development and pregnancy following in vitro fertilization and embryo transfer. Fertil Steril 1998;70:1022–29.
48. Dumoulin JC, Coonen E, Bras M, van Wissen LC, Ignoul-Vanvuchelen R, Bergers-Jansen JM, et al. Comparison of in-vitro development of embryos originating from either conventional in-vitro fertilization or intracytoplasmic sperm injection. Hum Reprod 2000;15:402–9.
49. Blake M, Garrisi J, Tomkin G, Cohen J. Sperm deposition site during ICSI affects fertilization and development. Fertil Steril 2000;73:31–37.
50. Sakkas D, Manicardi GC, Bizzaro D, Bianchi PG. Possible consequences of performing intracytoplasmic sperm injection (ICSI) with sperm possessing nuclear DNA damage. Hum Fertil 2000;3:26–30.
51. Evenson DP, Jost LK, Marshall D, Zinaman MJ, Clegg E, Purvis K, et al. Utility of the sperm chromatin structure assay as a diagnostic and prognostic tool in the human fertility clinic. Hum Reprod 1999;14:1039–49.
52. Spano M, Bonde JP, Hjollund HI, Kolstad HA, Cordelli E, Leter G. Sperm chromatin damage impairs human fertility. The Danish First Pregnancy Planner Study Team. Fertil Steril 2000;73:43–50.
53. Matsuda Y, Tobari I. Chromosomal analysis in mouse eggs fertilized in vitro with sperm exposed to ultraviolet light (UV) and methyl and ethyl methanesulfonate (MMS and EMS). Mutat Res 1988;198:131–44.
54. Sakkas D, Manicardi GC, Tomlinson M, Mandrioli M, Bizzaro D, Bianchi PG, et al. The use of density gradient centrifugation techniques and the swim-up method to separate spermatozoa with chromatin and nuclear DNA anomalies. Hum Reprod 2000;15:1112–16.

Part II

Physiology of the Embryo

5

The Cell Biology of Preimplantation Development

RICHARD J. TASCA

There are many aspects of the cell biology of preimplantation development. This chapter will focus upon several important cell membrane functions that appear as the egg develops into the blastocyst. Cell membrane functions reflect the interactions between an embryo and its fluid and cellular environment while it resides in the oviduct and uterus. In the context of this book, better knowledge of these interactions may provide new ideas for the improvement of culture conditions from egg to blastocyst. I shall first provide a brief overview of the cell biology of preimplantation development (PD), then a discussion of amino acid transport (AAT) in preimplantation embryos (PE), and finally a brief survey of the roles in blastocyst formation of three other cell membrane proteins, Na^+/K^+ATPase (NKA), the Na^+/H^+ exchangers (NHE), and the aquaporins (AQP).

Overview

PD is a cell biologist's dream because it is a period of dynamic reconstruction. At the morphological level, the single large egg cell is reconstructed by multiple cleavage divisions into the multicellular, fluid filled blastocyst that has properties that differ greatly from those of the egg cell. Two major morphological events called *compaction* and *cavitation* are conspicuous and are essential for successful progression through development (1–3). In the mouse, between the early eight-cell stage and the late eight-cell stage, the rounded blastomeres squeeze against each other (the compaction process) and intercellular junctions begin to form between the cells. This is followed by the morula stage with 16–32 cells in which the outer cells that squeeze together form tight junctions, thus creating an inside and an outside of the embryo. As the NKA pumps Na^+ into the small spaces between the inner cells, water follows through a local osmosis phenomenon. This inward pumping of Na^+ followed by water results in the formation of the blastocoelic cavity (the cavitation process), which is the central, fluid compartment of the blastocyst. The epithelial outer wall of the blastocyst is the *trophectoderm*.

The reconstruction is also obvious at the ultrastructural level by following the dramatic changes that occur in the mitochondria and the nucleolus during PD (4). Changes in both the localization and temporal appearance of other cellular organelles can be readily seen as part of this dynamic reconstruction. Then, at the level of cell membrane function, AAT and nucleoside transport increase tremendously between the early cleavage stages and the blastocyst stage (5). In the early cleavage stages, although inward AAT rates are slow, the egg seems to release huge quantities of taurine and glycine, which are two nonessential amino acids that are present in large concentrations (6).

Finally, the key reconstruction element is the regulation of gene expression. All of the discussed changes plus the many others that have not been mentioned are directed by the program of gene expression that consists of two major components (7–9). First, proteins, messenger RNAs, and other molecules inherited from the egg are used during the early cleavages and then decrease greatly by the two-cell stage or later. Then, at the two-cell stage in the mouse and at other stages in other species, there is the onset of a massive synthesis of messenger RNAs in addition to the ribosomal RNAs. By the blastocyst stage, there are many thousands of additional mRNAs than in the two-cell stage. This pattern has several elements to it, including the transient expression and degradation of some messages that occurs only at one stage or another (10). Some mRNAs appear to be synthesized in coordination with each other at a particular stage. The genes for some of these are clustered together on one chromosome perhaps to coordinate their synthesis. Thus, nuclear reprogramming is the hallmark of regulation of gene expression in PD.

The program of gene expression is of the utmost importance in the context of embryo culture because there have been several reports showing that inferior culture conditions can lead to abnormal levels of specific mRNAs. In one of these cases, it is shown that an inferior culture medium (Whitten's) leads to significantly decreased levels of mRNAs for insulinlike growth factors and their receptors in embryos cultured from the two-cell stage to the blastocyst stage (11). In KSOM/AA, however, a new medium proven to be superior to Whitten's, the levels of these same mRNAs are equivalent to fresh control blastocysts taken directly from the uterus. The other case shows very dramatically that culture in Whitten's medium causes the "erasure" of a genomic imprint on the H19 gene, a trophectoderm specific gene (12). Again, in KSOM/AA medium, the proper imprint is retained such that the pattern of gene expression for H19 closely resembles the fresh blastocyst control taken directly from the uterus. In both the growth factor and the H19 experiments, the culture conditions have their effect upon specific genes rather than globally, possibly operating on genes that are particularly sensitive to the culture conditions at a particular time during development. It is now well known that the particular culture conditions present during PD can have long-term effects upon fetal stages and after birth, especially in livestock (13–15). These experiments point very sharply to the need to design and improve our culture conditions for blastocyst formation so that the fidelity of the program of gene expression is maintained.

Amino Acid Transport (AAT)

Dramatic and specific changes in AAT rates occur during this period of dynamic reconstruction and represent an outstanding reflection of an embryo interacting with its environment. AAT is a particularly interesting current topic because the addition of amino acids to culture media is now widely acknowledged to have beneficial effects on development to the blastocyst and blastocyst quality, as well as in postimplantation embryo and fetal development (16–20). It is important to review some of the known roles of amino acids quickly because it is highly likely that (1) many of these functions for amino acids will occur in PE and (2) AAT mechanisms will be involved in regulation of these functions. Amino acids are well known: As precursors for the synthesis of proteins and play an important role in growth control; as precursors for hormones, neurotransmitters, nucleotides, and other amino acid derivatives; as sources of energy, nitrogen, and carbon. In addition, amino acids serve as osmolytes, anti-oxidants, pH regulators, chelators, and signaling molecules (e.g., nitric oxide). With this wide array of functions and with more than 20 amino acids, it should be no surprise that amino acids are beneficial in embryo culture media.

In view of these beneficial effects and the probable role of AAT in these effects, there is one experiment that is particularly important (21). When mouse blastocysts were incubated in 0.1 mM methionine for 1 or 2 hours, methionine accumulated in the embryos to 20–30 times the normal intracellular concentration. This abnormal accumulation depleted the blastocysts of nearly the entire intracellular pool of the other essential amino acids, probably through AAT exchange. At lower external concentrations of single amino acids, the internal essential amino acid pools can be spared (21,22). These results provide an extreme example of the danger of using high or unbalanced external concentrations of amino acids in the culture media. Thus, it seems reasonable that future embryo culture media should continue to include the full range of amino acids, but with relative proportions of amino acids reflecting the proportions found in the oviductal and uterine fluids. In these fluids, from a number of a species, only three or four amino acids constitute 50–90% of the total amino acid pool (Hassan, Leanez, Tasca, Wu, Watson, and Westhusin; unpublished observations). These are consistently the nonessential amino acids glycine, glutamate, taurine, and sometimes aspartate and alanine. Media with correct proportions, but with lower concentrations, should provide an appropriate environment for maintenance of intracellular pools through AAT.

Discovery of Na^+-Dependent AAT in Blastocysts

We initially found that AAT rates increase dramatically between mouse early cleavage embryos and blastocysts (5). We then discovered that on Na^+-dependent mechanism exists in blastocysts for transport of the essential amino acids leucine, methionine, and phenylalanine that did not resemble the classical AAT systems that had been described up to that time (23,24). A survey of 11 amino acids indicated that this Na^+ dependency is massive and extends to nearly all essential and nonessential amino acids (22,25). This same survey for earlier stages revealed a gradual onset of Na^+-dependent AAT. The transport of glycine, a small, neutral, and nonessential amino acid, is strongly Na^+ dependent from the mouse unfertilized egg stage through the blastocyst stage. Other nonessential amino acids such as alanine begin Na^+ dependency as early as the four-cell stage and glutamate as early as the eight-cell stage. Then, by the morula stage, Na^+ dependency begins for some of the essential amino acids, such as methionine, threonine, leucine and valine. Finally, by the blastocyst stage, major components of the transport of the essential and bulkier amino acids (i.e., phenylalanine, tyrosine, and tryptophan) are added to the Na^+-dependent group such that more than 50% of the total AAT in blastocysts is Na^+ dependent. It is interesting that this order of onset of Na+ dependency appears linked to amino acid structure that is reflected by the fact that nonessential amino acids are more lipophobic and most essential amino acids are more lipophilic.

Characterization of AAT Systems

An extensive characterization of AAT systems in mouse PE was then carried out over many years (26). This characterization indicated that the dynamic reconstruction of AAT during PD is reflected in the patterns of as many as 15 different AAT systems. These systems follow unique and sometimes dramatically changing patterns of expression. Some, such as the Xc (Na^+-independent glutamate transport) and the Gly system (glycine and alanine) are present in the zygote, but then disappear by the two-cell stage and the end of the morula stage, respectively. The remarkable Na^+-dependent AAT in blastocysts described earlier for nonessential and essential amino acids has been defined and characterized by Van Winkle as a novel system and named $B^{o,+}$ (B for blastocyst because the system was first discovered in the blastocyst). As noted earlier, this Na^+-dependent system has a gradual onset and eventually serves to transport most amino acids at the blastocyst stage, except glutamate, arginine, taurine and aspartate. Glutamate and aspartate transport are increased dramatically between the morula and blastocyst stage through the X_{AG}

system, a major excitatory AAT system in nervous tissue. Arginine, on the other hand, is transported by the Na^+ independent $b^{0,+}$ system that increases some 30-fold between the one-cell stage and the blastocyst stage (26).

Even though the program of gene expression for AAT systems in early embryos is largely unknown and there has been no AAT protein biochemically identified in these embryos, such data are beginning to emerge (26). It is now known that the disappearance of the Gly system is directly correlated with an enormous decrease in the intracellular glycine content between the one-cell and the blastocyst stage, as well as with the parallel presence and then disappearance of the mRNA for the Gly transport system. It is also known that the mRNA for the excitatory AAT system also parallels the dramatic onset of the X_{AG} transport system in PE. It is most important that the 15 or more AAT systems exhibit the element of redundancy in that most amino acids are taken up by more than one transport system. For example, arginine and tryptophan can each be taken up by at least five different systems. This provides the blastocyst with much versatility such that it can respond to changes in its in vivo environment (e.g., hormonal and other influences that may be present in the uterus). The AAT systems can serve to protect and replenish the intracellular amino acid pools, especially for the essential amino acids, to the extent that protein synthesis is also protected. This is of critical importance because the embryo sensation of lack of a needed amino acid would probably result in protein degradation.

Summary of Important and Potential Roles for AAT in Mouse PE

The changes in pool sizes and dramatic changes in AAT systems reviewed herein bear a strong relationship to the beneficial effects of amino acids in PE culture media. The nonessential amino acids seem to be most beneficial during early cleavage and the essentials, at least in higher concentrations, can be toxic, but there are species differences (27). Prior to the eight-cell stage, there is already substantial evidence that nonessential amino acids participate significantly in volume regulation (28,29), pH regulation (30), and intracellular metabolism (31). It is possible, but there is no direct evidence, that massive efflux and lowered intracellular concentrations of certain amino acids [e.g., taurine and glycine (6)], between the one-cell and eight-cell stages are necessary for the onset of embryonic genome activation that begins at the two-cell stage in the mouse. After the eight-cell stage, the essential amino acids seem to be especially important for development of high-quality blastocysts and even for postimplantation development, whereas the nonessential amino acids are also beneficial. After the eight-cell stage, it is likely that there are important and specific roles for essential AAT. It is already known that there is a net accumulation of essential amino acids between the eight-cell and blastocyst stages despite the abundance of nonessential amino acids in uterine fluid (6), presumably owing to high affinity AAT systems for these amino acids that are needed for the onset of growth that occurs after the morula stage (23).

We have already noted the influence of inferior culture media upon mRNA transcription. It is likely that the control levels of mRNAs, at least for certain transcripts, require the presence of certain levels of essential and/or nonessential amino acids. Some of the amino acids we have discussed are well known for their intercellular signaling properties in other types of tissues (e.g., aspartate and glutamate in nervous tissue). In this context, it is possible that AAT and secretion in blastocysts will provide critical signaling elements for the embryonic-maternal dialogue during early implantation phases.

$Na^+/K^+ATPase$ (NKA)

The NKA, or Na^+ pump, is an ubiquitous cell surface enzyme that is responsible for maintaining the steep gradient of high extracellular Na^+ and high intracellular K^+ that seems essential for cell survival and function. The enzyme also hydrolyzes ATP to produce energy in the form of high energy phosphate. The NKA also serves in a morphogenetic role during blastocyst formation because it is responsible for the vectorial transport of Na^+ and water that is essential for the initiation and formation of blastocoelic fluid as well as for the maintenance of the fluid-filled blastocyst. The location of the NKA on the inner cell membranes of the morula and blastocyst is the key to this role.

The latest evidence from murine and bovine embryos is that the enzyme and its mRNA are present from the one-cell through blastocyst stages (32). In the early cleavage stages, the protein is present as determined by enzymatic activity, but the abundance of the protein is either too low to be detected by antibodies or is masked (33). Later, the enzyme is present on the internal cell membranes of the four-cell and later stages, and becomes localized on the basolateral surface of the blastocyst. When it is coupled with other Na^+ transport systems (e.g., the NHE3 that is localized on the apical surface of the blastocyst, which will be discussed shortly) the blastocyst has powerful control over the inward transport of Na^+ towards the blastocoel, which in turn drives the strong influx of water in formation and maintenance of the blastocyst. The α-1 and β-1 subunits are the most prevalent forms of the NKA in PE, and both of these are needed for activity. They are both localized on the basolateral surface of the blastocyst (34). The α-1 form is the major catalytic subunit and the β-1 subunit may be necessary for full function of the α-1 form, but may be primarily needed for insertion of the subunits into the cell membrane.

It is difficult to study its functionality with the protected site of localization of the NKA inside of the blastocyst. For example, ouabain, which is the most specific and effective inhibitor of NKA activity, cannot reach the NKA in mouse blastocysts. For this reason, we utilized cytochalasin B to weaken the intercellular junctions between trophectodermal cells, causing collapse of the blastocyst that then allows ouabain to reach the internalized sites of NKA localization (25). This enabled us to prove directly that the massive Na^+-dependent AAT system that is present in blastocysts is largely dependent upon the activity of the NKA. Others have used the cytochalasin collapse of blastocysts in order to show the role of the NKA in Na^+ and in water transport. These and other experiments prove that the NKA plays an indispensable role in blastocyst formation and function and qualify it as one of the most important morphogenetic proteins in early development.

Na^+/H^+ Exchanger 3 (NHE3)

It has been proven that this cell surface protein is a key apical transporter of Na^+ in the blastocyst (35). It is also involved in pH control, serves as a cell volume regulator, and is involved in other cell types as a regulator of signal transduction in cell proliferation. The mRNA for NHE3 is found only in the oocyte. The protein, however, is found localized on the exterior cell membranes of the oocyte and all of the PE stages, culminating with its localization only on the apical surface of the blastocyst. As noted earlier, the NHE3 most likely works in consort with the NKA in the strong vectorial transport of Na^+ during blastocyst formation and maintenance. Because there is no detectable mRNA for NHE3 during PD, NHE3 can be classified as an oogenetic protein. As such, it is synthesized during oogenesis and then inserted into the cell membranes of the oocyte, where it remains throughout PD. It may be the first oogenetic protein discovered with a known function in the blastocyst stage.

Aquaporins

With our most recent knowledge of the mRNAs and protein localizations for the NKA and for NHE3 we are beginning to assemble a diagram of the trophectodermal apical and basolateral surfaces that is consistent with a true water transporting epithelium; however, our understanding of the actual mechanism by which water moves across the trophectoderm is still weak. Neither a diffusional mechanism nor a co-transport mechanism seems to be a major route for transtrophectodermal water transport; however, a family of at least 10 water channel proteins, called *aquaporins*, has been discovered in many adult tissues (36,37). Several aquaporin mRNAs have been found throughout murine and bovine egg to blastocyst stages, and the aquaporin 3 protein has been found on the basolateral surface of bovine blastocysts (Offenberg, Barcroft, Betts, Watson; unpublished observations). This work is quite new, but it provides very encouraging results that may lead to a more complete picture of the mechanism of water transport in trophectoderm.

Conclusion

One can see from this chapter that we are just beginning to assemble a functional and structural map of the cell surfaces of the blastocyst, particularly the apical and basolateral surfaces of the trophectoderm or fluid transporting epithelium of the blastocyst. The transport systems for amino acids are clearly the most well-characterized cell membrane functions in these embryos. It is possible that this knowledge can be used to select several amino acids carefully and to develop a panel of noninvasive amino acid transport tests for the evaluation of blastocyst quality. As emphasized, cell membrane functions such as AAT reflect events taking place inside the embryo and the nature of the interaction between the embryo and its environment. We have also emphasized the central role of the NKA in blastocyst formation and function. The NKA notably plays a major role in AAT and thus a panel of amino acid transport tests will simultaneously reflect NKA functions that are not revealed by the NKA role in water and ion transport. Other cell membrane functions (i.e., the NHE3 and aquaporins) were mentioned because they also seem to play integral and interactive roles with the NKA. Beyond the scope of this chapter, growth factor receptors, calcium channels, and integrins are among other important cell membrane molecules that appear in the trophectoderm as part of a precise cascade of carefully timed events that culminate in successful implantation of the blastocyst in the uterus (38).

References

1. Wiley LM. Cavitation in the mouse preimplantation embryo: Na/K-ATPase and the origin of nascent blastocoelic fluid. Dev Biol 1984;105:330–42.
2. Watson AJ. The cell biology of blastocyst development. Mol Reprod Dev 1990;33:492–504.
3. Watson AJ, Kidder GM, Schultz GA. How to make a blastocyst. Biochem Cell Biol 1992;70:849–55.
4. Hillman N, Tasca RJ. Ultrastructural and autoradiographic studies of mouse cleavage stages. Am J Anat 1969;126:151–74.
5. Tasca RJ, Hillman N. Effects of actinomycin D and cycloheximide on RNA and protein synthesis in cleavage stage mouse embryos. Nature 1970;225:1022–25.
6. Schultz GA, Kaye PL, McKay DJ, Johnson MH. Endogenous amino acid pool size in mouse eggs and preimplantation embryos. J Reprod Fertil 1981;61:387–93.
7. Kidder GM. The genetic program for preimplantation development. Dev Genet 1992;13:319–25.
8. Latham KE. Mechanisms and control of embryonic genome activation in mammalian embryos. Int Rev Cytol 1999;193:71–124.
9. DeSousa PA, Watson AJ, Schultz GA, Bilodeau-Goeseels S. Oogenetic and zygotic gene expression directing early bovine embryogenesis: a review. Mol Reprod Dev 1998;51:112–21.
10. Ko MS, Kitchen JR, Wang X, Threat TA, Wang X, Hasegawa A, et al. Large-scale cDNA analysis reveals phased gene expression patterns during preimplantation mouse development. Development 2000;127:1737–49.
11. Ho Y, Wigglesworth, K, Eppig JJ, Schultz RM. Preimplantation development of mouse

embryos in KSOM: augmentation by amino acids and analysis of gene expression. Mol Reprod Dev 1995;41:232–38.
12. Doherty AS, Mann MRW, Tremblay KD, Bartolomei MS, Schultz RM. Differential effects of culture on imprinted H19 expression in the preimplantation mouse embryo. Biol Reprod 2000;62:1526–35.
13. Thompson JG, Gardner DK, Pugh PA, McMillan WH, Tervit HR. Lamb birth weight is affected by culture system utilized during in vitro pre-elongation development of ovine embryos. Biol Reprod 1995;53:1385–91.
14. Blondin P, Farin PW, Crosier AE, Alexander JE, Farin CE. In vitro production of embryos alters levels of insulin-like growth factor-II messenger ribonucleic acid in bovine fetuses 63 days after transfer. Biol Reprod 2000;62:384–89.
15. Young LE, Fairburn HR. Improving the safety of embryo technologies: possible role of genomic imprinting. Theriogenology 2000;53:627–48.
16. Han H-D, Kiessling AA. In vivo development of transferred mouse embryos conceived in vitro in simple and complex media. Fertil Steril 1988;50:159–63.
17. Mehta TS, Kiessling AA. Development potential of mouse embryos conceived in vitro and cultured in ethylenediamine tetraacetic acid with or without amino acids or serum. Biol Reprod 1990;43:600–6.
18. Lane M, Gardner DK. Differential regulation of mouse embryo development and viability by amino acids. J Reprod Fertil 1997;109:153–64.
19. Lane M, Gardner DK. Amino acids and vitamins prevent culture-induced metabolic perturbations and associated loss of viability of mouse blastocysts. Hum Reprod 1998;13:991–97.
20. Biggers JD, McGinnis LK, Raffin M. Amino acids and preimplantation development in the mouse in protein-free potassium simplex optimized medium. Biol Reprod 2000;63:281–93.
21. Kaye PL, Schultz GA, Johnson MH, Pratt HPM, Church RB. Amino acid transport and exchange in preimplantation mouse embryos. J Reprod Fertil 1982;65:367–80.
22. DiZio SM. Amino acid transport, development of cell membrane function, and growth control in early mouse embryogenesis. Ph.D. Dissertation 1978; University of Delaware.
23. Borland RM, Tasca RJ. Activation of a Na^+-dependent amino acid transport system in preimplantation mouse embryos. Dev Biol 1974;36:169–82.
24. Borland RM, Tasca RJ. Na^+-dependent amino acid transport in preimplantation mouse embryos. II. Metabolic inhibitors and the nature of the cation requirement. Dev Biol 1975;46:192–201.
25. DiZio SM, Tasca RJ. Na^+-dependent amino acid transport in preimplantation mouse embryos. III. Na^+-K^+-ATPase linked mechanism in blastocysts. Dev Biol 1977;59:198–205.
26. Van Winkle LJ. Amino acid transport regulatioon and early embryo development. Biol Reprod 2001;64:1–12.
27. Steeves T, Gardner DK. Temporal and differential effects of amino acids on bovine embryo development in culture. Biol Reprod 1999;61:731–40.
28. Dawson KM, Baltz JM. Organic osmolytes and embryos: substrates of the Gly and β transport systems protect mouse zygotes against the effects of raised osmolarity. Biol Reprod 1997;56:1550–58.
29. Kolajova M, Baltz JM. Volume-regulated anion and organic osmolyte channels in mouse zygotes. Biol Reprod 1999;60:964–72.
30. Edwards LJ, Williams DA, Gardner DK. Intracellular pH of the mouse preimplanta-

tion embryo: amino acids act as buffers of intracellular pH. Hum Reprod 1998;13: 3441–48.
31. Chatot CL, Tasca RJ, Ziomek CA. Glutamine uptake and utilization by preimplantation mouse embryos in CZB medium. J Reprod Feril 1990;89:335–46.
32. MacPhee DJ, Jones DH, Barr KJ, Betts DH, Watson AJ, Kidder GM. Differential involvement of Na^+,K^+-ATPase isozymes in preimplantation development of the mouse. Dev Biol 2000;222:486–98.
33. Baltz JM, Smith SS, Biggers JD, Lechene C. Intracellular ion concentrations and their maintenance by Na^+/K^+-ATPase in preimplantation mouse embryos. Zygote 1997; 5:1–9.
34. Watson AJ, Westhusin ME, De Sousa PA, Betts DH, Barcroft LC. Gene expression regulating blastocyst formation. Theriogenology 1999;51:117–33.
35. Barr KJ, Garrill A, Jones DH, Orlowski J, Kidder GM. Contributions of NA^+/H^+ Exchanger isoforms to preimplantation development of the mouse. Mol Reprod Dev 1998;50:146–53.
36. Zeidel ML. Recent advances in water transport. Semin Nephrol 1998;18:167–77.
37. Verkman AS. Lessons on renal physiology from transgenic mice lacking aquaporin water channels. J Am Soc Nephrol 1999;10:1126–35.
38. Wang J, Mayernik L, Schultz JF, Armant DR. Acceleration of trophoblast differentiation by heparin-binding EGF-like growth factor is dependent on the stage specific activation of calcium influx by ErbB receptors in developing mouse blastocysts. Development 2000;127:33–44.

6

Metabolism of the Early Embryo: Energy Production and Utilization

HENRY J. LEESE, ISABELLE DONNAY, DONALD A. MACMILLAN, AND FRANCHESCA D. HOUGHTON

Embryo Metabolism: Energy Production

The vast majority of studies on early mammalian embryo metabolism have been concerned with the generation, rather than the fate, of ATP. Thus, research has focused on the uptake or metabolism of energy sources added to embryo culture media. There have been an even greater number of studies in which metabolism as such has not been measured, but rather where blastocyst formation has been used as an endpoint to assess the effect of different energy sources. It is generally agreed that the early phases of mammalian preimplantation development are relatively quiescent metabolically, relying on substrates such as pyruvate, lactate, or amino acids, which are metabolized aerobically (1–5).

The later preimplantation period is characterized by an increase in glucose uptake at around the morula stage (6), a proportion of which is converted to lactate by aerobic glycolysis, depending on the species (1–5,7). It should be realized that the early embryo has the capacity to adapt its metabolism to the availability of substrates. For example, mouse embryos consume glucose in preference to pyruvate in the later preimplantation stages, but they can continue to consume pyruvate at high rates in the absence of glucose (6). In other words, it is better to think of embryos as having "preferred" rather than "obligatory," metabolic pathways. Such flexibility may have survival value for embryos in the female reproductive tract. It is also important to caution against thinking we know most of what there is to know about early embryo metabolism; in fact, we know rather little. This is illustrated by the case of pyruvate. A few years ago, most would have said that pyruvate, which is required for the first cleavage division in the mouse and is added to virtually all embryo culture medium, is used as an oxidizable energy source. We now know that pyruvate has at least two further functions. In mouse embryos (8) and in all probability human (9) embryos it has a role in intracellular pH regulation. It may also be important in the scavenging of free radicals and in the disposal of ammonia derived from amino acid breakdown (10,11).

There is interest in the metabolism of endogenous fuels. Thus, eggs and embryos are very large cells and are likely to have considerable energy reserves, notably triglyceride, which may be important in cattle and sheep embryos, and, possibly, the human (12,13).

Energy Metabolism: Energy Utilization

Studies on the fate of ATP generation are few and far between. In somatic cells, it has been quantitatively shown that ATP has two major uses (14):

1. protein synthesis
2. Na^+,K^+ ATPase

and a number of minor ones:

3. substrate cycling
4. RNA and DNA turnover
5. enzyme phosphorylation
6. signal transduction

Adult cells obviously have tissue-specific requirements for ATP (eg., 6% of the ATP requirement of resting skeletal muscle is for the Ca^{++}-ATPase; 12% of the liver's basal requirement is for urea synthesis) (14), but these considerations are not relevant for undifferentiated early embryos.

Estimates of the relative ATP use by a cellular process are made either by measuring the rate of the process and calculating the oxygen consumption required to account for that rate or by specifically inhibiting the process and measuring the fractional change in oxygen consumption. Thus, ouabain can be used to inhibit the Na^+,K^+ATPase, and cycloheximide can be used to inhibit protein synthesis. Even though this approach has been used on adult cells for many years, there are four potential problems: (1) inhibitors are rarely specific, (2) inhibiting fundamental processes such as ion transport may affect energy metabolism at multiple sites, (3) inhibiting a major ATP-consuming process may raise the ATP–ADP ratio and stimulate other ATP-consuming processes (14), and (4) oxygen consumption is not exclusive to mitochondria.

To the best of our knowledge, the first report of such experiments in early embryos is due to Benos and Balaban (15), who used the rabbit blastocyst and measured the proportion of oxygen consumption devoted to the activity of the Na^+,K^+ATPase on Days 4–7 postcoitus. On Days 4–6, the values were in the range expected for somatic cells, whereas the ouabain-sensitive component of oxygen consumption fell to 16% on Day 7. This was attributed to a shift in metabolism in preparation for implantation. In a subsequent paper, Benos and Balaban (16) adopted a different approach to determine the proportion of energy consumption used for active Na^+ transport. This was based on an increase in ATP production (i.e., oxygen consumption and lactate production) after Na+ transport had been stimulated by the addition of Amphotericin B. This method gave a value of only 6% of energy devoted to the Na^+,K^+ATPase. The authors accounted for this puzzling finding in terms of Na^+ influx into the blastocyst through a leakage pathway requiring the Na^+ pump to turn over faster than was apparent from transepithelial Na^+ flux measurements.

We have revisited the question of the fate of ATP using mouse and bovine embryos and a novel method to measure oxygen consumption (7). Donnay and Leese (17) collapsed bovine blastocysts with cytochalasin D and allowed them to re-expand for 4 hours in the presence and absence of ouabain. It was necessary to collapse the blastocysts to allow ouabain access to the basal/lateral surfaces of the trophectoderm cells on which the Na^+,K^+ATPase are localized. Oxygen consumption directly correlated with the degree of re-expansion of the blastocyst (Fig. 6.1). Control embryos recovered 54% of their volume in 4 hours, whereas blastocysts expanded in the presence of 1 nM and 1 μM ouabain recovered 5.5% and 0% of their volume, respectively. ATP production for control embryos was 1435 pmol/4 hours and 1284 and 648 pmol/4 hours for embryos treated with 1 nM and 1 μM ouabain, respectively. These calculations suggest that at these two concentrations of ouabain, 10.5% and 44% of the energy generated by the bovine blastocyst is used by the Na^+,K^+ATPase. Because ATP may also be generated by aerobic glycolysis, we also measured glucose consumption and lactate production in the presence and absence of ouabain; however, neither parameter was significantly affected by ouabain. This was a surprising result because bovine blastocysts collapsed with cytochalasin D were able to expand at control rates even in the presence of 0.1 and 0.01 mM KCN and 2,4 Dinitrophenol, which are concentrations that totally inhibit blastocyst expansion in the mouse. This indicates that bovine blastocysts are tolerant to anoxia, a conclusion confirmed by Thompson et al. (18), and that it can derive sufficient ATP from glycolysis as is the case for late preimplantation rat embryos (19). Ouabain addition inhibits re-expansion of cytochalasin D-collapsed blastocysts in the mouse; however, it is notable that in this species a higher concentration of ouabain (0.5 mM) is required to inhibit re-expansion. Values for oxygen consumption by mouse blastocysts +/– ouabain are given in Figure 6.2. These data are difficult to interpret. At a concentration of 0.5 mM, ouabain gave a small, but nonsignificant decrease in oxygen consumption; however, oxygen consumption increased at higher concentrations probably due to nonspecific, toxic effects. In no case was glucose consumption or lactate production affected by ouabain, which is a result similar to that obtained for the bovine.

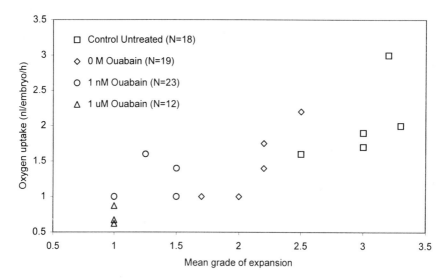

FIGURE 6.1. Relationship between oxygen uptake and degree of (re-)expansion of bovine blastocysts. n = total number of embryos. Each point represents the mean of three to four embryos. Expansion following cytochalasin D treatment evaluated as follows: grade 1 = collapsed embryo (no visible cavity); grade 2 = expanding/collapsing embryo; grade 3 = (re-)expanded blastocyst (no visible space between the zona pellucida and the trophectoderm); grade 4 = hatching or hatched blastocyst. Oxygen consumption was measured by the method of Houghton et al. (7). Regression: all conditions: $R^2 = 0.63$; $p = 0.0001$; 0 M ouabain: $R^2 = 0.82$; $p = 0.0036$. Reproduced with permission from Ref. (17).

Energy Cost of Protein Synthesis

The best data regarding the energy cost of protein synthesis are available for the bovine blastocyst. The early bovine blastocyst has a mass of 350 ng (including the zona pellucida); the expanded blastocyst, 24 hours later, has a protein content of 420 ng, also including the zona; an increase of 70 ng. Oxygen consumption rises from 1.0 nl/embryo/hour to 1.7 nl/embryo/hour during this time (Ferguson and Leese, unpublished). There are then two ways of calculating the energy cost of this increase in protein, depending on the assumptions made.

First, if it is assumed that all of the "extra" oxygen consumed is used in protein synthesis, and that 1 nl oxygen can give rise to 225 pmol ATP (17,20), then the net synthesis of 1 ng protein requires 23 pmol ATP. This assumption is unlikely to be valid because a fraction of the "extra" oxygen could equally be used in Na^+ pumping required for blastocyst expansion. This would make the energy cost of protein synthesis even lower—say 10 pmol ATP/ng protein.

Second, if the calculation is based on the total oxygen consumed over this time, the figure is 104 pmol ATP/p ng protein synthesised. This figure is likely to be an overestimate for the same reason as that given earlier (the need of oxygen for Na^+ pumping) as well as the consumption of ATP by the minor components of energy utilization. The true figure is therefore likely to lie between 10 and 104 pmol ATP/ng net protein synthesis. In this context, it is interesting that theoretical calculations indicate that the synthesis of 1 ng protein requires the expenditure of 40 pmoles ATP (21), or midway between these two extreme values.

These calculations ignore the existence of protein turnover. Thus, the protein content of a cell represents the difference between the rate of synthesis and that of degradation. It is possible that an increase in protein content could be due, in part, to a reduced rate of degradation as well as an increase in protein synthesis. The position is also complicated by the yield of ATP arising from protein degradation.

Nevertheless, it is reasonable to conclude that the formation of 1 ng protein by the bovine blastocyst requires an ATP expenditure quite similar to the theoretical value.

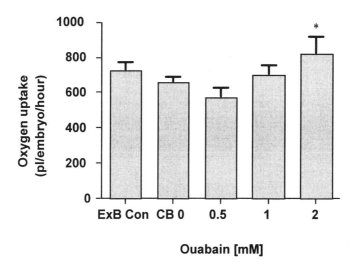

FIGURE 6.2. The effect of ouabain on oxygen uptake by re-expanding mouse blastocysts (± SEM). ExB Con = Intact Control Blastocysts (not treated with cytochalasin D). CB 0 = Re-expanding blastocysts in absence of ouabain. (0.5; 1; 2) = Re-expanding blastocysts incubated with 0.5, 1 and 2 mM ouabain. Blastocysts were collapsed with Cytochalasin D [0.5 µg(ml)] and allowed to expand for 3–5 hours in the presence and absence of ouabain. Oxygen consumption was measured by the method of Houghton et al. (7). *Significantly different from ExB Con ($p < 0.05$).

What Do Oxygen Consumption Measurements Tell Us?

Nonmitochondrial oxygen consumption (mainly due to oxidase enzymes) has been estimated as 21% in liver cells, 14% in skeletal muscle, 2% in thymocytes, and 3% in heart, with an average figure of 10% for the body as a whole. Moreover, around 1–2% of oxygen consumption by mitochondria results in the production of hydrogen peroxide. These data are interesting in view of the work of Manes and Lai (22) on nonmitochondrial oxygen utilization by Day 6 rabbit blastocysts. It was found that cyanide-insensitive oxygen consumption accounted for about half of the total and that about half of the cyanide-resistant fraction was due to superoxide production by an NADPH oxidase on the trophoblast cell surface. The data suggest a role for superoxide in the initiation of implantation in this species as well as providing a caution against uncritically ascribing the whole of oxygen consumption by the blastocyst in any species to mitochondrial energy production.

There is a further potential confounding factor. Working on the mouse blastocyst, Hewitson and Leese (23) found that the glucose metabolism of isolated trophectoderm (TE) and inner cell mass (ICM) differed. Isolated ICMs consumed almost three times more glucose per cell than TE, and all the glucose consumed by the ICM could be accounted for in terms of lactate appearance; the figure for TE was 55%. In other words, both the ICM and the TE can derive energy by aerobic glycolysis, but they differ in their capacity to do so. When cell number is taken into account, about 40% of the total lactate formed by a mouse blastocyst is due to the ICM and 60% to the TE.

These data are consistent with those of Barnett et al. (24) who showed in hamster blastocysts that active mitochondria were largely distributed in the TE rather than by the ICM. These findings are also interesting in the context of work by Lane and Gardner (25), who showed that mouse blastocysts with a high glucose consumption and low glycolysis were the most viable after embryo transfer. This raises the question: What constitutes a "good blastocyst" metabolically?

The problem in answering this question for the species of most interest medically or commercially; the human, cow, sheep and pig, is that in each case, glycolytic rates for intact blastocysts approach, or exceed, 100%, ruling out diagnosis of embryo health on this basis. Experimental data reinforce this conclusion (26). The use of oxygen consumption, which might seem intuitively to be the ideal marker of embryo health, becomes complicated by the existence of nonmitochondrial consumption and the capacity of embryos to generate ATP by aerobic glycolysis. It should be emphasized however, that data on the metabolism of separated ICM and TE are not available for species other than mouse and that in the absence of such data, speculation on the best marker(s) for the health of intact blastocysts, and the extent to which it reflects the health of the ICM and the TE, is unwise.

The Blastocyst as a Model System for Functional Genomics in Humans

As genome sequencing continues apace, there will become a need for a simple cellular system in mammals, including man, with which to understand the role of genes and their products. The blastocyst is ideal for such an analysis. It is relatively simple, consisting of 100 cells or so, devoid of circulatory, endocrine, or nervous influences that complicate the study of tissue–organ function. The blastocyst is still relatively autonomous and free-living; attributes essential for ease of generation, maintenance, and study in vitro. It contains the first epithelium and the progenitors of all the 200 tissues in the adult. In summary, the blastocyst can be considered as an intact mammalian organism—the simplest there is, and therefore the easiest with which to begin the task of unravelling the control of gene expression and its phenotypic consequences. Part of this task will be to provide a quantitative description of the phenotype of the blastocyst—ultimately, everything the blastocyst is doing at a given moment. Generating and using energy, which is the focus of this chapter, is one part of this.

Acknowledgments. Supported by the U.K. Medical Research Council, Biotechnological and Biological Sciences Research Council and European Commission.

References

1. Barnett DK, Bavister BD. What is the relationship between the metabolism of preimplantation embryos and their developmental competence? Mol Reprod Dev 1996;43:105–33.
2. Gardner DK. Changes in requirements and utlization of nutrients during mammalian preimplantation embryo development and their significance in embryo culture. Theriogenology 1998;49:83–102.
3. Leese HJ. Metabolism of the preimplantation mammalian embryo. In: Milligan SR, ed. Oxford Reviews of Reproductive Biology 13. London: Oxford University Press, 1991:35–72.
4. Leese HJ. Metabolic control during preimplantation mammalian development. Hum Reprod Update 1995;1:63–72.
5. Rieger D. Relationship between energy metabolism and development of the early embryo. Theriogenology 1992;37:75–93.
6. Martin KL, Leese HJ. Role of glucose in mouse preimplantation embryo development. Mol Reprod Dev 1995;40:436–43.
7. Houghton FD, Thompson JG, Kennedy CJ, Leese HJ. Oxygen consumption and energy metabolism of the early mouse embryo. Mol Reprod Dev 1996;44:476–85.
8. Gibb CA, Poronnik P, Day ML, Cook DI. Control of cytosolic pH in two cell mouse embryos: role of H^+-lactate cotransport and Na^+/H^+ exchange. Am J Physiol 1997;273:C404–19.

9. Butcher L, Coates A, Martin KL, Rutherford AJ, Leese HJ. Metabolism of pyruvate by the early human embryo. Biol Reprod 1998;58:1054–56.
10. Van Winkle LJ, Dickinson HR. Differences in amino acid content of preimplantation mouse embryos that develop in vitro versus in vivo: in vitro effects of five amino acids that are abundant in oviductal secretions. Biol Reprod 1995;52:96–104.
11. Partridge RJ, Leese HJ. Consumption of amino acids by bovine preimplantation embryos. Reprod Fertil Dev 1996;8:945–50.
12. Leese HJ, Ferguson EM. Embryo metabolism. In: Jansen R, Mortimer D, eds. Towards reproductive certainty. New York: Parthenon Publishing Group, 1999:360–66.
13. Ferguson EM, Leese HJ. Triglyceride content of bovine oocytes and early embryos. J Reprod Fertil 1999;116:373–78.
14. Rolfe DFS, Brown GC. Cellular energy utilization and molecular origin of standard metabolic rate in mammals. Physiol Rev 1997;77:731–58.
15. Benos DJ, Balaban RS. Energy requirements of the developing mammalian blastocyst for active ion transport. Biol Reprod 1980;23:941–47.
16. Benos DJ, Balaban RS. Energy metabolism of preimplantation mammalian blastocysts. Am J Physiol 1983;245:C40–C45.
17. Donnay I, Leese HJ. Embryo metabolism during the expansion of the bovine blastocyst. Mol Reprod Dev 1999;53:171–78.
18. Thompson JG, McNaughton C, Gasparrini B, McGowan LT, Tervit HR. Effect of inhibitors and uncouplers of oxidative phosphorylation during compaction and blasatulation of bovine embryos cultured in vitro. J Reprod Fertil 2000;118:47–55.
19. Brison DR, Leese HJ. Blastocoel cavity formation by preimplantation rat embryos in the presence of cyanide and other inhibitors of oxidative phosphorylation. J Reprod Fertil 1994;101:305–9.
20. Thompson JG, Partridge RJ, Houghton FD, Cox CI, Leese HJ. Oxygen uptake and carbohydrate metabolism by in vitro derived bovine embryos. J Reprod Fertil 1996;106:299–306.
21. McDonald P, Edwards RA, Greenhalgh JFD, Morgan CA. Animal nutrition, 5th ed. Harlow Essex, UK: Addison Wesley Longman, 1998:209.
22. Manes C, Lai NC. Nonmitochondrial oxygen utilization by rabbit blastocysts and surface production of superoxide radicals. J Reprod Fertil 1995;104:69–75.
23. Hewitson LC, Leese HJ. Energy metabolism of the trophectoderm and inner cell mass of the mouse blastocyst. J Exp Zool 1993;267:337–43.
24. Barnett DK, Kimura J, Bavister BD. Translocation of active mitochondria during hamster preimplantation embryo development studied by confocal laser scanning microscopy. Dev Biol 1996;205:64–72.
25. Lane M, Gardner DK. Selection of viable mouse blastocysts prior to transfer using a metabolic criterion. Hum Reprod 1996;11:1975–78.
26. Jones GM, Trounson AO, Vella FJ, Thuoas GA, Lolatgis N, Wood C. Glucose metabolism cannot be used as a biomarker of viability to select human blastocysts for transfer. Proceedings of the eleventh world congress on in vitro fertilization and human reproductive genetics, Sydney, Australia, 1999:143.

7

Blastomere Homeostasis

MICHELLE LANE AND DAVID K. GARDNER

Cellular homeostasis is defined as the ability of the cell to regulate key processes such as intracellular levels of calcium ($Ca^{2+}i$), pH (pHi), and metabolic parameters such as energy charge and redox potential. Cellular homeostasis regulates a multitude of cell functions such as cell division, protein synthesis, differentiation, cell–cell communication, cytoskeletal dynamics, and metabolism. In addition, calcium is a universal trigger for many cell functions. Changes in metabolic homeostasis (e.g., energy charge or redox potential) are also key regulators of enzyme function and therefore metabolic activity and energy production. Small changes in levels of pHi or $Ca^{2+}i$ can also regulate enzyme activity and energy production; therefore, it is a prerequisite for normal cell development that both ionic and metabolic homeostasis are tightly regulated. Aberrations in cellular homeostasis result in perturbed cell function and a loss in developmental competence.

Intracellular pH

Levels of Intracellular pH

When discussing pHi, the first concept that must be discussed is the relationship between pHi and external pH (pHo). External pH rarely equates to pHi. Cells have the ability to buffer pHi changes themselves. In addition, most cells possess membrane transport systems that control levels of pHi. Studies on mammalian embryos have demonstrated that there is no effect of pHo over a range of 7.0–7.4 on the ability to maintain pHi (1). Under normal circumstances, therefore, pHo does not affect embryo pHi. Studies investigating pHi in mammalian embryos from several species such as mice (2,3), hamster (4,5), cow (6), and human (7) have revealed that pHi of embryos is relatively constant at around pH 7.2 in a bicarbonate/CO_2 buffer system; therefore the dogma that media for the development of the mammalian embryo should be set at 7.4 means that the embryo must work to maintain intracellular pH at the physiological level of 7.2 against a gradient. As physiological pHi is 7.2 it would seem more advisable for media to be at that same external pH to prevent the embryo from having to maintain pHi against a gradient, thereby inducing unnecessary stress.

In direct contrast to the lack of effect of pHo on embryo pHi, some components of culture media (e.g., lactate concentration) can have dramatic effects on pHi. Incubation of embryos in a media containing only 5 mM D/L-lactate resulted in a significant reduction in pHi of around 0.15 pH units (1,8). Although L-lactate is the only isomer that can be metabolized by the embryo, both D- and L-lactate can have a significant effect on pHi (1,8). It is therefore important to know the lactate concentration in the medium that is used as well as whether the medium contains both D- and L-lactate because this will further reduce pHi. With this in mind it makes little sense to prepare embryo culture media with a lactate preparation of D- and L-isomers.

Regulation of pHi

Intracellular pH is regulated by several mechanisms, intrinsic buffering capacity, external buffering such as that supplied by amino acids, and, most effectively, by specific transport proteins in the cell membrane. An inability to regulate pHi leaves the cell/embryo susceptible to challenges to pHi such as that from acidic by-products of metabolism (i.e., lactate and protons that result from ATP hydrolysis) (9). It has been demonstrated in several species that embryos with disrupted levels of pHi exhibit severely retarded development in culture, mouse (10,11), hamster (4,5), and cow (6). The ability of hamster pronucleate stage embryos to regulate pHi has been positively correlated with the ability to develop to the blastocyst stage in culture (Fig. 7.1). The ability to regulate pHi is therefore essential for maintenance of developmental competence.

Intrinsic Buffering Capacity

To understand the regulation of pHi in cells it is essential to consider the contribution of intracellular buffering by the cytoplasm and organelles. The intrinsic buffering capacity of cells is the non-CO_2 contribution to minimizing changes in pH caused by changes in proton concentrations. When the term *intrinsic buffering* is applied to whole cells it usually refers to physiochemical and organelle buffering because these occur simultaneously and are therefore difficult to distinguish. Intracellular intrinsic buffering occurs in a matter of seconds, and thus can be distinguished from recovery from a pH challenge by membrane transport proteins that takes several minutes. Intrinsic buffering capacity can be measured and expressed as the mM of protons that can be buffered by the cell. A higher value indicates an increased ability of the cytoplasm of the cell to buffer against a pH challenge. Intrinsic

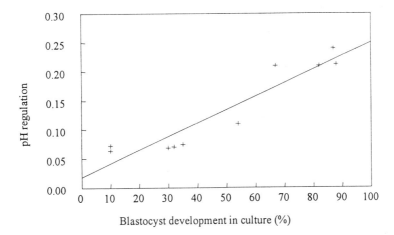

FIGURE 7.1. Correlation of ability to regulate pH and development in culture of hamster embryos. pH regulation is the ability to recover from an acid load in pH units/minute. There is a significant positive correlation between ability to regulate pH and to develop to the blastocyst stage in culture ($r = 0.94$; $p < 0.05$).

buffering of mammalian embryos has been reported to range from 12 to 30 mM/ΔpH. This is similar to the range reported for other cell types.

External Buffering

Regulation of pHi can also be assisted by external factors (e.g., the buffering capacity of amino acids). A proportion of specific amino acids (e.g., taurine and glycine) exist as zwitterions at physiological pH. Zwitterions are able to move readily across the cell membrane and are negatively charged so that they are able to bind protons. A high concentration of these types of amino acids may therefore be able to buffer against an increase in protons in the cell. The amino acids that can buffer protons, taurine, glycine, and glutamine are the amino acids present at high concentrations in the female reproductive tract (12). It is therefore likely that in vivo these amino acids are able to act to help regulate pHi. The capacity of amino acids in the culture medium to buffer pHi has been demonstrated in mouse pronucleate stage embryos. Incubation of embryos in the presence of the weak acid DMO results in a significant decrease in pHi. Addition of nonessential amino acids (which contains glycine) to the culture medium containing DMO reduced the resultant acidification and therefore increased the ability of the embryos to buffer protons and maintain pHi (13). Furthermore, the addition of amino acids to the culture medium prevents the efflux of endogenous amino acids (14) and would therefore assist in maintaining the intrinsic buffering capacity of the cytoplasm.

Transport Proteins

The most robust mechanism for the regulation of pHi is by transport proteins on the cell membrane that transport either protons or bicarbonate from the cell in response to a challenge to pHi. The two most common transport systems reported for the regulation of pHi are the Na^+/H^+ antiporter and the HCO_3^-/Cl^- exchanger. The Na^+/H^+ antiporter transports protons out of the cell in exchange for Na^+ ions and regulates pHi in the acid to neutral range, whereas the HCO_3^-/Cl^- exchanger transports bicarbonate out of the cell in exchange for Cl^- and regulates pHi in the neutral to alkaline range.

Na^+/H^+ Antiporter

The Na^+/H^+ antiporter is ubiquitously found in mammalian nucleated cells; however, early studies on the preimplantation mouse embryo reported that the Na^+/H^+ antiporter activity was absent in the cleavage-stage mouse embryo (15,16). It is now clear that Na^+/H^+ antiporter activity is present in cleavage-stage mammalian embryos. Na^+/H^+ antiporter activity has been demonstrated in embryos from several strains of mice (8; Baltz and Lane, unpublished observations), hamster (4,5), cow (6), and human (7). In addition, the mRNA for the antiporter has been detected in cleavage mouse embryos (17). The activity of the Na^+/H^+ antiporter in embryos differs both between species as well as between the different strains of mice. Mice embryos from some strains appear to have a mechanism for passive recovery from an acid load that can obscure the measurement of the Na^+/H^+ antiporter activity. This observation may explain the early studies that failed to detect Na^+/H^+ antiporter activity in BDF mice, whereas investigators using a different strain of mice (Quackenbush) where able to detect sizable Na^+/H^+ antiporter activity. In the mammalian embryo, Na^+/H^+ antiporter activity is activated by a decrease in pHi from the physiological set point of around 7.1. Activity of the antiporter increases exponentially as the acidification from pHi increases (4).

HCO_3^-/Cl^- Exchanger

When pHi of the cell rises above the physiological set-point the HCO_3^-/Cl^- exchanger acidifies the cytoplasm by exporting bicarbonate in exchange for chloride entering the cell until pHi is restored to physiological levels (18). Like the Na^+/H^+ antiporter, activity of the HCO_3^-/Cl^- exchanger is increased the further pHi deviates from the physiological set point. HCO_3^-/Cl^- exchanger is utilized by mouse (2), hamster (19), cow (6), and human (7) embryos to regulate intracellular pH in the alkaline range.

Intracellular pH and Fertilization

In addition to controlling cell division and differentiation, pHi in sea urchin (20,21) and Xenopus (22–24) controls egg activation and subsequent initiation of development. In these species there is significant rise in pHi in eggs after activation by spermatozoa. This alkalization with an accompanying spike in intracellular Ca^{2+} levels is necessary for subsequent development to proceed. It initiates both protein and DNA synthesis as well as other biosynthetic processes (25–27). In the sea urchin (20,28,29) and surf clam (30) the increase in pHi is due to the activity of the Na^+/H^+ antiporter. In contrast, however, the increase in pHi after activation in the Xenopus egg is not due to activity of the Na^+/H^+ antiporter, although the transporter is present in the egg (22,23).

Unlike marine species or Xenopus, oocytes from mammalian species do not appear to change pHi following activation and/or fertilization. Studies on oocytes of mice (31,32), rats (33), and human (34) did not detect any change in pHi during egg activation or fertilization. An explanation for this lack of change in pHi with activation is that mammalian oocytes appear to lack any transport mechanisms for regulating pHi. Studies on the mouse and hamster oocyte failed to detect either Na^+/H^+ antiporter (5) or HCO_3^-/Cl^- exchanger (3,19) activity; however, mRNA for both transporters were present (3,5). Activity of these two pHi regulatory systems was not detected until several hours after egg activation (3,5). Activity of the transport systems appeared gradually until maximum activity was reached around 8–10 hours after egg activation (Fig. 7.2). Activity was not associated with protein synthesis or cytoskeletal movement for both the Na^+/H^+ antiporter and the

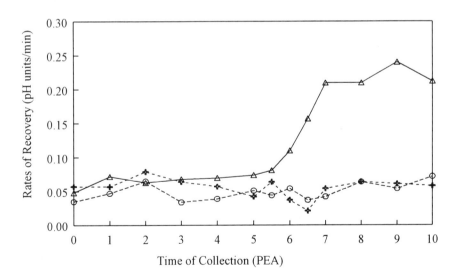

FIGURE 7.2. Activation of Na^+/H^+ antiporter activity in hamster oocytes following fertilization. Rates of recovery in control medium (triangle). Rates of recovery in the absence of Na+ (cross). Rates of recovery in the presence of EIPA which inhibits Na^+/H^+ antiporter activity (circle). Rates of recovery are significantly increased at 6 hours post-egg activation and this increase in ability to recover pH is both sodium dependent and EIPA sensitive indicating that recovery is due to Na^+/H^+ antiporter activity. Reproduced with permission from Lane et al. (5).

HCO_3^-/Cl^- exchanger; rather the calcium oscillations initiated by activation of the egg that continue for around 5–6 hours after fertilization (35–37) appear to be involved in the activation of the transporters. These calcium oscillations signal second messenger systems that result in activation of existing protein. For the Na^+/H^+ antiporter, activity is activated by a calcium-dependent protein kinase C pathway (5).

It is apparent that the mammalian oocyte and early embryo do not have any mechanism for the regulation of pHi prior to around 6–10 hours after fertilization. It is interesting that hamster oocyte cytoplasm had an increased intrinsic buffering capacity (51 mM/pH) compared with that of cleavage-stage embryos of 17–35 mM/pH (4,19). This increased intrinsic buffering capacity by the oocytes may be an evolutionary mechanism to compensate for the reduced capacity to restore pHi due to a lack of a functional Na^+/H^+ antiporter or HCO_3^-/Cl^- exchanger.

Role of Cumulus Cells

Although it is apparent that the oocyte and early embryo lack a robust mechanism for the regulation of pHi, it is important to consider that in vivo the oocyte and early embryo are surrounded by the cumulus, which persists for several hours after fertilization. The cumulus layer persists for around 15 hours in the mouse and around 10 hours in the hamster. There is considerable communication between the cumulus cells and oocytes during early development through cumulus cell processes that extend into the oocyte itself. In addition, the cumulus cells are surrounded by a matrix of glycoproteins and glycsoaminoglycans (e.g., hyaluronate) that would produce a gellike protective layer around the oocyte itself (38,39). We therefore postulate that in vivo the oocyte and early embryo are protected by the surrounding cumulus and are not required to regulate pHi themselves until after the transport systems are initiated at around 8 hours after egg activation. The cumulus may therefore play a significant protective role to the oocyte and embryo that is lost when embryos are denuded and placed in culture. This will have a significant impact on procedures in the IVF laboratory that involve denuding oocytes and early embryos (see later).

Effect of pHi on Embryo Development

Intracellular pH regulates many cell processes (e.g., cell division, differentiation, cytoskeletal dynamics). Cyclic changes in pHi also control mitotic divisions in many cell types (40). In sea urchin oocytes changes in pHi affects sperm aster formation and pronuclear movements (41), as well as microvilli elongation (42,43). Alteration of pHi is known to be a mechanism used by some cells to regulate intracellular organelle distribution. In hyphae, a reduction in pHi results in the migration of mitochondria toward the apex (44), although changes in fibroblast pH_i alter the distribution of lysosomes in the cells by microtubule function (45). In the case of the Xenopus oocyte, increases in pHi result in a general disruption in the organization of endoplasmic reticulum (46).

Analysis of effects of pH on cytoskeleton of hamster two-cell embryos revealed that the actin network is dramatically altered by both acidic and alkaline pHi. When the pHi is decreased the microfilament network becomes dissociated from the perinuclear region, whereas an increase in pH_i results in an increase in actin aggregation throughout the cytoplasm (47). Actin organization is known to be controlled by changes in pHi in sea urchins (42,43) and fungi (44,48). This disruption in cytoskeletal arrangement in hamster embryos also results in a disruption of the mitochondrial distribution from around the nucleus to a more homogeneous distribution in the cytoplasm (47). In hamster embryos, a disruption in mitochondrial distribution is associated with developmental arrest in culture (49).

Intracellular pH and Control of Embryo Metabolism

Intracellular pH is a powerful regulator on many key enzyme pathways and reactions that control both oxidative metabolism and glycolysis. pHi must therefore be controlled in a very precise manner in order for cells to maintain normal growth, development, and differentiation. Increases in pHi above the physiological level of 7.2 are known to stimulate activity of a flux-generating enzyme of glycolysis, phosphofructokinase (PFK) (50). Small increases in PFK activity can cause disproportionately large increases in glycolytic pathway activity. In some cells, PFK activity can be altered 10- to 20-fold by a pH change of only around 0.1 units (51,52). Studies on the effects of pH on the activity of PFK isolated from mouse two-cell embryos indicates that the activity of PFK can be significantly altered by increasing the external pH by only 0.2 units (Gardner et al., unpublished observations; Fig. 7.3). Glycolytic activity have similarly been shown to be abnormally increased in both mouse (13) and hamster two-cell embryos (53) by changes in pHi induced by incubation with the weak base trimethylamine (TMA). In both of these species this premature activation of glycolysis is associated with developmental arrest in culture (54,55).

Like somatic cells, changes in pHi have therefore been shown to have a significant effect on essential cellular process such as regulation of the cytoskeleton. Furthermore, regulation of ionic homeostasis is central to the ability of the preimplantation embryo to regulate enzyme activity and therefore metabolism and energy production.

Intracellular pH and Cryopreserved Embryos

Ability to maintain homeostatic control is especially important for cells that are stressed (e.g., during cryopreservation). Embryos that are cryopreserved

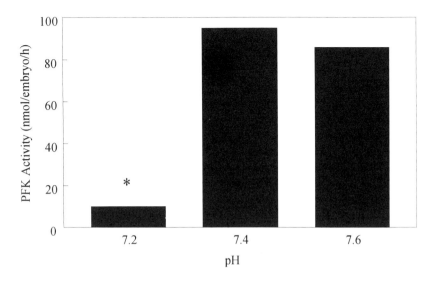

FIGURE 7.3. Effect of pH on PFK activity. PFK was isolated from mouse zygotes. *Significantly different from other treatments ($p < 0.05$).

have a reduced developmental competence compared with fresh embryos as evidenced by lower rates of implantation and fetal development after transfer. Investigation of cryopreserved cleavage-stage embryos revealed an inability to maintain physiological levels of pHi of around 7.2. Embryos that were cryopreserved had elevated levels of pHi immediately following thawing (53) and reduced rates of both Na^+/H^+ antiporter and HCO_3^-/Cl^- exchanger activity. Furthermore, intrinsic buffering capacity of cryopreserved embryos was also reduced immediately following warming. Normal activities of both the Na^+/H^+ antiporter and HCO_3^-/Cl^- exchanger were not re-established until between 4 and 6 hours after thawing; therefore, for this period following thawing embryos could not regulate pHi appropriately and pH_i rose by around 0.2 units. This increase in pH results in a significant increase in glycolytic activity, which is a pathway that is not preferentially used by the cleavage-stage embryo (53). An abnormal increase in glycolytic activity in cleavage-stage embryos results in a concomitant reduction in oxidative metabolism (54,55). This severely reduces the ability of the embryo to produce energy to sustain normal development. As mentioned previously the addition of Eagle's nonessential amino acids increases the ability of mouse cleavage stage embryos to buffer pHi (13). It may therefore be prudent to include these amino acids in the culture medium for embryos following cryopreservation when the embryo has a reduced ability to regulate pHi.

Intracellular Calcium

Calcium is the universal regulator in all cells. Like pHi, changes in intracellular calcium levels ($Ca^{2+}i$) trigger many cell functions, including the initiation of development following fertilization by calcium oscillations in both Xenopus (56), sea urchin (57), and mammals (58–61). Aberrations in cellular regulation of $Ca^{2+}i$ concentrations can result in perturbations in protein synthesis, DNA replication, mitochondrial function, and cell–cell communication (62–65). In the majority of cells, the most common mechanisms for the maintenance of this $Ca^{2+}i$ levels involve either sequestering into intracellular stores [e.g., the endoplasmic reticulum, mitochondria or nucleus, (which together contain around 90% of the cell calcium)] (66), or by membrane transport via Na^+-Ca^{2+} or Mg^{2+}-Ca^{2+} ATPases, which extrude calcium ions from the cytoplasm (67), or by calcium channels (64). Many of these mechanisms require expenditure of energy to maintain calcium levels low and constant. It is interesting that cells that are undergoing stress due either to cell injury or metabolic perturbation exhibit increased levels of intracellular calcium due to disruptions in subcellular handling of calcium or alterations in membrane transport (68).

Effect of Culture on $Ca^{2+}i$ Levels

The concentration of calcium present in the oviduct and uterus is 1.13 and 1.42 mM for human (69,70), and 1.04 and 1.94 mM for the mouse (71); however, the $Ca^{2+}i$ level in embryos is many orders of magnitude lower than that in the reproductive tract environment. Intracellular calcium levels of hamster two-cell embryos is 129 nM, which is around 1000 times lower than the calcium concentration reported for the oviduct. Preimplantation embryos must therefore maintain their low intracellular levels of calcium against a large electrochemical gradient. Examination of the ability of hamster preimplantation stage embryos to regulate $Ca^{2+}i$ revealed that embryos cultured for 24 hours from the one-cell to the two-cell stage resulted in a threefold increase in $Ca^{2+}i$ concentration compared with in vivo developed embryos (72). Furthermore, culture of pronucleate stage hamster embryos for just 3 hours also resulted in a significant increase in $Ca^{2+}i$ levels. These embryos also exhibited lower rates of metabolism and perturbed organelle distribution compared with in vivo–developed embryos. The stress of removing the early embryo from the reproductive tract and placing it into culture appears to disrupt one or more of the mechanisms of calcium regulation in the embryo, thereby perturbing calcium homeostasis. The level of increase (around 200 nM) in intracellular calcium levels in cultured embryos would be sufficient to activate many potentially destructive enzymatic pathways (e.g., proteases, phospholipases, and endonucleases) that can further diminish cell function (68).

Role of Magnesium for Regulation of $Ca^{2+}i$ Levels

In addition to specific transport mechanisms for the regulation of calcium, magnesium plays an important regulatory role in the control of calcium uptake, release, and homeostasis in many cell types (73). The magnesium and calcium ratio (Mg:Ca) is very important for the control of membrane stability and ion-channel permeability in somatic cells (74). In cardiac cells increasing extracellular magnesium concentration linearly decreases intracellular calcium concentrations (75). Magnesium also appears to be an important counter ion for calcium in the preimplantation embryo because hamster embryos cultured in the presence of an increased Mg:Ca ratio had an increased ability to regulate $Ca^{2+}i$ levels when placed in culture (72). Increasing the magnesium concentration in the culture medium linearly decreased the $Ca^{2+}i$ levels in the two-cell embryos, whereas changing the extracellular calcium levels did not affect $Ca^{2+}i$ levels. This increased ability to regulate $Ca^{2+}i$ by increasing the external magnesium concentration was associated with increased development in culture and increased viability after transfer (72). This highlights that the ability to regulate calcium homeostasis by the early cleavage stage embryo is essential for normal development.

Calcium Channels

One of the mechanisms that allows magnesium to reduce intracellular calcium levels in somatic cells is by inhibiting L-gated calcium channels (64). Addition of nifedipine and verapamil, which inhibit slow inward L-gated channels, to the culture medium increased the ability of embryos to regulate $Ca^{2+}i$ levels. These inhibitors also increased embryo development in culture as well as energy production and mitochondrial distribution (76). It therefore appears that the inability of embryos to regulate $Ca^{2+}i$ levels in culture is due to an inability to regulate these voltage-gated calcium channels. The stress induced on the embryo by removing it from the reproductive tract results in the embryo being unable to regulate these calcium channels. As a result, intracellular calcium levels become elevated; however, increasing the magnesium level in the medium can minimize this induced stress. It is of interest to note that in cardiac cells calcium influx through these channels is regulated by intracellular pH (77,78), highlighting the interactions that are present between intracellular levels of ions (H^+, Ca^{2+} and Mg^{2+}) within the cell.

Embryo Metabolism

The mammalian oocyte and early embryo develop from a quiescent cell with very low biosynthetic activity to a rapidly dividing, highly metabolic and biosynthetically active group of cells with a metabolic rate or QO_2 similar to that of a tumor cell. In addition, at the blastocyst stage there is differentiation into two distinct cell types: the trophectoderm and inner cell mass. These two cell types are known to differ in their energy production (79,80) and likely utilize different mechanisms for the control and regulation of growth.

Somatic cells maintain their energy requirements from the metabolism of glucose by the Embden-Meyerhof pathway and the tricarboxylic acid cycle; however, the preimplantation mammalian embryo has an unusual and continually changing nutrient requirement and energy metabolism (81,82). Glucose cannot support development until the eight-cell stage (83). Instead pyruvate is required for cleavage of the zygote, whereas lactate can be used as an energy source from the two-cell stage onward (84). Later studies on the nutrient uptake of embryos developed in vivo and in vitro demonstrated that nutrient uptake by the embryo mirrors these earlier culture experiments. The cleavage-stage embryo takes up pyruvate preferentially until compaction. Glucose uptake remains low up to the morula stage and then increases significantly at the blastocyst stage (82,85,86). A similar pattern of nutrient uptakes has been reported for the sheep (87), cow (88,89), and human embryo (90).

Glycolysis is therefore not a pathway preferentially utilized by the cleavage stage embryo. This inability of glucose to support development of the early mouse embryo has been attributed to a blockade of glycolysis (91,92). PFK is specifically thought to be allosterically inhibited by a high ATP:ADP ratio, which exists in the cleavage-stage embryo (93). This high ATP:ADP ratio in the embryo is most likely the result of low biosynthetic activity of the oocyte and embryo prior to genome activation (94).

Effect of Culture on Embryo Metabolism

In poor culture conditions, preimplantation embryos lose the ability to regulate their metabolism; however, the mechanism behind this inability to regulate metabolism is unknown. Mouse embryos derived from outbred strains of mice arrest development at the two-cell stage in a simple medium (e.g., MTF) (95). Analysis of the metabolism of arrested embryos revealed an elevated level of glycolysis with a concomitant reduction in pyruvate oxidation when compared with in vivo–developed two-cell embryos (55). In contrast, embryos cultured in a more complex medium designed to support development to the blastocyst stage (medium with EDTA and amino acids) have lower levels of glycolysis and normal levels of pyruvate metabolism (Fig. 7.4a). Conditions that allow limited development beyond the two-cell block (EDTA or amino acids) had intermediate levels of glycolysis and pyruvate metabolism (Fig. 7.4a). Glycolytic activity of two-cell embryos was therefore negatively correlated with their subsequent development in culture, whereas pyruvate oxidation was positively correlated with development. Embryos with a metabolic profile more similar to in vivo–developed embryos had a higher rate of development in culture. In contrast to the embryos of outbred

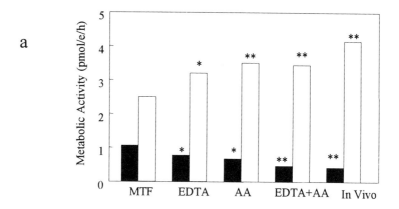
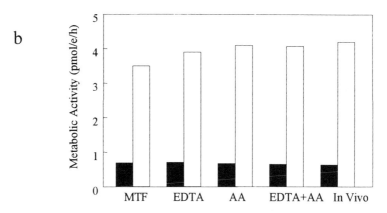

FIGURE 7.4. Effect of culture conditions on embryo metabolism of two-cell mouse embryos. (a) CF1 embryos. (b) F1 embryos. Closed bars represent pyruvate oxidation (pmol/embryo/h). Open bars represent glycolysis (pmol/embryo/h). MTF, mouse tubal fluid medium, AA, amino acids. *Significantly different from embryos cultured in MTF ($p < 0.05$). **Significantly different from embryos cultured in MTF ($p < 0.01$). Data from Gardner (55).

strains of mice, embryos collected from an F1 hybrid strain that do not exhibit the two-cell block in culture did not exhibit significant alteration in embryo metabolism compared with in vivo–developed embryos (Fig. 7.4b).

ATP:ADP Ratio

ATP:ADP ratio is an important regulator of carbohydrate metabolism by the regulation of key enzymes in metabolic pathways. Change in the ATP:ADP ratio is a major controlling mechanism of glycolytic activity. A high ATP:ADP ratio allosterically inhibits the enzyme PFK, resulting in an inhibition in glycolysis. A decrease in this ratio results in an increase in PFK activity and therefore glycolysis. In the in vivo–developed cleavage stage mouse embryo both citrate levels (90,91) and the ATP:ADP ratio are high (93), which inhibits PFK activity; therefore, glycolytic flux is reduced. The early embryos instead oxides pyruvate, lactate, or amino acids as the preferred energy substrates.

Comparison of the levels of ATP:ADP ratio of embryos from the two strains of mice CF1 and F1 cultured in the simple medium revealed that while the ATP:ADP ratio in embryos from the F1 strain did not alter, the ratio in the CF1 embryos decreased significantly. This decrease in ATP:ADP ratio in the two-cell embryos causes elevated PFK activity and increased rates of glycolysis (96); however, the CF1 embryos cultured in the more complex medium that is able to support high rates of development had normal ATP:ADP ratios. The ability to maintain developmental competence, therefore is related to the ability to regulate the ATP:ADP ratio. This ratio is disrupted in conditions that retard development. The ability to control this ratio in culture is essential for normal metabolic patterns and energy production. It is currently unknown why the embryo is unable to maintain this ratio in culture.

Regulation of Energy Metabolism by Ionic Homeostasis

As mentioned earlier changes in level of pHi has a significant effect on the ability of embryos to regulate energy metabolism. This is particularly important for the early embryos as the ability to regulate pHi is increased with the formation of the transporting epithelium at the morula stage (1). A small change in pHi (e.g., the 0.2 unit increase observed following cryopreservation) would result in a substantial increase in PFK activity and subsequently glycolytic activity. As glycolytic activity is not the preferred pathway for the cleavage-stage embryo this would result in a loss in viability. It is currently unknown as to the effect of pH on the metabolism of the blastocyst; however, following compaction of the embryo and the formation of a transporting epithelium the ability to regulate pH is significantly enhanced and may therefore prevent much change in pHi.

In addition to pHi, both intracellular levels of calcium and magnesium are regulators of metabolism. The level of $Ca^{2+}i$ in the cytoplasm is thought to influence the regulation and levels of Ca^{2+} in the mitochondria (62). Calcium is a key regulator of the mitochondrial enzymes, pyruvate dehydrogenase (through action on phosphate phosphatase, isocitrate dehydrogenase, and α-ketoglutarate dehydrogenase) (97). Increases in mitochondrial calcium levels stimulate the activity of these enzymes. Although little is known about the regulation of enzymes in embryos, it is proposed that the regulation of cytosolic calcium affects the levels of intramitochondrial calcium levels as seen in other cell types. It may also alter levels of mitochondrial metabolism.

Magnesium is also an important ion in metabolism as it is the most prevalent enzyme co-factor (98). Magnesium is an essential co-factor of metabolic kinases (e.g., hexokinase, PFK, phosphoglycerate kinase, and pyruvate kinase), which regulate embryo metabolism. It is only by Mg^{2+} binding to the co-factor ATP reacting in a conformational change that enables ATP to bind to the correct site on the enzyme complex to activate the enzyme. Chelation of the intracellular magnesium, such as what occurs when EDTA is added to the culture media, results in an inhibition of glycolysis due to an inhibition of the glycolytic kinases (99). In addition, magnesium also affects the activity of phosphorylation in cells (100). A correct balance of magnesium levels in the cytoplasm, therefore, is essential for the maintenance of enzyme activity and energy metabolism in embryos. It has been demonstrated in hamster two-cell embryos that the cytosolic concentration of magnesium is directly affected by the concentration of magnesium in the culture medium (72).

Redox Potential

Redox potential is a measure of the reducing power of a cell and can be thought of as the NAD^+:NADH ratio. The NAD^+:NADH ratio in cells is controlled by the pyruvate:lactate ratio within the cytosol. There is a marked increase in lactate formation from pyruvate when cytosolic the NAD^+:NADH ratio is low. Redox potential, therefore, can substantially affect the fate of pyruvate metabolism. This also has consequences for the glucose metabolism because glucose is converted to pyruvate via the Embden-Meyerhof pathway before entry into the tricarboxylic acid cycle.

The effect of redox potential in controlling metabolism of embryos can be assessed by determining the fate of pyruvate metabolized by the embryo (percentage of pyruvate uptake that is oxidized compared with the percentage that is converted to lactate) in the presence of increasing lactate concentrations. Analysis of pyruvate metabolism in the mouse zygote and blastocyst in response to increasing lactate concentrations revealed a striking difference (86). For the zygote, increasing the lactate concentration decreased the percentage of total pyruvate that was oxidized by the TCA cycle, whereas the percentage of pyruvate that was oxidized by the blastocyst increased with increasing lactate concentration (Fig. 7.5). More pyruvate is therefore converted at the zygote to lactate via the enzyme lactate dehydrogenase, whereas this enzyme converts less pyruvate to lactate at the blastocyst stage. As LDH in the zygote and the blastocyst are the same isoform of the enzyme, the differences in the activity of LDH at the different stages of development must result from regulation in situ (86). Analysis of redox potential in the zygote in the presence of increasing lactate concentrations resulted in a decrease in the NAD^+:NADH ratio, whereas redox potential was not altered in the later stages. Redox potential, which is an intracellular regulator of LDH activity, therefore differs between the zygote and the blastocyst and results in the differences in pyruvate metabolism in the two stages of development. The ability to regulate redox potential is important to maintain normal cell metabo-

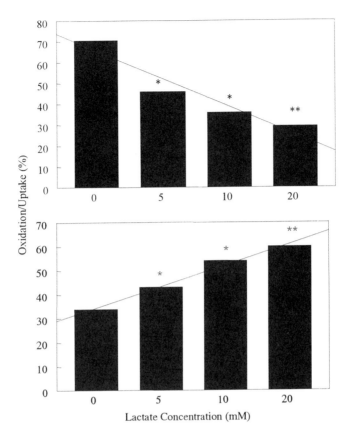

FIGURE 7.5. Effect of lactate concentration on pyruvate metabolism. (top) Zygote ($r = 0.96$). (bottom) Blastocyst ($r = 0.97$). Data expressed as pyruvate oxidation as a percentage of pyruvate uptake. *Significantly different from 0 mM lactate ($p < 0.05$). **Significantly different from 0 mM lactate ($p < 0.01$). Reproduced with permission from Lane and Gardner (86).

lism and prevent an increase in lactate production from either glucose or pyruvate, and to prevent a decrease in the yield of ATP. The reason for the difference in ability to regulate redox potential in the zygote is not known; however, redox potential in somatic cells is controlled by the activity of reducing equivalent shuttles in the mitochondrial membrane. Whether these shuttles also have a role in the regulation of embryo metabolism is currently unknown.

Implications for the IVF Laboratory

The main focus of the IVF laboratory is maintaining the viability of the gametes and embryos until they are replaced into the mother. Reducing intracellular stress and the maintenance of cellular homeostasis, therefore, are essential to maintaining developmental competence. The protection of the gametes and embryos must therefore be of the highest priority in the laboratory. Specific media designed with the theme of protection and reduction of intracellular stress for development to the blastocyst stage have been developed (see Chap. 10). There are still specific procedures in the laboratory, however, that induce considerable intracellular stress.

ICSI

In most clinics around one third of the patients require the use of ICSI to attain adequate fertilization rates (101); however, it has been reported in several laboratories that the use of ICSI for fertilization results in a reduction in subsequent blastocyst development (101,102). Furthermore, some laboratories also report such a decrease in blastocyst development following ICSI that all ICSI patients are forced to have a Day 3 cleavage-stage transfer. Although some of the reduction in development may be due to poor genetics and quality of the sperm, the variation in ability to produce blastocysts following ICSI between programs is likely to represent different orders of stress induced on the oocyte. The ICSI procedure itself requires that oocytes are stripped from their surrounding cumulus. As mentioned earlier, the cumulus provides both a protective and potentially regulatory mechanism for maintaining ionic homeostasis in the oocyte. The oocyte does not have any robust mechanism to regulate intracellular ionic homeostasis and the removal of the cumulus renders the oocyte increasingly susceptible to the surrounding environment. This may be further exacerbated by the common use of PBS for the incubation of the egg during the ICSI procedure. The use of a phosphate-buffered medium would increase proton flux across the plasma membrane of which the oocyte has no mechanism to protect against. It therefore appears to be advisable that oocyte or early embryos not be exposed to phosphate-buffered media. Media with a buffering system of HEPES or MOPS would be a more appropriate medium. Furthermore, as mentioned earlier, addition of nonessential amino acids to culture medium increases the buffering capacity of the cytoplasm to protect against changes in pHi. It is prudent, therefore, to add these amino acids to any medium for the handling or manipulation of the denuded oocyte or early embryo.

Cryopreservation

It is also evident from studies on animal embryos that the ability to regulate pHi is substantially reduced for around 6 hours after thawing. This observation may in part explain the reduction in developmental competence following cryopreservation because the embryo would be highly susceptible to its surrounding environment. Much like the oocyte for ICSI, therefore, care should be taken to handle the embryo following cryopreservation. The use of phosphate-buffered medium should likewise be avoided and media should be supplemented with the amino acids that are shown to increase buffering capacity. It would also seem advisable to use a medium with a high magnesium:calcium ratio to assist with the regulation of $Ca^{2+}i$ levels.

Conclusions

The ability to maintain embryo development in culture depends upon the ability of the embryo to maintain both ionic and metabolic homeostasis. Disruptions in the ability to regulate cellular homeostasis results in reduced rates of development in culture and a reduced ability to establish and maintain a pregnancy following transfer. It is important, therefore, that in vitro conditions are designed to minimize stress on the embryo and maximize the ability to maintain cellular homeostasis as the ability to regulate pHi, $Ca^{2+}i$, and metabolism are intimately linked both to each other and to cellular processes such as energy production, cell division, and differentiation as well as regulation of cytoskeleton. It has significantly also been demonstrated that the stress of growing embryos in the absence of amino acids impairs gene expression in the developing embryos (103,104). The role of the IVF laboratory therefore has to be in reducing cellular stress in order to maintain developmental competence. This important concept should be applied to every step of the IVF procedure from the handling of the gametes until the time the embryo is replaced in the mother. An awareness of the effect of each procedure on the gametes/embryos may well separate the clinics with poor results from more successful programs.

References

1. Edwards LJ, Williams DA, Gardner DK. Intracellular pH of the preimplantation mouse embryo: effects of extracellular pH and weak acids. Mol Reprod Dev 1998;50:434–42.
2. Zhao Y, Chauvet PJ, Alper SL, Baltz JM. Expression and function of bicarbonate/chloride exchangers in the preimplantation mouse embryo. J Biol Chem 1995;270:24428–34.
3. Phillips KP, Baltz JM. Intracellular pH regulation by HCO3-/Cl- exchange is activated during early mouse zygote development. Dev Biol 1999;208:392–405.
4. Lane M, Baltz JM, Bavister BD. Regulation of intracellular pH in hamster preimplantation embryos by the Na^+/H^+ antiporter. Biol Reprod 1998;59:1483–90.
5. Lane M, Baltz, JM, Bavister BD. Na+/H+ antiporter activity in hamster embryos is activated during fertilization. Dev Biol 1999;208:244–52.
6. Lane M, Bavister BD. Regulation of intracellular pH in bovine oocytes and cleavage stage embryos. Mol Reprod Dev 1999;54:396–401.
7. Phillips KP, Leveille MC, Claman P, Baltz JM. Intracellular pH regulation in human preimplantation embryos. Hum Reprod 2000;15:896–904.
8. Gibb CA, Poronnik P, Day ML, Cook DI. Control of cytosolic pH in two-cell mouse embryos: roles of H^+-lactate cotransport and Na^+/H^+ exchange. Am J Physiol 1997;273:C404–19.

9. Busa WB, Nuccitelli R. Metabolic regulation via intracellular pH. Am J Physiol 1984;246:R409–38.
10. Leclerc C, Becker D, Buehr M, Warner A. Low intracellular pH is involved in the early embryonic death of DDK mouse eggs fertilized by alien sperm. Dev Dyn 1994;200:257–67.
11. Zhao Y, Baltz JM. Bicarbonate/chloride exchange and intracellular pH throughout preimplantation mouse embryo development. Am J Physiol 1996;271:C1512–20.
12. Miller JGO, Schultz GA. Amino acid content of preimplantation rabbit embryos and fluids of the reproductive tract. Biol Reprod 1987;36:125.
13. Edwards LJ, Williams DA, Gardner DK. Intracellular pH of the mouse preimplantation embryo: amino acids act as buffers of intracellular pH. Hum Reprod 1998;13:3441–48.
14. Kolajora M, Baltz JM. Volume-regulated anion and organic osmolyte channels in mouse zygotes. Biol Reprod 1999;60:964–72.
15. Baltz JM, Biggers JD, Lechene C. Apparent absence of the Na^+/H^+ antiport activity in the two-cell mouse embryo. Dev Biol 1990;138:421–29.
16. Baltz JM, Biggers JD, Lechene C. Two-cell stage mouse embryos appear to lack mechanisms for alleviating intracellular acid loads. J Biol Chem 1991;266:6052–57.
17. Barr KJ, Garrill A, Jones DH, Orlowski J, Kidder GM. Contributions of Na+/H+ exchanger isoforms to preimplantation development of the mouse. Mol Reprod Dev 1998;50:146–53.
18. Olsnes S, Tonessen TI, Sandvig K. pH regulated anion antiport in nucleated mammalian cells. J Cell Biol 1986;102:967–71.
19. Lane M, Baltz JM, Bavister BD. Bicarbonate/chloride exchange regulates intracellular pH of embryos but not oocytes of the hamster. Biol Reprod 1999;61:452–57.
20. Johnson JD, Epel D, Paul M. Intracellular pH and activation of sea urchin eggs after fertilization. Nature 1976;262:661–64.
21. Dube F, Epel D. The relation between intracellular pH and rate of protein synthesis in sea urchin eggs and the existence of a pH-independent event triggered by ammonia. Exp Cell Res 1986;162:191–204.
22. Nuccitelli R, Webb DJ, Lagier ST, Matson GB. 31P NMR reveals increased intracellular pH after fertilization in Xenopus eggs. Proc Natl Acad Sci USA 1981;78:4421–25.
23. Webb DJ, Nuccitelli R. Direct measurements of intracellular pH changes in Xenopus eggs at fertilization and cleavage. J Cell Biol 1981;91:562–67.
24. Towle DW, Baksinski A, Richard NE, Kordylewski M. Characterization of an endogenous Na+/H+ antiporter in Xenopus laevis oocytes. J Exp Biol 1991;159:359–69.
25. Vacquier VD. The isolation of intact cortical granules from sea urchin eggs: calcium lons trigger granule discharge. Dev Biol 1974;43:62–74.
26. Grainger JL, Winkler MM, Shen SS, Steinhardt RA. Intracellular pH controls protein synthesis rate in sea urchin egg and early embryo. Dev Biol 1979;68:396–406.
27. Winkler MM, Steinhardt RA. Activation of protein synthesis in a sea urchin cell-free system. Dev Biol 1981;84:432–39.
28. Shen SS, Steinhardt RA. Direct measurement of intracellular pH during metabolic derepression of the sea urchin egg. Nature 1978;272:253–54.
29. Dube F, Schmidt T, Johnson CH, Epel D. The hierarchy of requirements for an elevated pHi during development of sea urchin embryos. Cell 1985;40:657–66.
30. Dube F, Eckberg WR. Intracellular pH increase driven by an Na^+/H^+ exchanger upon activation of surf clam oocytes. Dev Biol 1997;190:41–54.

31. Kline D, Zagray JA. Absence of an intracellular pH change following fertilization of the mouse egg. Zygote 1995;3:305–11.
32. Phillips KP, Baltz JM. Intracellular pH change does not accompany egg activation in the mouse. Mol Reprod Dev 1996;45:52–60.
33. Ben-Yosef D, Oron Y, Shalgi R. Intracellular pH of rat eggs is not affected by fertilization and the resulting calcium oscillations. Biol Reprod 1996;55:461–68.
34. Dale B, Menezo Y, Cohen J, DiMatteo L, Wilding M. Intracellular pH regulation in the human oocyte. Hum Reprod 1998;13:964–70.
35. Miyazaki S, Igusa Y. Fertilization potential in golden hamster eggs consists of recurring hyperpolarizations. Nature 1981;290:706–7.
36. Jones KT, Carroll J, Merriman JA, Whittingham DG, Kono T. Repetitive sperm-induced Ca2+ transients in mouse oocytes are cell cycle dependent. Development 1995;121:3259–66.
37. Bos-Mikich A, Whittingham DG, Jones KT. Meiotic and mitotic Ca^{2+} oscillations affect cell composition in resulting blastocysts. Dev Biol 1997;182:172–79.
38. Salustri A, Yanagishita M, Underhill CB, Laurent TC, Hascall VC. Localization and synthesis of hyaluronic acid in the cumulus cells and mural granulosa cells of the preovulatory follicle. Dev Biol 1992;151:541–51.
39. Laurent C, Hellstrom S, Engstrom-Laurent A, Wells AF, Bergh A. Localization and quantity of hyaluronan in urogenital organs of male and female rats. Cell Tissue Res 1995;279:241–48.
40. Grandin N, Charbonneau M. Cycling of intracellular free calcium and intracellular pH in Xenopus embryos: a possible role in the control of the cell cycle. J Cell Sci 1991;99: 5–11.
41. Schatten G, Bestor T, Balczon R, Henson J, Schatten H. Intracellular pH shift leads to microtubule assembly and microtubule-mediated motility during sea urchin fertilization: correlations between elevated intracellular pH and microtubule activity and depressed intracellular pH and microtubule disassembly. Eur J Cell Biol 1985;36:116–27.
42. Begg DA, Rebhun LI. pH regulates the polymerization of actin in the sea urchin egg cortex. J Cell Biol 1979;83:241–48.
43. Begg DA, Wong GK, Hoyle DH, Baltz JM. Stimulation of cortical actin polymerization in the sea urchin egg cortex by NH4Cl, procaine and urethane: elevation of cytoplasmic pH is not the common mechanism of action. Cell Motil Cytoskeleton 1996;35:210–24.
44. Bachewich CL, Heath IB. The cytoplasmic pH influences hyphal tip growth and cytoskeleton-related organization. Fungal Genet Biol 1997;21:76–91.
45. Heuser J. Changes in lysosome shape and distribution correlated with changes in cytoplasmic pH. J Cell Biol 1989;108:855–64.
46. Charbonneau M. The organization of the cortical endoplasmic reticulum in Xenopus eggs depends on intracellular pH: artefact of fixation or not? Cell Differ Dev 1990;30:171–79.
47. Squirrell JM, Lane M, Bavister BD. Development and cellular organization in preimplantation hamster embryos are disrupted by altering intracellular pH. Dev Dyn 2001 (in press).
48. Yokoyama K, Kaji H, Nishimura K, Miyaji M. The role of microfilaments and microtubules during pH-regulated morphological transition in Candida albicans. Microbiology 1994;140:281–87.
49. Barnett DK, Bavister BD. Inhibitory effect of glucose and phosphate on the second

cleavage division of hamster embryos: is it linked to metabolism? Hum Reprod 1996;11:177.
50. McKhann GM, Tower DB. Ammonia toxicity and cerebral oxidative metabolism. Am J Physiol 1960;200:420–24.
51. Danforth WH. Activation of glycolytic pathway in muscle. In: Chance B, Estabrook RW, Williamson JB, eds. Control of energy metabolism. New York: Academic Press, 1965:287–98.
52. Trivedi B, Danforth WH. Effect of pH on the kinetics of frog muscle phosphofructokinase. J Biol Chem 1966;241:4110–12.
53. Lane M, Lyons EA, Bavister BD. Cryopreservation reduces the ability of hamster 2-cell embryos to regulate intracellular pH. Hum Reprod 2000;15:389–94.
54. Seshagiri PB, Bavister BD. Glucose and phosphate inhibit respiration and oxidative metabolism in cultured hamster eight-cell embryos: evidence for the "Crabtree effect." Mol Reprod Devel 1991;30:105–11.
55. Gardner DK. Changes in requirements and utilization of nutrients during mammalian preimplantation embryo development and their significance in embryo culture. Theriogenology 1998;49:83–102.
56. Nuccitelli R, Yim DL, Smart T. The sperm-induced Ca2+ wave following fertilization of the Xenopus egg requires the production of Ins(1,4,5)P3. Dev Biol 1993;158:200–12.
57. Poenie M, Alderton J, Tsein RY, Steinhardt RA. Changes in free calcium with stages of the cell division cycle. Nature 1985;315:147–49.
58. Miyazaki S, Igusa Y. Ca-mediated activation of a K current at fertilization of golden hamster eggs. Proc Natl Acad Sci USA 1982;79:931–35.
59. Mitani S. The reduction of calcium current associated with early differentiation of the murine embryo. J Physiol 1985;363:71–86.
60. Ben-Yosef D, Oron Y, Shalgi R. Prolonged, repetitive calcium transients in rat oocytes fertilized in vitro and in vivo. FEBS Lett 1993;331:239–42.
61. Taylor CT, Lawerence YM, Kingsland CR, Biljan MM, Cuthbertson KSR. Oscillations in intracellular free Ca2+ induced by spermatozoa in human oocytes at fertilization. Hum Reprod 1993;8:2174–79.
62. McCormack JG, Halestrap AP, Denton RM. Role of calcium ions in regulation of mammalian intraitochondrial metabolism. Physiol Rev 1990;70:391–425.
63. Lazrak A, Peracchia C. Gap junction gating sensitivity to physiological internal calcium regardless of pH in Novikoff hepatoma cells. Biophys J 1993;65:2002–12.
64. Herman B. Regulation of calcium metabolism in cells. In: Anderson JJB, Garner SC, eds. "Calcium and phosphorus in health and disease." Boca Raton: CRC Press, 1995:83–93.
65. Ishide N. Intracellular calcium modulators for cardiac muscle in pathological conditions. Jpn Heart J 1996;37:1–17.
66. Campbell AK. Intracellular calcium: its universal role as a regulator. Chichester: John Wiley & Sons; 1983.
67. Eisner DA, Lederer WJ. Na-Ca exchange: stoichiometry and electrogenicity. Am J Physiol 1985;248:C189–202.
68. Parratt JR. Control and manipulation of calcium movements. New York: Raven Press, 1985.
69. Borland RM, Biggers JD, Lechene CP, Taymour ML. Elemental composition of fluid in the human fallopian tube. J Reprod Fertil 1980;58:479–82.
70. Casslen B, Nilsson B. Human uterine fluid, examined in undiluted samples for osmo-

larity and the concentrations of inorganic ions, albumin, glucose and urea. Am J Obstet Gynecol 1984;150:877–81.
71. Borland RM, Hazra S, Biggers JD, Lechene CP. The elemental composition of the environments of the gametes and preimplantation embryo during the initiation of pregnancy. Biol Reprod 1977;16:147–57.
72. Lane M, Boatman DE, Albrecht RM, Bavister BD. Intracellular divalent cation homeostasis and developmental competence in the hamster preimplantation embryo. Mol Reprod Dev 1998;50:443–50.
73. Altura BM, Altura BT, Carella A, Turlapaty PD. Ca^{2+} coupling in vascular smooth muscle: Mg^{2+} and buffer effects on contractility and membrane Ca^{2+} movements. Can J Physiol Pharmacol 1982;60:459–82.
74. Wacker WEC, Williams RJP. Magnesium/calcium balances of a biological system. J Theor Biol 1968;20:65–78.
75. Altura BM, Zhang A, Altura BT. Exposure of piglet coronary arterial muscle cells to low concentrations of Mg^{2+} found in blood of ischemic heart disease patients result in rapid elevation of cytosolic Ca^{2+}: relevance to sudden infant death syndrome. Eur J Pharmacol 1997;338:R7–R9.
76. Lane M, Bavister BD. Calcium homeostasis in early hamster preimplantation embryos. Biol Reprod 1998;59:1000–7.
77. Kaibara M, Mitarai S, Yano KA, Kameyama M. Involvement of Na^+-H^+ antiporter in regulation of L-type Ca^{2+} channel current by angiotensin II in rabbit ventricular myocytes. Circ Res 1977;75:1121–25.
78. Irisawa H, Sato R. Intra and extracellular actions of proton on the calcium current of isolated guinea pig ventricular cells. Circ Res 1986;59:348–55.
79. Hewitson LC, Leese HJ. Energy metabolism of the trophectoderm and inner cell mass of the mouse blastocyst. J Exp Zool 1993;267:337–43.
80. Hewitson LC, Martin KL, Leese HJ. Effects of metabolic inhibitors on mouse preimplantation embryo development and the energy metabolism of isolated inner cell masses. Mol Reprod Dev 1996;43:323–30.
81. Leese HJ. Metabolism of the preimplantation mammalian embryo. In: Milligan SR, ed. Oxford Reviews of Reproductive Biology. Oxford: Oxford University Press, 1992:35.
82. Gardner DK, Leese HJ. Non-invasive measurement of nutrient uptake by single cultured pre-implantation mouse embryos. Hum Reprod 1986;1:25–27.
83. Brinster RL, Thomson JL. Development of eight-cell mouse embryos in vitro. Exp Cell Res 1966;42:308–15.
84. Biggers JD, Whittingham DG, Donahue RP. The pattern of energy metabolism in the mouse oocyte and zygote. Proc Natl Acad Sci USA 1967;58:560–67.
85. Leese HJ, Barton AM. Pyruvate and glucose uptake by mouse ova and preimplantation embryos. J Reprod Fertil 1984;72:9–13.
86. Lane M, Gardner DK. Lactate regulates pyruvate uptake and metabolism in the preimplantation mouse embryo. Biol Reprod 2000;62:16–22.
87. Gardner DK, Lane M, Spitzer A, Batt PA. Enhanced rates of cleavage and development for sheep zygotes cultured to the blastocyst stage in vitro in the absence of serum and somatic cells: amino acids, vitamins and culturing embryos in groups stimulate development. Biol Reprod 1994;50:390.
88. Rieger D, Loskutoff NM, Betteridge KJ. Developmentally related changes in the metabolism of glucose and glutamine by cattle embryos produced and co-cultured in vitro. J Reprod Fertil 1992;95:585–95.

89. Steeves TE, Gardner DK. Temporal and differential effects of amino acids on bovine embryo development in culture. Biol Reprod 1999;61:731–40.
90. Hardy K, Hooper MAK, Handyside AH, Rutherford AJ, Winston RML, Leese HJ. Non-invasive measurement of glucose and pyruvate uptake by individual human oocytes and preimplantation embryos. Hum Reprod 1989;4:188.
91. Barbehenn EK, Wales RG, Lowry OH. The explanation for the blockade in glycolysis in early mouse embryos. Proc Nat Acad Sci USA 1974;71:1056.
92. Barbehenn EK, Wales RG, Lowry OH. Measurement of metabolites in single preimplantation embryos; a new means to study metabolic control in early embryos. J Embryol Exp Morphol 1978;43:29.
93. Leese HJ, Biggers JD, Mroz EA, Lechene C. Nucleotides in a single mammalian ovum or preimplantation embryo. Anal Biochem 1984;140:443–48.
94. Biggers JD, Gardner DK, Leese HJ. Control of carbohydrate metabolism on preimplantation embryos. In: Rosenblum IY, Heyner S, eds. Growth factors in mammalian development. Boca Raton: CRC Press, 1989:19.
95. Gardner DK, Leese HJ. Concentrations of nutrients in mouse oviduct fluid and their effects on embryo development and metabolism in vitro. J Reprod Fert 1990;88:361–68.
96. Gardner DK, Lane M. Developmental arrest is associated with altered ATP:ADP ratios and PFK activity. Biol Reprod 1997;56(Suppl. 1):216.
97. Denton RM, McCormack JG, Edgell NJ. Role of calcium ions in the regulation of intramitochondrial metabolism. Effects of Na+, Mg2+, and ruthenium red on the Ca2+-stimulated oxidation of oxoglutarate and on pyruvate dehydrogenase activity in intact rat heart mitochondria. Biochem J 1985;190:107–17.
98. Wyatt HV. Cations, enzymes and control of cell metabolism. J Theor Biol 1964;6:441–70.
99. Lane M, Gardner DK. EDTA stimulates development of cleavage stage mouse embryos by inhibiting the glycolytic enzyme phosphoglycerate kinase. Biol Reprod 1997;56(Suppl. 1):193.
100. Cockcroft S, Gromerts BD. Activation and inhibition of calcium-dependent histamine secretion by ATP ions applied to rat mast cells. J Physiol 1979;29:222–43.
101. Schoolcraft WB, Gardner DK, Lane M, Schlenker T, Hamilton F, Meldrum DR. Blastocyst culture and transfer: analysis of results and parameters affecting outcome in two in vitro fertilization programs. Fertil Steril 1999;72:604–9.
102. Shoukir Y, Chardonnens D, Campana A, Sakkas D. Blastocyst development from supernumerary embryos after intracytoplasmic sperm injection: a paternal influence? Hum Reprod 1998;13:1632–37.
103. Ho Y, Wigglesworth K, Eppig JJ, Schultz RM. Preimplantation development of mouse embryos in KSOM: augmentation by amino acids and analysis of gene expression. Mol Reprod Dev 1995;41:232–38.
104. Doherty AS, Mann MR, Tremblay KD, Bartolomei MS, Schultz RM. Differential effects of culture on imprinted H19 expression in the preimplantation mouse embryo. Biol Reprod 2000;62:1526–35.

8

Cell Junctions and Cell Interactions in Animal and Human Blastocyst Development

Tom P. Fleming, M. Reza Ghassemifar, Judith Eckert,
Aspasia Destouni, Fay Thomas, Jane E. Collins,
and Bhavwanti Sheth

The first differentiation event in mammalian development is the generation of the outer trophectoderm epithelium of the blastocyst, which is responsible for blastocoel cavity formation and for vectorial transport between the maternal environment and the embryo interior where the inner cell mass (ICM) resides. Blastomeres within the trophectoderm lineage interact via four types of epithelial intercellular junctions: the E-cadherin/catenin (or adherens junction) system, gap junctions, tight junctions (or zonula occludens), and desmosomes. These membrane complexes collectively contribute to the integrity, signaling activity, polarized functioning, and stability of the developing epithelium, therefore, they are crucial elements in blastocyst morphogenesis and viability. Moreover, particularly in the mouse model, analysis of the mechanisms of junction formation and activation, commonly regulated by the pattern of cell interactions provides insight into the timing and coordination of epithelial differentiation.

Human blastocyst formation in vitro is known to be a highly sensitive and susceptible period of morphogenesis. On average, only a minority of human embryos will reach the blastocyst stage in vitro for a variety of perceived reasons ranging from chromosomal imbalance to inadequate culture conditions (1). As a result, procedures in assisted conception treatment have included routine transfer of usually two or three early cleavage stage embryos. This practice, however, has not resulted in any significant improvement in the live birth rate per treatment (around 15%) and can enhance the risk of multiple pregnancy. Although blastocyst culture and transfer of single embryos may improve success rates, this strategy requires further understanding of cellular mechanisms controlling human blastocyst development. Here, key aspects of epithelial junction formation and cell interactions in mammalian embryos are reviewed with emphasis on their contribution to blastocyst morphogenesis. We will consider first the expression and experimental data from the mouse model before analysis of our limited understanding of these processes during early human development.

E-Cadherin Adhesion and Compaction

In the mouse, compaction occurs during the eight-cell stage and represents the activation of the E-cadherin/catenin calcium-dependent adherens junction adhesion system (2) (Fig. 8.1), which causes blastomeres to convert from a loose aggregation of separated cells into a morula of tightly adherent cells. E-cadherin, and the catenin proteins with which it interacts for cytoskeletal linkage, are distributed uniformly on blastomere surfaces throughout early cleavage and relocalize to regions of intercellular contact as adhesion initiates (3). This process coincides with each blastomere changing from a nonpolar to polar phenotype. This is most clearly evident in the formation of a pole of microvilli on the apical (outer) surface and the clustering of endocytic organelles and cytoskeletal elements in the subjacent apical cytoplasm (4). Each blastomere therefore contributes to a radially organized protoepithelial polarity for the entire embryo, representing the origin of trophectoderm differentiation. Experimental analysis has shown that it is the adhesive component of compaction that is responsible for catalyzing and coordinating cellular polarization. Moreover, E-cadherin and α-catenin null mutant embryos show

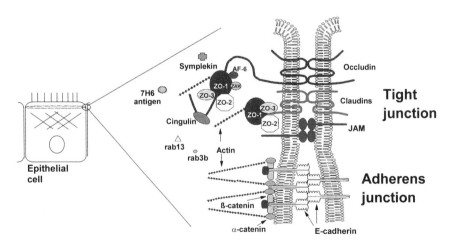

FIGURE 8.1. Diagram of the organization of the apicolateral region of contact between epithelial cells showing the multiprotein constituents of the tight junction and the adherens junction.

developmental lethality with trophectoderm differentiation effectively abolished (5).

What initiates E-cadherin adhesivity at compaction? Because expression and membrane localization of E-cadherin–catenin complex proteins are readily detectable throughout cleavage (3), posttranslational control of adhesivity is implied. Thus, use of biosynthetic inhibitors has shown that protein translation necessary for compaction to occur is completed during the four-cell stage. Moreover, activation of protein kinase C (PKC) induces premature compaction in four-cell embryos, whereas inhibition of kinases blocks natural and premature compaction (6). One candidate for the substrate of PKC activation is E-cadherin itself because it becomes phosphorylated for the first time in the early eight-cell embryo. The timing of this event, however, is unaltered under conditions where compaction is either prematurely induced or inhibited (7). It has been shown that β-catenin becomes phosphorylated at serine/threonine residues at the time of both normal and prematurely induced compaction (8), which strongly implicates this member of the adhesion complex as a substrate for PKC. Moreover, the phosphorylating kinase may be the PKCα isoform because it relocates to cell contact sites as compaction occurs (8). Downstream of the kinase cascade to activate adhesion, the reorganization of the actin cytoskeleton required to initiate blastomere polarization has been shown to be regulated by the rho family of GTPases (9).

E-cadherin adhesion, activated posttranslationally, therefore has an important role in initiating and organizing epithelial polarity and tissue formation in the early embryo, but it is not restricted to the trophectoderm lineage. Thus, following the next two rounds of cytokinesis, during which differentiative divisions of certain blastomeres lead to segregation of outer trophectoderm and inner ICM cell lineages, E-cadherin adhesion is maintained in both cell populations up to and during blastocyst formation and expansion.

Gap Junctions

Gap junctions are intercellular communication channels composed of oligomeric connexin protein units that permit exchange of ions and small signaling molecules (< 1kDa) between cells and which regulate and coordinate diverse cellular processes, including proliferation, differentiation, and apoptosis (10). It is during compaction that gap junction communication is first evident between mouse blastomeres (11). Like the E-cadherin protein complex, synthesis of gap junction proteins takes place well in advance of compaction and is regulated by DNA replication during the two-cell stage (12). There are more than 20 different connexin genes identified (10). The principal connexins found in mouse embryos at compaction are Cx32 and Cx43; Cx32 is a maternal gene product, whereas Cx43 is zygotically expressed and increases in proportion at later stages. Membrane assembly of

Cx43 at gap junctions occurs from compaction onward, forming a zonular distribution pattern between outer trophectoderm cells and discontinuous, plaquelike localizations between ICM cells (13). In addition, other members of the connexin family, notably Cx31, 31.1 and 45, contribute to gap junctional assembly in the preimplantation mouse embryo (14). As a result, despite reduced gap junctional communication occurring in null mutant Cx43 embryos, other connexins can replace Cx43 to maintain blastocyst viability (15).

Gap junctional coupling between blastomeres has been inhibited by injection of antibody against either gap junction protein or Cx32- and Cx43-specific peptide domains, resulting in decompaction and extrusion of antibody-containing cells (16). These data indicate that gap junctional coupling is required for blastomere adhesion to be maintained and for the continued participation of cells in trophectoderm differentiation. DDK strain mouse eggs, fertilized by foreign sperm, similarly fail to develop gap junctional coupling at compaction, resulting in de-adhesion and extrusion of cells at the morula stage and embryo lethality. This condition, and gap junctional communication in normal embryos, is induced by low intracellular pH (17).

Tight Junctions

The tight junction, or zonula occludens, is a beltlike site of close intercellular contact circumscribing the apicolateral border between epithelial cells. This junction is responsible for both the adhesive permeability seal of epithelial sheets that control paracellular solute diffusion and transepithelial resistance (barrier function) and for the maintenance of distinct apical and basolateral membrane domains (fence function) (18). The tight junction is composed of multiple proteins, including transmembrane proteins that engage in intercellular sealing (occludin, claudins, JAM) and cytoplasmic plaque proteins (e.g., ZO-1, ZO-2, ZO-3, cingulin, rab13 and others; Fig. 8.1) (18). Occludin and claudin family members span the membrane four times with both N- and C-terminal domains being cytoplasmic. Occludin and claudin C-termini interact with the three related ZO proteins (19,20) with ZO-1 binding actin to permit cytoskeletal anchorage. ZO-1 also occurs in two alternatively spliced isoforms either with or without a C-terminal 80 amino acid α domain (ZO-1α-, ZO-1α+) (21).

The development of the tight junction in the mouse embryo initiates from compaction and has been shown to involve a complex zygotic expression program that coordinates membrane assembly of components at the apicolateral region of contact between outer cells in three phases corresponding to 8-, 16- and early 32-cell stages, respectively. Within 1–2 hours of compaction, the tight junction plaque protein, ZO-1α- isoform, is detectable at the apicolateral junction site (22,23). ZO-1α- mRNA and protein are detectable by RT-PCR and immunoblotting throughout cleavage, but membrane assembly is dependent upon prior activation of E-cadherin adhesion. When E-cadherin adhesion at compaction is blocked (e.g., by neutralizing antibody), ZO-1α- membrane assembly is delayed and randomly distributed (22,23).

We have found that ZO-1a- assembly initiating tight junction formation at compaction is associated with membrane delivery of the rab protein, rab13, the two proteins colocalizing precisely at the apicolateral contact site (B. Sheth et al., unpublished observations). Rab proteins are part of the Ras superfamily of small GTPases, and are involved in the regulation and targeting of intracellular transport (24). Certain rab proteins have been implicated to have a role in epithelial polarity including rab13, which has been proposed to target newly synthesized constituents to the tight junction (25). Thus, the early assembly of rab13 at the apicolateral site between blastomeres after compaction may act to define the site of tight junction formation.

Tight junction formation continues during the 16-cell stage in outer blastomeres by apicolateral membrane assembly of the plaque protein, cingulin, which colocalizes with ZO-1α-(26). This pool of cingulin is expressed from the embryonic genome, whereas a pool of cingulin expressed from the maternal genome localizes to the egg cytocortex and, during cleavage, is depleted by turnover within endocytic vesicles. The importance of E-cadherin adhesion in tight junction formation has also been shown by its effect on the stability of newly synthesized cingulin. Once adhesion initiates, the level of cingulin detectable by immunoprecipitation increases markedly due to a longer turnover time, as revealed in pulse-chase experiments (27).

The last phase of tight junction formation begins during the 32-cell stage. During this cell cycle, apicolateral membrane assembly of the ZO-1α+ isoform occurs for the first time following de novo transcription and translation during the late 16-cell stage (23). The synthesis and assembly of this isoform appears to be regulatory for completion of tight junction formation because the establishment of a permeability seal and blastocoele cavitation rapidly follow this event (Fig. 8.2A–C). One important component of this mechanism is that newly synthesised ZO-1α+ first appears to associate with the tight junction transmembrane protein, occluding, at perinuclear Golgi sites before the two proteins are delivered to the membrane together (23). We have found that occludin is expressed at mRNA and protein levels throughout cleavage, but it does not assemble at the membrane and link to the cytoskeleton (detergent insoluble) until after ZO-1α+ is expressed (28). Occludin assembly is also regulated by posttranslational mechanisms. At least four forms of occludin are detectable by immunoblotting throughout cleavage, representing distinct posttranslational states or possibly splicing variants, each of which increase or decrease in relative amount at each stage of cleavage (28). It is interesting that one form (occludin band 2) increases in amount during the morula stage, undergoes phosphorylation, and exclusively becomes detergent-insoluble, which indicates that it is the

96   T.P. Fleming et al.

target of ZO-1α+ and is utilized to complete tight junction formation. In ongoing studies, we have further evidence that other tight junction proteins (claudins, ZO-2) may also assemble at this late stage and be part of the ZO-1α+/occludin complex (F. Thomas, R. Nowak, T.P. Fleming and colleagues, unpublished observations).

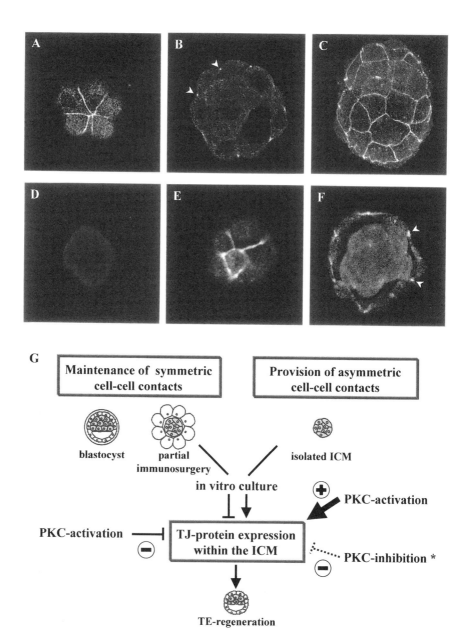

Desmosomes

Desmosomes are spotlike multimolecular membrane complexes that provides intercellular adhesion and intermediate filament anchorage in epithelial cell. They also contribute toward tissue integrity (29). These junctions comprise transmembrane desmosomal cadherins, the desmocollins and the desmogleins, which mediate adhesion at desmosomes and are encoded by two sets of three differentially expressed genes (Dsc1, 2 and 3; Dsg1, 2 and 3), with each Dsc gene encoding a pair of isoforms, a and b, generated by alternate splicing, that differ in their C-termini (29). The desmosomal cadherin cytoplasmic domains contain binding sites for plakoglobin, desmoplakin, and plakophilins. Desmoplakin and plakophilins also interact with the intermediate filament system (29).

Desmosomes first form in the mouse late morula or nascent blastocyst (30). The timing of desmosome assembly appears to be regulated by the pattern of expression of the desmosomal cadherins. Thus, the cytoplasmic plaque proteins, plakoglobin and desmoplakin, can be detected by immunoprecipitation at 8- and 16-cell stages, respectively, but desmocollins and desmogleins are not detectable until late morula or early blastocyst stages (30). In a detailed study of desmocollin expression, it was found that only Dsc2 transcripts were detectable during preimplantation development, including both a and b isoforms (31). Significantly, zygotic expression of Dsc2 was not detected until late cleavage, implicating this desmocollin as regulatory in permitting desmosome formation to occur (31). Thus, the embryo appears to regulate the timing of completion of both tight and desmosome junction biogenesis by delayed expression of perhaps one gene product (ZO-1α+, Dsc2), which acts as a limiting factor. We have proposed that desmosomes are required to stabilize the trophectoderm during blastocyst expansion (30,31).

←
___

FIGURE 8.2. (A–C). Immunolocalization of ZO-1α+ within wholemount mouse blastocysts using confocal microscopy. (A) Tangential plane of trophectoderm showing ZO-1α+ localized to cell borders. (B) Midplane of blastocyst showing spot-like ZO-1α+ at the apicolateral region of contact between trophectoderm cells (arrowheads), but absent from the internal ICM. (C) Z-series image showing ZO-1α+ at trophectoderm contact sites. (D–E) ICM isolated from early blastocyst and culture for 0 hours (D) or 6 hours (E) and immunolabeled for ZO-2. Upregulation and membrane assembly of ZO-2 occurs during culture. (F) Partial immunosurgery of 2 hours cultured ICM in which the lysed trophectoderm layer is not removed and showing absence of ZO-2 staining in the ICM; arrowheads show ZO-2 staining in the trophectoderm layer. (G) Diagram illustrating the role of cell contact patterns and PKC signaling on the expression of tight junction (TJ) proteins in the ICM; *although PKC inhibition generally leads to suppression of expression, use of different inhibitors shows a complex reaction.

Cell–Cell Interactions

The pattern of cell contacts regulate epithelial differentiation and the segregation of trophectoderm and ICM lineages in the early embryo. Thus, asymmetric contacts (i.e., lateral cell contacts, but with one face contact-free), mediated through E-cadherin, coordinate polarization at compaction and initiate subsequent maturation of the trophectoderm phenotype (see earlier discussion). Our data similarly suggest that contact symmetry (i.e., total enclosure) acts to suppress epithelial differentiation in the ICM lineage.

The ICM does not exhibit tight junctions or desmosomes (Fig. 8.2B). RT-PCR and in situ hybridization studies, however, have shown that transcripts for the tight junction proteins ZO-1α-, ZO-1α+, occludin, and rab13 are all present within ICM cells (23,28) (B. Sheth et al., unpublished observations). ICM cells, however, translate cingulin protein at a significantly lower rate than trophectoderm cells (27). This would indicate that suppression of the epithelial phenotype is achieved posttranscriptionally, but confirmation by semi-quantitative techniques is required. In addition, both mRNA and protein for tight junction components may enter the ICM lineage by inheritance during differentiative division (32). In contrast, Dsc2 mRNA is only detectable within a minority (~25%) of ICM cells, and there is evidence that these cells may inherit Dsc2 mRNA during differentiative division (31). Taken together, suppression of epithelial differentiation within the ICM may be regulated at transcriptional or posttranscriptional levels, depending on gene product.

Suppression of the epithelial phenotype within the ICM is at least partially regulated by the transcription factor Oct-4 and its downstream genetic pathway required for maintenance of totipotency (33). However, continued cell contact symmetry is also required. Thus, if ICM cells experience cell contact asymmetry for even very short periods (e.g., following their immunosurgical isolation from early blastocysts) this process may be reversed. In such circumstances, ZO-1, ZO-2 and other tight junction proteins rapidly assemble at the apicolateral contact sites between outer ICM cells in a sequence similar to that occurring during trophectoderm differentiation in intact embryos, leading ultimately to cavitation (32) (Fig. 8.2D,E; J. Eckert, unpublished observations). The same upregulation of Dsc2 and desmoplakin membrane assembly during desmosome formation occurs in isolated ICMs (31). It is interesting that ZO-1 assembly in isolated ICMs occurs in the presence of transcriptional inhibitor, but not protein synthesis inhibitor, which indicates that the endogenous ZO-1 transcripts are available for expression (32). In the case of Dsc2, ICM isolation causes upregulation of Dsc2 mRNA detection, suggesting transcriptional activation is also involved (31).

We have begun to investigate the processes linking cell contact asymmetry with junctional protein assembly in isolated ICMs. If immunosurgery by complement-mediated lysis is performed but the dead trophectoderm shell is not removed (partial immunosurgery), junctional protein assembly in the

ICM is inhibited (Fig. 8.2F). Moreover, PCK activation stimulates the assembly process, whereas PKC inhibition tends to slow it down (J. Eckert, unpublished observations). In addition to intracellular signaling cell contact patterns appear to regulate the expression level and assembly of junctional gene products in the embryo (Fig. 8.2G).

Human Embryos

To date, our understanding of the role of intercellular junctions and cell interactions in human early development is very sparse. Human embryos express E-cadherin (34), show evidence of cadherinlike adherens junctions at contact sites (35), and engage in compaction during day 4 of development corresponding approximately with the 16-cell stage (36). Similar to the mouse embryo, compaction coincides with cell polarization and the establishment of a protoepithelial phenotype (36). Given the importance of E-cadherin adhesion in subsequent epithelial differentiation (see earlier), however, one future goal should be to investigate the frequency of compaction and potential mechanisms of its activation (e.g., β-catenin phosphorylation). Are human embryos deficient in PKC-mediated signaling activity?

Human embryos engage in gap junctional communication, show the presence of gap junctions ultrastructurally, and assemble connexins at cell contact sites at different stages of cleavage (35,37,38). Cx43 is the predominant connexin expressed, together with Cx32 and Cx26 (38). The extent of blastomere decompaction and exclusion evident in human embryos is excessive, however, provoking the suggestion that deficient connexin expression and gap junction communication may be responsible (38). Again, this is an important area for future analysis.

Tight junctions and desmosomes in the human trophectoderm layer have been reported (37–39). In our work, we have investigated the expression of selected junction genes and found evidence of ZO-1α-, ZO-1α+, occludin, JAM and Dsc2 mRNAs in humans embryos (Fig. 8.3A; M.R. Ghassemifar, unpublished observations). Moreover, the differential timing of mRNA expression of ZO-1α- and ZO-1α+ isoforms previously shown to be critical in regulating tight junction assembly in the mouse embryo (23) also occurs in the human embryo (Fig. 8.3B; M.R. Ghassemifar, unpublished observations). However, the level of detection of junctional transcripts in human embryos may be low compared with the mouse. In addition, analysis of tight and desmosome junction protein localization during human trophectoderm formation indicates that membrane assembly of proteins may be frequently impaired when compared with the mouse embryo (Fig. 8.3C,D). Thus, junctional proteins are commonly detected in the cytoplasm rather than specifically at membrane contact sites.

Studies on a limited number of cultured human embryos collectively suggest that events associated with trophectoderm epithelial differentiation may be defective and may contribute to the poor rate of blastocyst development in culture.

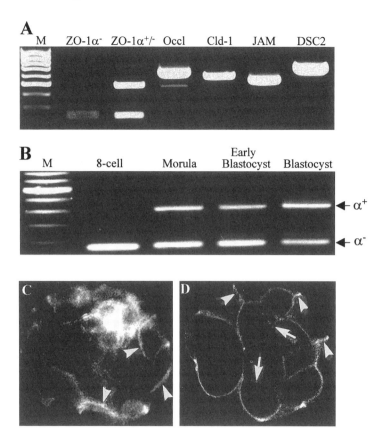

FIGURE 8.3. (A) Detection of tight and desmosome junction gene expression in single human embryos following RT-PCR (M = markers). (B) Differential timing of expression of ZO-1α- and ZO-1α+ mRNAs in human embryos over eight-cell to blastocyst stages. (C,D) Immunostaining of human (C) and mouse (D) blastocysts for junction adhesion molecule (JAM); note the poor level of membrane assembly of JAM (arrowheads, arrows) in the human versus the mouse blastocyst.

Further research is required to determine the molecular/cellular processes that may account for these abnormalities.

Acknowledgments. We are grateful to the Medical Research Council, the Wellcome Trust, and the European Union for research funding to TPF for epithelial differentiation studies in both animal and human embryos.

References

1. Trounson A, Bongso A. Fertilization and development in humans. Curr Top Dev Biol 1996;32:59–101.

2. Yeaman C, Grindstaff KK, Nelson WJ. New perspectives on mechanisms involved in generating epithelial cell polarity. Physiol Rev 1999;79:73–98.
3. Ohsugi M, Hwang SY, Butz S, Knowles BB, Solter D, Kemler R. Expression and cell membrane localization of catenins during mouse preimplantation development. Dev Dyn 1996;206:391–402.
4. Fleming TP, Butler E, Collins JE, Sheth B, Wild AE. Cell polarity and mouse early development. Adv Mol Cell Biol 1998;26:67–94.
5. Torres M, Stoykova A, Huber O, Chowdhury K, Bonaldo P, Mansouri A, et al. An α-E-catenin gene trap mutation defines its function in preimplantation development. Proc Natl Acad Sci USA 1997;94:901–6.
6. Winkel GK, Ferguson JE, Takeichi M, Nuccitelli R. Activation of protein kinase C triggers premature compaction in the four-cell stage mouse embryo. Dev Biol 1990;138:1–15.
7. Sefton M, Johnson MH, Clayton L, McConnell JM. Experimental manipulations of compaction and their effects on the phosphorylation of uvomorulin. Mol Reprod Dev 1996;44:77–87.
8. Pauken CM, Capco DG. Regulation of cell adhesion during embryonic compaction of mammalian embryos: roles for PKC and β-catenin. Mol Reprod Dev 1999;54:135–44.
9. Clayton L, Hall A, Johnson MH. A role for rho-like GTPases in the polarisation of mouse eight-cell blastomeres. Dev Biol 1999;205:322–31.
10. Simon AM, Goodenough DA. Diverse functions of vertebrate gap junctions. Trends Cell Biol 1998;8:477–83.
11. Lo CW, Gilula NB. Gap junctional communication in the preimplantation mouse embryo. Cell 1979;18:399–409.
12. Valdimarsson G, Kidder GM. Temporal control of gap junction assembly in preimplantation mouse embryos. J Cell Sci 1995;108:1715–22.
13. De Sousa PA, Valdimarsson G, Nicholson BJ, Kidder GM. Connexin trafficking and the control of gap junction assembly in mouse preimplantation embryos. Development 1993;117:1355–67.
14. Davies TC, Barr KJ, Jones DH, Zhu D, Kidder GM. Multiple members of the connexin gene family participate in preimplantation development of the mouse. Dev Genet 1996;18:234–43.
15. De Sousa PA, Juneja SC, Caveney S, Houghton FD, Davies TC, Reaume AG, et al. Normal development of preimplantation mouse embryos deficient in gap junctional coupling. J Cell Sci 1997;110:1751–58.
16. Becker DK, Evans WH, Green CR, Warner A. Functional analysis of amino acid sequences in connexin43 involved in intercellular communication through gap junctions. J Cell Sci 1995;108:1455–67.
17. Leclerc C, Becker D, Buehr M, Warner A. Low intracellular pH is involved in the early embryonic death of DDK mouse eggs fertilized by alien sperm. Dev Dyn 1994;200:257–67.
18. Matter K, Balda MS. Occludin and the functions of tight junction. Int Rev Cytol 1999;186:117–46.
19. Furuse M, Itoh M, Hirase T, Nagafuchi A, Yonemura S, Tsukita S, et al. Direct association of occludin with ZO-1 and its possible involvement in the localisation of occludin at tight junctions. J Cell Biol 1994;127:1617–26.
20. Itoh M, Furuse M, Morita K, Kubota K, Saitou M, Tsukita S. Direct binding of three tight junction-associated MAGUKs, ZO-1, ZO-2, and ZO-3, with the COOH termini of claudins. J Cell Biol 1999;147:1351–63.

21. Balda MS, Anderson JM. Two classes of tight junctions are revealed by ZO-1 isoforms. Am J Physiol 1993;264:C918–24.
22. Fleming TP, McConnell J, Johnson MH, Stevenson BR. Development of tight junctions de novo in the mouse early embryo: control of assembly of the tight junction-specific protein, ZO-1. J Cell Biol 1989;108:1407–18.
23. Sheth B, Fesenko I, Collins JE, Moran B, Wild AE, Anderson JM, et al. Tight junction assembly during mouse blastocyst formation is regulated by late expression of ZO-1α+ isoform. Development 1997;124:2027–37.
24. Novick P, Zerial M. The diversity of rab proteins in vesicle transport. Curr Opin Cell Biol 1997;9:496–504.
25. Zahraoui A, Joberty G, Arpin M, Fontaine J-J, Hellio R, Tavitian A, et al. A small rab GTPase is distributed in cytoplasmic vesicles in non-polarised cells but colocalised with the tight junction marker ZO-1 in polarised epithelial cells. J Cell Biol 1994;124:101–15.
26. Fleming TP, Hay M, Javed Q, Citi S. Localisation of tight junction protein cingulin is temporally and spatially regulated during early mouse development. Development 1993;117:1135–44.
27. Javed Q, Fleming TP, Hay M, Citi S. Tight junction protein cingulin is expressed by maternal and embryonic genomes during early mouse development. Development 1993;117:1145–51.
28. Sheth B, Moran B, Anderson BM, Fleming TP. Post-translational control of occludin membrane assembly in mouse trophectoderm: a mechanism to regulate timing of tight junction biogenesis and blastocyst formation. Development 2000;127:831–40.
29. Garrod D, Chidgey M, North A. Desmosomes: differentiation, development, dynamics and disease. Curr Opin Cell Biol 1996;8:670–78.
30. Fleming TP, Garrod DR, Elsmore AJ. Desmosome biogenesis in the mouse preimplantation embryo. Development 1991;112:527–39.
31. Collins JE, Lorimer JE, Garrod DR, Pidsley SC, Buxton RS, Fleming TP. Regulation of desmocollin transcription in mouse preimplantation embryos. Development 1995;121:743–53.
32. Fleming TP, Hay MJ. Tissue-specific control of expression of the tight junction polypeptide ZO-1 in the mouse early embryo. Development 1991;113:295–304.
33. Nichols J, Zevnik B, Anastassiadis K, Niwa H, Klewe-Nebenius D, Chambers I, et al. Formation of pluripotent stem cells in the mammalian embryo depends on the POU transcription factor Oct4. Cell 1998;95:379–91.
34. Campbell S, Swann HR, Seif MW, Kimber SJ, Aplin JD. Cell adhesion molecules on the oocyte and preimplantation human embryo. Hum Reprod 1995;10:1571–78.
35. Tesarik J. Involvement of oocyte-coded message in cell differentiation control of early human embryos. Development 1989;105:317–22.
36. Nikas G, Ao A, Winston RM, Handyside AH. Compaction and surface polarity in the human embryo in vitro. Biol Reprod 1996;55:32–37.
37. Dale B, Gualtieri R, Talevi R, Tosti E, Santella L, Elder K. Intercellular communication in the early human embryo. Mol Reprod Dev 1991;29:22–28.
38. Hardy K, Warner A, Winston RM, Becker DL. Expression of intercellular junctions during preimplantation development of the human embryo. Mol Hum Reprod 1996;2:621–32.
39. Gualtieri R, Santella L, Dale B. Tight junctions and cavitation in the human pre-embryo. Mol Reprod Dev 1992;32:81–87.

Part III

Blastocyst Development in Culture

9

Blastocyst Development in Culture: The Role of Macromolecules

THOMAS B. POOL

Developmental plasticity—the ability of an embryo to retain viability in the face of environmental fluctuation and challenge—is the biological quality that has facilitated the success of clinical in vitro fertilization. Plasticity, however, can be foe as well as friend because it is a major confounder in experimental efforts to define the nutritional requirements of preimplantation embryos. For example, the range in latitude we are afforded by plasticity in one embryo may not be the same that is available in a sibling embryo. Patient age, diagnosis, and ovarian stimulation protocol all impinge upon plasticity, so producing a cohort of embryos with developmental tolerances similar to another cohort is difficult at best. Optimization requires us to find the middle of the range of tolerances. This approaches impossibility without quantitative measures in vitro that relate directly to viability after transfer.

Despite these limitations, we have a history of being able to produce livebirth following the transfer of embryos grown in media of widely varying and, often, inappropriate composition. Can this range in forgiveness to environmental impropriety that is expressed by embryos be due solely to mechanisms resident within the embryo? Can plasticity of the embryo alone account for the retention of viability following culture in a medium as simple as a dilute solution of salts or in complex media laden with a complete array of amino acids, vitamins, trace elements, antioxidants, and energetic substrates? Perhaps, but a more reasonable explanation is that developmental resilience is imparted by modulators found in the external environment of the embryo, in addition to those mechanisms functioning within the embryo, that these modulators acting in vitro are less effective surrogates of those found in vivo and that they act through physical as well as chemical means.

This chapter will consider the possibility that macromolecules in the embryonic environment, as well as those used to supplement culture media, serve this role. One must realize that these functions are distinct from those of polypeptide growth factors that act through specific receptors to affect developmental competence and progression through both autocrine and paracrine mechanisms. It is not the intent of this chapter to address specific macromolecular interactions (e.g., growth factors and their specific receptors), but rather to examine how macromolecules might act through nonspecific ways, modifying the exposure of embryos to nutrients, anions, cations, and even water, to potentiate preimplantation development, with special emphasis upon blastocyst production in vitro.

The Use of Whole Serum as a Macromolecular Supplement

The addition of serum as a supplement to embryo culture medium is not a practice dictated by any demonstrated obligate requirement for exogenous protein by blastomeres; rather, it simply is a relic from the somatic cell culture technology that was borrowed in the early days of in vitrofertilization (IVF). In reality, it was shown decisively by Caro and Trounson (1) that fertilization, cleavage, and pregnancy could be achieved by transferring embryos produced completely under protein-free culture conditions. The use of serum or other sources of protein, therefore, improves the performance characteristics of culture medium instead of satisfying a nutritional requirement (see Pool et al. 1998 [2] for a review). The sources of serum that have been used for embryo culture supplementation are varied and a representation is given in Table 9.1. Saito et al. (3) compared embryo development in Ham's F10 medium supplemented with either whole fetal cord serum (FCoS), a high molecular weight fraction from FCoS, a low molecular weight fraction from FcoS, or human serum albumin (HSA). Both whole FCoS and the high-molecular weight fraction were superior to the low-molecular weight fraction or HSA. Leung et al. (4) likewise compared fertilization, cleavage, and pregnancy rates between modified Ham's F10 medium supplemented with maternal serum (MS) or FCoS. Although fertilization and cleavage rates were the same between the two supplements, the pregnancy rate achieved was significantly higher in the

TABLE 9.1. Sources of serum used for supplementation of embryo culture medium.

Year	Source	Investigators
1965	Fetal calf serum	Edwards (5)
1980	Maternal serum	Edwards et al. (6)
1983	Fetal cord serum, high and low molecular weight fractions, albumin	Saito et al. (3)
1984	Fetal cord serum, maternal serum	Leung et al. (4)

TABLE 9.2. Effects of using whole serum as a supplement to embryo culture medium.

Observation	Investigators
1. Dark, granular morphology of blastocysts	Gardner et al. (7)
2. Granular vesicles present in trophectoderm	
3. Excess production of lactate by blastocysts	
4. Mitochondrial degeneration in blastocysts observed with transmission electron microscopy	Dorland et al. (8)
5. Production of large offspring in sheep and cattle following ET	Walker et al. (9)
6. Trophectodernal vesicles determined to be lipid through osmium fixation and transmission electron microscopy	Thompson et al. (10)
7. Significant extension of gestational period	
8. Increased birth weight attributable to whole serum; restoration of normal birth weight by replacing serum with BSA	

FCoS group. These studies are important because they demonstrate that the beneficial effects of serum can be mediated by a subset of whole serum (i.e., the high molecular weight fraction). They show, more importantly, that the quality of the supplement can be manifest postembryo transfer in the pregnancy rate, not in embryo performance or appearance in culture as are most often scored in studies that address components of culture media. These data represent some of the earliest evidence that macromolecular components of human embryo culture medium can influence eventual viability, as reflected by pregnancy, even though the basic culture medium used, Ham's F10, was the same in all experiments.

Although supplementation with serum was the norm for embryo growth in clinical assisted reproductive technology (ART) programs for 10–12 years, it was not without major drawbacks. As Gardner (7) has indicated, serum is produced only after clotting and is a pathological fluid. It is a complex mixture containing a number of undefined or ill-defined components that can vary from patient to patient or within an individual under differing physiological conditions. The use of whole serum both thwarts the formulation of culture medium with lot to lot consistency, and it induces more dire metabolic and developmental consequences for embryos and resulting fetuses. Some cumulative observations from using whole serum in domestic animal culture systems are summarized in Table 9.2.

Albumins and Plasma Protein Fractions

The trend has been to avoid the use of whole serum and, instead, to use HSA or a commercially available plasma protein fraction that is predominately HSA, but with varying amounts of contaminating α and β globulins. A summary of the application of this form of protein supplementation is given in

TABLE 9.3. Use of albumins and plasma protein fractions as supplements for embryo culture medium.

Year	Supplement	Investigators
1969	Bovine serum albumin (BSA)	Edwards et al. (11)
1984	Human serum albumin (HSA)	Menezo et al. (12)
1989	HSA (Albuminar-5)	Ashwood-Smith et al. (13)
1990	HSA (Albuminar-20)	Staessen et al. (14)
1993	HSA (Plasmanate)	Adler et al. (17)
1994	HSA/globulins (Plasmatein)	Pool, Martin (15)
1995	HSA/globulins (SSS)	Weathersbee et al. (16)

Table 9.3. Although bovine serum albumin (BSA) had been used experimentally in human embryo culture in 1969 (11), Menezo et al. (12) were the first to use it as a component of a culture medium formulated specifically for human in vitro fertilization and embryo culture. This medium, B-2, later became commercially available and is still in wide use today.

Ashwood-Smith et al. (13) raised concerns about using animal products in human embryo culture medium because it increases the risk of introducing animal viruses into patients or of sensitizing them to foreign proteins. They therefore considered using a commercial source of HSA (Albuminar 5) that was licensed for intravenous infusion as a vascular volume expander and compared the fertilization and pregnancy rates obtained through using this product with those obtained with the use of patient serum. No differences were seen in fertilization rates, even though sperm survival was less in Albuminar-supplemented media. In addition, no blastocysts were seen to form from extra embryos in Albuminar-supplemented medium, but the basal medium used in these experiments was Earle's balanced salt solution, a medium devoid of amino acids. In a subsequent study of Albuminar versus whole serum (14) as the protein supplement to modified Earle's medium, it was seen that both the percentage of cleaved embryos and pregnancy rates were significantly higher in the Albuminar group, even though the fertilization rates were the same. This, again, demonstrates that the qualitative form of macromolecular supplementation can modulate the effects of the basal culture medium to affect embryo behavior significantly, both pre- and posttransfer.

Pool and Martin (15) studied the effects of another plasma volume expander, Plasmatein. This product, like other expanders, is produced from cold ethanol precipitation of whole, pooled plasma. It is predominately HSA, but with more contaminating globulins than other commercial expanders. Up to 18% of the total protein can be in the form of α and β globulins in Plasmatein. The use of Plasmatein as a supplement to culture medium resulted in high continuing pregnancy rates upon embryo transfer. Good outcomes aside, the use of plasma protein fractions has drawbacks. First, they are products prepared for intravenous volume expansion that act by raising vascular oncotic pressure and were never designed to be used as a culture medium supplement. The amount of globulins varies from lot to lot, they contain preservatives, and the fluid vehicle has been optimized chemically for vascular physiology, not embryo growth. Weathersbee et al. (16) recognized these drawbacks and, thus, constructed a protein supplement designed specifically for embryo culture by adding traceable components in defined quantities, a macromolecular solution named Synthetic Serum Substitute (SSS). This solution, when added to culture medium to produce a final protein concentration of 6 mg/mL, produced rapid cleavage rates, both in mouse and in human embryos (16), and yielded pregnancy rates equivalent to those seen with Plasmatein (15).

Alternatives to Protein Supplementation

Several efforts have been made to develop alternatives, either to proteins or to macromolecules in general, with most investigators pointing out the dangers of using natural products in the clinical setting (e.g., the potential transmission of viruses or prions). In reality, the desire for alternatives has been less toward addressing safety issues and more toward removing complication; therefore, experiments designed to unravel the complexities of embryo physiology can be interpreted less ambiguously.

Polyvinylalcohol

Bavister (18) used polyvinylalcohol (PVA) in place of BSA in medium used to study sperm motility, acrosome reaction, and fertilizing ability. Although motility was maintained by supplementation with PVA, no acrosome reactions were detected, and sperm failed to penetrate oocytes. The mechanism of action of PVA is unknown, but it may relate to the surface active properties of this molecule (18). In subsequent work, PVA was added to culture medium in lieu of protein and used to support the growth of both hamster (19) and bovine embryos (20). The bovine embryos, however, resulted from oocytes exposed to protein in the in vitro maturation medium (10% bovine calf serum) and IVF medium (BSA) prior to replacement with PVA. Embryos grew in protein-free medium, but significantly fewer reached the blastocyst stage than those grown in medium containing protein (20). The capacity of PVA to replace protein in all of the media required for IVF, embryo culture, and ET has yet to be demonstrated.

Dextran

Pool and Martin (15) and Pool et al. (2), seeking to explain why glycoprotein-rich PPFs produce faster cleavage rates over albumin alone, postulated that one particular way in which macromolecules could exert the observed modulatory behavior on culture medium is through a physical interaction with water. This was based upon the following: (1) fertilization and embryogenesis occur in a hydrated, anatomical potential space, not in a fluid-filled cavity, where macromolecular–water interactions should be pronounced, (2) tubal and uterine water are exposed to a very high density of polyhydroxylated compounds in the forms of mucopolysaccharides, glycosaminoglycans, and mucins, and (3) proteins of the circulation, including albumin and other globulins, control colloid osmotic pressure by specific interactions with water. These are the same proteins that effectively improve the performance characteristics of culture medium during embryo culture. If this interaction with water is involved in the mechanism whereby macromolecules induce their effects in embryo culture, then they proposed that a nonproteinaceous polyhydroxy compound with a high oncotic efficiency, like dextran, might produce similar effects in culture medium. Subsequent experiments with both mouse and with human embryos showed that supplementation with dextran could support rapid cleavage in early embryos and could be used in combination with albumin to produce growth rates equivalent to those obtained with PPF-supplemented media (15).

Hyaluronan

Dextran is essentially linear polymeric glucose with few branches. It is a structure that is known to interact even more strongly with water than with albumin, but not one that is likely to be encountered in the reproductive tract as a component of glycosylated proteins or mucoproteins. Gardner et al. (21), however, examined the effects of using a molecule that occurs naturally in the reproductive tract—the glycosaminoglycan hyaluronan—which is a polymer formed by repeats of D-glucuronic acid and N-acetyl-D-glucosamine. In this study, the effects of supplementation with BSA, PVA, dextran, and hyaluronan were compared. It is of interest that the highest rates of implantation and fetal development were seen from the use of hyaluronan, but additional experiments demonstrated that the effect could be isolated to including hyaluronan to the transfer medium. This is an interesting observation because both bovine and human embryos are known to have the receptor for hyaluronan, CD44, throughout preimplantation embryogenesis.

Agarose

Another potential molecule for medium supplementation is agarose, a polymer consisting of a basic agarobiose repeat of 1,3 linked β-D-galactopyranose and 1,4-linked 3,6-anhydro-a-galactopyran. We have examined agaroses, kindly supplied by FMC BioProducts, with the following properties: BRE 1673, gelling temperature (Tg) of 36°C, and low electroendosmosis (EEO);

BRE 1674, Tg of 36°C, but with high EEO; BRE 1675 with a low Tg of 11.5°C, and BRE 1676 with a reduced Tg of 30°C. Experiments were conducted with frozen mouse embryos in an attempt to determine the effect of agarose on generation times of early cleavage-stage embryos and upon the rate of blastocyst formation. Studies were conducted over a range of agarose concentrations, both in the absence and presence of small amounts of HSA (0.05%). There was some slight beneficial effect of agarose BRE 1674 on early cleavage and blastocyst formation in the presence of albumin, but none that was significant. From this work, we concluded that there is no advantage to using agarose over HSA/dextran or BSA/hyaluronan at the present time, although the flexibility in gel induction and the potential for chemical modification of agarose may prove useful as new information about macromolecular functions in culture emerge.

Macromolecular-Embryo Interactions In Vivo

The trend in culture medium design has been to model media composition to reflect the specific changing requirements of the preimplantation period, an evolution that has given rise to the current sequential culture systems (see Chap. 10). The efforts that have been directed toward the definition of energetic and amino acid requirements, however, ones that have made sequential culture possible, have not spilled over into the arena of macromolecules. The trend in macromolecular supplementation has not been one of definition; rather, it has been in overt simplification, resulting in an in vitro milieu that bears no resemblance to the chemical environment in vivo. This is not to say that all macromolecules encountered in the female reproductive tract are involved mechanistically in embryogenesis. They are clearly not and this is one of the pitfalls of blindly mimicking nature; however, but even the use of a complex fluid such as whole serum is a gross oversimplification of what occurs in vivo. It is evident that work to find alternatives to proteins as medium supplements has not been initiated with the broad goal of supporting embryogenesis, but of fulfilling isolated needs instead, such as fostering sperm motility or controlling extracellular hydration states. The fact that viable human blastocysts can be generated in vitro with very simple forms of macromolecular supplementation (e.g., HSA or SSS) signifies how important it has been to rectify the energetic and amino acid presentations in vitro with those produced in vivo and to do so in a temporally correct manner; however, can the full developmental potential of a cohort of embryos be realized by such simplification of macromolecular components? Perhaps, but despite the reported effectiveness of sequential media by a number of investigators, it appears in some situations that the transfer of embryos on Day 3 can produce blastocysts, as evidenced by pregnancy, where continued sequential culture does not.

Racowsky et al. (22) have shown that if no eight-cell embryos are formed by Day 3, continued culture in a sequential system and blastocyst transfer on Day 5 resulted in no fetal heartbeats, whereas ET on Day 3 resulted in fetal heartbeat in 9 out of 27 patients. From these data, it seems that the crucial conditions for continued embryogenesis to the blastocyst stage are met in the uterus, but not in the culture dish during the second interval because embryos from both arms of the study encountered the same conditions in the first culture interval. We are faced, then, with the following questions: What roles do macromolecules play in vivo that are related to embryogenesis? What molecules are the best candidates to fulfill those roles? Can we replicate the complexity of macromolecular function seen in vivo in our culture systems and, if so, then how?

The most common category of macromolecule found in the reproductive tract is not protein per se; rather, it is carbohydrate in the form of glycosaminoglycans, acid mucopolysaccharide, and highly acidic mucus glycoprotein. Many molecules serve important functions in vivo that are not required in vitro. For example, work from Oliphant (23) has shown that specific materials purified from the rabbit oviduct inhibit immunological complement from oviductal fluid. These materials were demonstrated to be sulfated glycoproteins and function, in general, to protect sperm and embryos from the maternal humoral immune system. Mucus glycoproteins can also function as lubricants (24), and the paucity of them in the human fallopian tube has even been postulated as the reason that humans are prone to tubal pregnancy (25). They are also known to have antibacterial properties and protect the reproductive tract epithelium from invasion by microorganisms (24). A host of uterine macromolecules, to include mucins, have been implicated in the mechanisms of implantation (26). Other macromolecules [e.g., oviductin (MUC 9)] serve to foster sperm viability and function in the reproductive tract.

Macromolecules and Embryo Growth: Estrogen-Dependent Oviduct Glycoproteins

Tubal-specific glycoproteins are synthesized in response to estrogen in a number of mammalian species, including humans (see Pool et al. [2]; Murray and Messinger [27]). Hunter (28) proposed that these compounds may be involved in modulating the microenvironment of developing embryos by affecting the concentration of cations, sugars, and other essential substrates presented to the surface of oocyte or embryonic membranes during development in vivo. In his words, estrus-enhanced glycoproteins may be contributing in some special way to the "economy of early embryonic development," a hypothesis that is completely consistent with observation on the modulatory behavior of macromolecules in vitro. His suggestion that these macromolecules may provide a sensitive means of regulating crucial concentrations of fluid constituents, perhaps by acting in the perivitelline space, is a strong possibility given the ratio of water to macromolecules in the reproductive tract. It is clear that E_2-dependent glycoproteins from the oviduct invade the perivitelline space. Murray and Messinger (27) used antiserum against the 90,000 molecular weight E_2-dependent oviduct secretory glycoprotein from sheep to identify an antigenically related protein (200,000 molecular weight) associated with developing embryos of the Djungarian hamster. The initial reticular intertwining of the protein in the zona pellucida of one- and two-cell embryos was replaced by more intense accumulation in four-, eight- and >16-cell embryos. In two-cell embryos, the glycoprotein associated with blastomere plasma membranes, forming patches in regions of membrane devoid of f-actin. These disappeared, giving rise to intense localization in areas of cell–cell contact. Verhage et al. (29) have described the details of similar E_2-dependent glycoproteins from humans.

Mucus Glycoproteins: The Mucins

The most ubiquitous macromolecules of the reproductive tract (i.e., the mucins) may have received the least attention with respect to its contribution to facilitating embryogenesis, which is a suspicious oversight given that one of the most universally studied animal embryos (e.g., the rabbit) is visibly encased in it early in embryogenesis. It is likely that the polydisperse nature of mucins, and other physicochemical properties that complicate their isolation and analysis have contributed greatly to this oversight. As Jansen (25) indicates, mucus glycoproteins can have apparent molecular weights in the millions and the use of relatively tight-packed polyacrylamide or other gels, as are routinely employed in protein biochemistry, will lead investigators to "miss the true molecular constituents of oviductal mucus" because they are excluded by such analytical gels. However, ten distinct mucin genes have now been identified in humans and many have been sequenced, at least in part (30). The occurrence and distribution of mucins in the human reproductive tract has been studied extensively by DeSouza et al. (24) and Gipson et al. (31), and has been reviewed by Lagow et al. (30). In addition, the chemistry and macrostructure of mucins in solution has been reviewed concisely by Harding (32).

Mucins occur in two forms, either as transmembrane molecules (e.g., MUC1) or as secreted molecules. They comprise only 0.5–1% of mucus gels, but they account largely for the properties of mucus. The molecule contains more than 80% carbohydrate and contains a single polypeptide backbone that is rich in threonine, serine and proline residues. The SER and THR residues serve as sites for O-linked glycosylation and occur in about every third residue. This creates a dense array of carbohydrate that protects the protein backbone from proteolysis and gives the molecule the appearance of a bottlebrush (33), with the bristles representing the oligosaccharide side chains. The molecules show quasi-continuous polydispersity, due to variable carbohydrate composition, as well as discrete polydispersity, a function of variable tandem repeats in sequence. The mucins collectively constitute a class of molecules that yield an environment, in association with water, salts, and other proteins, which is totally unlike that seen in contemporary embryo culture medium. In reality, no solution (i.e., thermodynamic ideality), but dilute solutions of salts and other charged species, such as amino acids, show at least some similarity of cohesive forces upon mixing. Mucins, to the contrary, are highly nonideal. They can bind entire proteins, ones that can retain enzymatic activity upon binding. They can function as polyelectrolytes, behave as a semi-permeable membrane and become hydrated following a Donnan equilibrium (34). Mucus gels, however, have the capacity to relax by varying local acidity or salt, thereby constituting a dynamic matrix that can react to different microenvironments. They can bind ions and metabolites and do so reversibly. Through an examination of the biochemical, structural, and, now, genetic studies of reproductive tract mucins, therefore we see the description, not of a static class of molecules, but of a dynamic matrix. It is one that controls hydration states of the embryonic microenvironment and, thus, controls local ionic strength and pH. It reversibly binds ions, metabolites and fully functional proteins such as enzymes. It behaves physically as a viscoelastic, nonideal entity in thermodynamic terms. These are the conditions in which the human blastocyst develops in vivo, not in a dilute solution of salts and metabolites with scant protein or glycoprotein.

Macromolecules and Future Considerations for the Production of Blastocysts In Vitro

The clinical embryologist faces a perplexing situation with the advent of commercially available sequential culture systems and the capacity to produce blastocysts in vitro. In certain patients, the marvel of this technology is evident by efficient production of a large number of fully expanded blastocysts by Day 5 of sequential culture. In the next patient, however, few or no blastocysts are produced, even in some patients who yield eight-cell embryos by Day 3 of the first culture interval. The embryologist is often left to account for this disparity but it becomes difficult or impossible to separate the potential effects of patient selection, stimulation protocol, and culture technology upon embryogenesis in vitro. It often seems that the size of the subset of embryos that fail to develop into blastocysts in culture exceeds what might be accounted for by embryonic genetics alone. The data of Racowsky et al. (22) imply that, at least to some degree, the culprit is the culture system, specifically that of the second interval, and it is manifest as an inability to support continued development in embryos that are slightly delayed developmentally on Day 3. These conclusions are derived from observing the capacity of the uterus to facilitate continued development and implantation of similarly delayed embryos upon transfer on Day 3, even though they experienced the same conditions in culture during the first interval of growth.

How might macromolecules relate to these observations? The most likely explanation is that specific macromolecules in the tube, produced in response to estrogen, work in concert with albumin and glycosaminoglycans to modulate the first phase of embryogenesis. The requirement for macromolecules appears to be more relaxed in the first interval and can be fulfilled in vitro by simple supplementation of media with albumin or PPF. In the second phase of embryogenesis, however, the uterus provides environmental plasticity to embryos, a plasticity that is eliminated by using a single macromolecule or a simple solution of macromolecules in the second culture interval. The chemistry and structure of mucus gels yields a dynamic matrix in vivo that does not exist currently in culture media used for the second interval. The embryo enters the second interval in vitro to face chemically and physically fixed conditions. If the physiological status of the embryo matches well with these fixed conditions, then a viable embryo is produced. If the match is less good but embryonic plasticity is not exceeded by the environmental challenge presented by fixed conditions, then a viable embryo is produced, but not with the "economy of development" described by Hunter (28). If, however, the physiological status of the embryo is compromised, as might be signified by developmental delay on Day 3, and the range of developmental plasticity is exceeded, then development arrests in the face of static culture conditions that are inappropriate for embryos in a physiologically compromised condition. There is little doubt that patient age, health, and stimulation protocol contribute materially to determining the physiological state of oocytes at the beginning of the first culture interval.

The value of blastocyst culture as a means to eliminate high-order multiple gestation, as demonstrated in the literature (35,36), is monumental and in the intensive work that has fostered our ability to produce blastocysts. The contributions made by macromolecules during embryogenesis have been woefully ignored and now need to enjoy the focus of future investigation. E_2-dependent glycoproteins and mucins must be studied in concert with an understanding that isolated molecules may produce no effect and that species-specific responses are not out of the question (37,38). A number of mucin-producing continuous cell lines from a variety of epithelia may be convenient source material for initial studies. It is conceivable that cloned mucin genes could be placed into appropriate expression vehicles. It is even possible that artificial genetic constructs could produce neoglycoproteins as a safe and reproducible way of adding macromolecular environmental plasticity to facilitate a predictable economy of blastocyst production in vitro.

References

1. Caro CM, Trounson A. Successful fertilization, embryo development, and pregnancy in human in vitro fertilization (IVF) using a chemically defined culture medium containing no protein. J In Vitro Fertil Embryo Transf 1986;3:215–17.
2. Pool TB, Atiee SH, Martin JE. Oocyte and embryo culture. Basic concepts and recent advances. In: May JV, ed. Assisted reproduction: laboratory considerations. Infert Reprod Med Clin N Am 1998;9:181–203.
3. Saito H, Marrs RP, Berger T, Brown J, Mishell DR, Jr. Enhancement of in vitro development by specific serum supplements. Fertil Steril (Abstr) 1983;39:423.
4. Leung PCS, Gronow MJ, Kellow GN, Lopata A, Speirs AL, McBain JC, et al. Serum

supplement in human in vitro fertilization and embryo development. Fertil Steril 1984;41:36–39.
5. Edwards RG. Maturation in vitro of mouse, sheep, cow, pig, rhesus monkey and human ovarian oocytes. Nature 1965;208:349–51.
6. Edwards RG, Steptoe PC, Purdy JM. Establishing full-term human pregnancies using cleaving embryos grown in vitro. Br J Obstet Gynaecol 1980;87:737–56.
7. Gardner DK. Mammalian embryo culture in the absence of serum or somatic cell support. Cell Biol Int 1994;18:1163–79.
8. Dorland M, Gardner DK, Trounson AO. Serum in synthetic oviduct fluid causes mitochondrial degeneration in ovine embryos. J Reprod Fertil Abstract Series 1994;13:70.
9. Walker SK, Heard TM, Seamark RF. In vitro culture of sheep embryos without co-culture: successes and perspectives. Theriogenology 1992;37:111–26.
10. Thompson JG, Gardner DK, Pugh PA, McMillan WH, Tervit HR. Lamb birth weight following transfer is affected by the culture system used for pre-elongation development of embryos. J Reprod Fertil Abstract Series 1994;13:69.
11. Edwards RG, Bavister BD, Steptoe PC. Early stages of fertilization in vitro of human oocytes matured in vitro. Nature 1969;221:632–35.
12. Menezo Y, Testart J, Perone D. Serum is not necessary in human in vitro fertilization and embryo development. Fertil Steril 1984;42:750–55.
13. Ashwood-Smith MJ, Hollands P, Edwards RG. The use of Albuminar (TM) as a medium supplement in clinical IVF. Hum Reprod 1989;4:702–5.
14. Staessen C, Van den Abbeel E, Carle M, Khan I, Devroey P, Van Steirteghem AC. Comparison between human serum and Albuminar-20 (TM) supplement for in vitro fertilization. Hum Reprod 1990;5:336–41.
15. Pool TB, Martin JE. High continuing pregnancy rates after in vitro fetilization-embryo transfer using medium supplemented with a plasma protein fraction containing α and β-globulins. Fertil Steril 1994;61:714–19.
16. Weathersbee PS, Pool TB, Ord T. Synthetic serum substitute (SSS): a globulin-enriched protein supplement for human embryo culture. J Assist Reprod Genet 1995;12:354–60.
17. Adler A, McVicker-Reing A, Bedford MJ, et al. Plasmanate as a medium supplement for in vitro fertilization. J Assist Reprod Genet 1993;10:67–71.
18. Bavister BD. Substitution of a synthetic polymer for protein in a mammalian gamete culture system. J Exp Zool 1981;217:45–51.
19. Schini SA, Bavister BD. Two-cell block to development of cultured hamster embryos is caused by phosphate and glucose. Biol Reprod 1988;39:1183–92.
20. Pinyopummintr T, Bavister BD. In vitro-matured/in vitro-fertilized bovine oocytes can develop into morulae/blastocysts in chemically defined, protein-free culture medium. Biol Reprod 1991;45:736–42.
21. Gardner DK, Rodriegez-Martinez H, Lane M. Fetal development after transfer is increased by replacing protein with the glycosaminoglycan hyaluronan for mouse embryo culture and transfer. Hum Reprod 1999;14:2575–80.
22. Racowsky C, Jackson KV, Ceklenik NA, Fox JH, Hornstein MD. The number of eight-cell embryos is a key determinant for selecting day 3 or day 5 transfer. Fertil Steril 2000;73:558–64.
23. Oliphant G. Biochemistry and immunology of oviductal fluid. In: Seigler AM, ed. The fallopian tube: basic studies and clinical contributions. New York: Futura Publishing Company, 1986:129–45.

24. DeSouza M, Lagow E, Carson D. Mucin function and expression in mammalian reproductive tract tissues. Biochem Biophys Res Commun 1998;247:1–6.
25. Jansen RPS. Ultrastructure and histochemistry of acid mucus glycoproteins in the estrous mammal oviduct. Microsc Res Tech 1995;32:29–49.
26. Aplin JD, Hey NA. MUC1, endometrium and embryo implantation. Biochem Soc Trans 1995;23:826–31.
27. Murray MK, Messinger SM. Early embryonic development in the Djungarian hamster (*Phodopus sungorus*) is accompanied by alterations in the distribution and intensity of an estrogen (E_2)-dependent oviduct glycoprotein in the blastomere membrane and zona pellucida and in its association with f-actin. Biol Reprod 1994;1126–39.
28. Hunter RHF. Modulation of gamete and embryonic microenvironments by oviduct glycoproteins. Mol Reprod Dev 1994;39:176–81.
29. Verhage HG, Fazleabas AT, Donnelly K. The in vitro synthesis and release of proteins by the human oviduct. Endocrinology 1988;122:1639–45.
30. Lagow E, DeSouza M, Carson DD. Mammalian reproductive tract mucins. Hum Reprod Update 1999;5:280–92.
31. Gipson I, Ho SB, Spurr-Michaud SJ, Tisdale AS, Zhan Q, Torlakovic E, et al. Mucin genes expressed by human female reproductive tract epithelia. Biol Reprod 1997;56: 999–1011.
32. Harding SE. The macrostructure of mucus glycoproteins in solution. Adv Carbohydr Chem Biochem 1989;47:345–81.
33. Allen A. Structure of gastrointestinal mucus glycoproteins and the viscous and gel-forming properties of mucus. Br Med Bull 1978;34:28–33.
34. Tam PY, Verdugo P. Control of mucus hydration as a Donnan equilibrium process. Nature 1981;292:340–42.
35. Gardner DK, Schoolcraft WB, Wagley L, Schlenker T, Stevens J, Hesla J. A prospective randomized trial of blastocyst culture and transfer in in-vitro fertilization. Hum Reprod 1998;13:3434–40.
36. Behr B, Pool TB, Milki AA, Moore D, Gebhardt J, Dasig D. Preliminary clinical experience with human blastocyst development in vitro without co-culture. Hum Reprod 1999;14:454–57.
37. Hill JL, Wade MG, Nancarrow CD, Kelleher DL, Boland MP. Influence of ovine oviducal amino acid concentrations and an ovine oestrus-associated glycoprotein on development and viability of bovine embryos. Mol Reprod Dev 1997;47:164–69.
38. Vansteenbrugge A, Van Langendonckt A, Massip A, Dessy F. Effect of estrus-associated glycoprotein and tissue inhibitor of metalloproteinase-1 secreted by oviduct cells on in vitro bovine embryo development. Mol Reprod Dev 1997;46:527–34.

10

Culture Systems and Blastocyst Development

DAVID K. GARDNER, MICHELLE LANE, AND WILLIAM B. SCHOOLCRAFT

Since the birth of the first in vitro fertilization (IVF) baby in 1978, there have been numerous developments in the field of human assisted reproductive technologies (ART), including the development of intracytoplasmic sperm injection (ICSI) to treat male factor infertility and the development and application of preimplantation genetic diagnosis. Implantation rate, however, which is one of the rate-limiting factors, has remained relatively static. Implantation rates of 10–30% have been reported in the literature for the transfer of cleavage stage embryos conceived through IVF. These values are somewhat below the 60% implantation rate reported by Buster and colleagues (1), who were able to transfer in vivo–developed human blastocysts to recipient patients. This therefore raises some important questions: Why is the implantation rate of the cleavage stage embryo so low and can it be improved? Second, does the blastocyst on Day 5 have a higher implantation rate than an embryo transferred between Days 1 and 3? If the latter is the case, then one should consider the move to blastocyst transfer in human IVF.

The issue of cleavage-stage embryo implantation potential has certainly been the recipient of attention. This stems from work by Scott and Smith (2), who performed a retrospective analysis of pronucleate polarity and timing of the first cleavage division and related this to implantation rate. A scoring system was developed that took pronucleus alignment, cytoplasmic appearance, and timing of cleavage into account. It was observed that those embryos with a high score gave rise to an implantation rate of 28%. These observations have been promoted by Edwards and Beard (3) with the emphasis on the significance of oocyte and pronucleate polarity. Gerris et al. (4) have similarly used a scoring system for use on Day 3 to increase implantation rates in a highly selected group of patients (<34 and no previous IVF attempts). Implantation rates of 48% were reported. It would therefore appear that implantation rates of the cleavage stage embryo can be improved by careful selection criteria; however, assessment of embryos at either the pronucleate or cleavage stages can at best be considered as an assessment of the oocyte. Up to the eight-cell stage only a limited number of embryonic genes have been transcribed (5,6); therefore, it is not possible to identify those embryos with the highest developmental potential from within a given cohort of cleavage-stage embryos. Only by culturing embryos past the maternal/embryonic genome transition and up to the blastocyst does it becomes possible to identify those embryos with limited or no developmental potential. The quality and polarity of an oocyte are certainly important because the quality of the developing embryo is ultimately dependent on the quality of the gametes from which it is derived (7), but it provides limited information regarding true embryo developmental potential as it only addresses the "quality" of one gamete. It has also been shown that there is a significant paternal contribution to embryonic development (8).

No matter how effective a given culture system or selection criteria are, the transfer of an embryo on Day 1–3 results in the premature placement of the embryo into the uterus. The human embryo would normally only enter the uterus sometime on Day 4 (9). The significance of this is that the environment within the human oviduct and uterus differ. The embryo, therefore, is exposed to gradients of nutrients as it progresses through the female tract (10; Table 10.1). These changes in nutrient levels within the female reproductive tract mirror changes in embryo requirements as it develops and differentiates (11). The premature placement of embryos in the uterus, therefore, will lead to some nutritional stress. Such stress adversely affects embryonic development and can compromise subsequent viability (11). In other words, no mater how good the culture medium that was used to support the development of the embryo up to Day 3, by placing the cleavage-stage embryo into a potentially compromising environment (the uterus) subsequent embryo development may be impaired. This is plausibly why it is hard to determine large differences between culture media used for the cleavage-stage embryo. Furthermore, when the issue is raised regarding whether it is better to return the embryos to the mother as soon as possible, it is frequently overlooked that the maternal environment of an IVF patient may be compromised after the patient has received exogenous gonadotropins during controlled ovarian hyperstimulation. It is known from animal studies that the hyperstimulated female tract is

TABLE 10.1. Concentration of carbohydrates in the human oviduct and uterus.

	Pyruvate (mM)	Lactate (mM)	Glucose (mM)
Oviduct (midcycle)	0.32	10.5	0.50
Uterus	0.10	5.87	3.15

Source: Data from Gardner et al. (10).
Lactate measured as the biologically active L-isoform[2]. The concentrations of carbohydrates present in the oviduct are used in medium G1; the concentrations of carbohydrates present in the uterus are those used in medium G2.

a less-than-optimal environment for the developing embryo, resulting in impaired embryo and fetal development (12–15). Statistical modeling has indicated that the human endometrial receptivity is significantly compromised after controlled ovarian hyperstimulation (16).

A further concern regarding the transfer of cleavage-stage embryos to the uterus is that uterine contractions have been negatively correlated with embryo transfer outcome, possibly by the expulsion of embryos from the uterine cavity (17). Uterine junctional zone contractions have been quantitated and found to be strongest on the day of oocyte retrieval (18). Patients exhibit such contractions on Day 2 and 3 after retrieval, but contractility decreases and is barely evident on Day 4. It is therefore feasible that the transfer of blastocysts on Day 5 is by default associated with reduced uterine contractions; therefore, there is less chance for embryonic expulsion and loss (18).

Data will be presented here to show that blastocyst culture and transfer can result in a significant increase in implantation rates compared with those obtained after the transfer of cleavage-stage embryos, and that implantation rates as high as 70% can be obtained in certain patients and in oocyte donor recipients.

How Can Viable Blastocysts Be Obtained in Culture?

It is important when discussing embryo culture to consider (1) the development of viable blastocysts and (2) the embryo culture system as a whole (19). First, human embryos can develop in a wide range of culture conditions, but the inherent viability of the resultant blastocysts are very different. This has led to a great deal of confusion regarding the role of the blastocyst in human ART. For example, in 1991 Bolton et al. (20) found that it was possible to obtain 40% blastocyst development using Earle's salts supplemented with pyruvate and 10% maternal serum. Resultant implantation and pregnancy rates, however, were only 7%. Such low rates have detered people from employing blastocyst culture and transfer clinically. Second, embryo culture media is but one part of the overall culture system, and although the composition of culture media is critical, all aspects of the culture system impact on how the media perform; therefore, all aspects of the system have to be optimized to get the best results.

Four key components of the culture system that are considered in detail here are:

1. Culture media
2. Gas phase
3. Incubation volume: embryo ratio
4. Macromolecules

Culture Media

There are several extensive treatises on the development and formulations of mammalian embryo culture media (19–25). Perhaps the most significant change to embryo culture media has been the inclusion of specific amino acids. The amino acids that have been shown to have a beneficial effect on the cleavage-stage mammalian embryo include alanine, asparate, asparagine, glutamate, glutamine, glycine, serine, taurine, and proline (25–30). It is significant that such amino acids are present at relatively high levels in oviduct fluid (31,32). It is interesting that this group of amino acids, with the exception of glutamine and taurine, share a striking homology with those present in Eagle's nonessential amino acids (33). Although this nomenclature has no bearing on embryology it has been a convenient way to catergorize amino acids broadly. Nonessential amino acids are those not required by somatic cells in culture. The significance of amino acids is that they have numerous niches in cellular physiology on top of their role as a biosynthetic precursor. The group of amino acids listed earlier have been shown to act as regulators of energy metabolism (11,34), osmolytes (35), and buffers of pHi (36) (i.e., they have been shown to reduce intracellular stress and help facilitate normal cell function and hence embryo development). Those amino acids defined by Eagle (33) to be required for the development of somatic cells, termed essential amino acids, have been found to negate the beneficial effects of the nonessential amino acids during the first few cleavage divisions in culture. This effect of the essential amino acids is plausibly through competition for specific transporters on the embryo's plasma membrane.

In parallel with changes in embryo physiology there is an increased demand for amino acids with development, so that by the blastocyst stage the embryo requires a more complete array of amino acids. Those amino acids classified as essential significantly stimulate the development of the inner cell mass, whereas the nonessential amino acids help in the development of the trophectoderm (37). In terms of embryo culture, therefore, the embryo should be exposed to one or more of the nonessential amino acids, glutamine and/or taurine for the first 48 hours. From around the eight-cell stage onward the embryo should be cultured in a more complete mix of amino acids.

The embryo similarly undergoes significant changes in carbohydrate uptake and utilization during the preimplantation period (11,19,21–23, 38–40). The changes in carbohydrate utilization significantly mirror the changes in the levels of carbohydrates within the human oviduct and uterus (10).

In light of the dynamics of the maternal environment and embryo physiology, it has therefore been proposed that optimal development of the mammalian embryo in culture will require more than one culture medium formulation. This cannot be considered a new idea because it was proposed in 1990 that: "It would seem likely that the optimal development of embryos in vitro could well occur in not one but possibly two or more media, each one reflecting the embryo's requirements as development proceeds" (41). Based upon the available data on maternal and embryo physiology, two culture media designated Growth 1 and 2 (G1 and G2) were therefore specifically formulated to support the growth of the human pronucleate embryo to the blastocyst stage (42). Medium G1 is based on the levels of carbohydrates present in the human Fallopian tube, and contains nonessential amino acids and glutamine that stimulate development of the cleavage-stage mammalian embryo. The chelator EDTA is also present, both to sequester any toxic divalent cations present in the system, as well as to help minimize glycolytic activity of the embryo, thereby minimizing metabolic perturbations and cellular stress (11).

In contrast, medium G2 is based on the levels of carbohydrates present in the human uterus and contains both nonessential and essential amino acids to facilitate both blastocyst development and differentiation. EDTA is not present in medium G2 because it appears to impair inner cell mass development and function selectively, culminating in a loss of viability. Both media are supple-

---

FIGURE 10.1. Effect of sequential culture media on the development of F1 (C57/BL6 x CBA/Ca) mouse zygotes in vitro. Zygotes were collected at 20 hours post-hCG. All media were supplemented with BSA (2 mg/ml). All embryos were transferred to fresh medium after 48 hours of culture, with the exception of embryos in medium G1, where the embryos were transferred to either medium G1 or G2. To compensate for this, twice the number of embryos were originally cultured in medium G1, although only a designated 50% of these embryos were used in the statistical analysis of the 44–52 hours data set. (a) Embryo cell number after 44, 48 and 52 h of culture. Values are mean ± sem. n = 200 embryos/medium. Media: G1 (solid bar); HTF (open bar); Ham's F-10 (hatched bar). Significantly different from other media; **, $p < 0.01$. (b) Embryo development after 72 hours of culture. $n = 150$ embryos/medium. G1/G2; embryos cultured for 48 hours in medium G1 and then transferred to medium G2. Blastocyst (solid bar), hatching blastocysts (as a percentage of total blastocysts; open bar). Like pairs are significantly different; a, c, d, $p < 0.05$; b, $p < 0.01$. (c) Embryo development after 92 hours of culture. $n = 150$ embryos/medium. G1/G2; embryos cultured for 48 hours in medium G1 and then transferred to medium G2. Blastocyst (solid bar), hatching blastocysts (as a percentage of total blastocysts; open bar). Like pairs are significantly different; a, b, c, $p < 0.05$. Significantly different from medium G1 and G1/G2; **, $p < 0.01$. (d) Cell allocation in the blastocyst after 92 hours of culture $n = 150$ embryos/medium. G1/G2; embryos cultured for 48 hours in medium G1 and then transferred to medium G2. Trophectoderm (solid bars), inner cell mass (open bars). Significantly different from other media; *, $p < 0.05$; **, $p < 0.01$. (e) Viability of cultured blastocysts $n =$ at least 60 blastocysts transferred per treatment. G1/G2; embryos cultured for 48 hours in medium G1 and then transferred to medium G2. Implantation (solid bar), fetal development per implantation (open bar). Like pairs are significantly different; a, d, $p < 0.05$; b, c, $p < 0.01$. From Gardner and Lane (22). Reproduced with permission from the European Society of Human Reproduction and Embryology. Reproduced with permission from Oxford University Press/Human Reproduction.

10. Culture Systems and Blastocyst Development   123

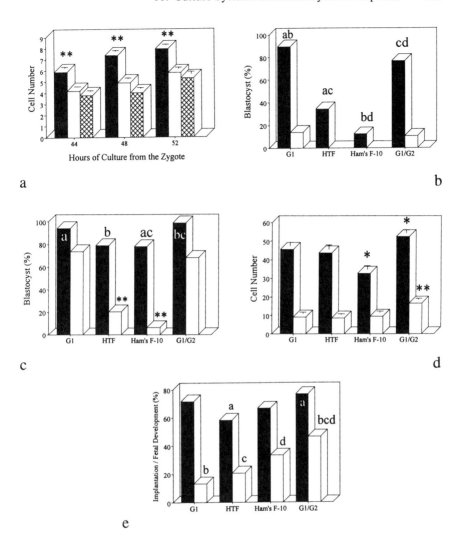

mented with serum albumin. Serum is not required or desired in embryo culture systems, especially those designed to support blastocyst growth (27). It has been demonstrated that culture conditions that support optimal blastocyst development and differentiation in the mouse are actually inhibitory to the development of the early cleavage-stage embryo. On the other hand, those conditions, which do support good growth of the zygote in culture, do not sustain optimal blastocyst development and differentiation (22) (Fig. 10.1). Other sequential media systems that have subsequently been developed have been used clinically with success (e.g., medium P1 and Ham's F-10 [Blastocyst medium]) (43,44).

Gas Phase

The concentration of oxygen in the lumen of the rabbit oviduct is reported to be 2–6% (45), and 8% in the oviduct of hamster, rabbit, and rhesus monkey (46). It is interesting that the oxygen concentration in the uterus is significantly lower than it is in the oviduct, ranging from 5% in the hamster and rabbit to 1.5% in the rhesus monkey (46,47). Studies on the embryos from different mammalian species have demonstrated that culture in a reduced oxygen concentration results in enhanced development in vitro. Several studies have shown that a reduced oxygen concentration between 5 and 8% enhances development to the blastocyst stage in the mouse (48–50). Studies on the rabbit (51) and on domestic animal species [e.g., sheep (52), goats (53), and cows (52)] have also demonstrated that an oxygen concentration of 7% results in increased development in vitro compared with 20% oxygen. It has subsequently been observed that human blastocysts cultured in a low oxygen environment (5%) have significantly more cells than those cultured in a high oxygen environment (20%) (54). As the human and mouse embryos can grow at elevated oxygen concentrations (albeit at a compromised level) there is some confusion regarding the optimal concentration for embryo culture; however, the available data indicate that it would be prudent to culture human embryos in a reduced oxygen concentration of between 5 and 7%. This is based on the low oxygen levels present in the female reproductive tract, and the fact that culture in a low oxygen environment is associated with an increase in cell number of the human blastocyst. That cell number is related to viability (37).

The concentration of CO_2 employed in the culture system has a direct impact on medium pH. Although most media work over a wide range of pH (7.2–7.4), it is preferable to ensure that pH does not go over 7.4 considering that pHi is actually 7.2 (see Chap. 7). It is advisable, therefore, to use a CO_2 concentration of between 6 and 7%.

Incubation Volume: Embryo Ratio

It has been reported for numerous mammalian species that the culture of embryos in reduced volumes of medium and/or in groups significantly increases blastocyst development (55–57) as well as blastocyst cell number (57). Futhermore, culturing embryos in reduced volumes increases subsequent viability after transfer (57). It has been proposed that the benefit of growing embryos in small volumes and/or in groups is due to the production of specific embryo-derived autocrine/paracrine factor(s) that stimulate development. The culture of embryos in large volumes will result in a dilution of the factor so that it becomes ineffectual (Fig. 10.2a,b) (58). This phenomenon is not confined to the mouse, in which several embryos reside in the female tract at one time, but it has been reported for the sheep and cow, which, like the human, are monovular (59–61). Such data has implications for human IVF, especially as there is a tendency to culture human embryos either individually in order to track the development of an embryo, or in

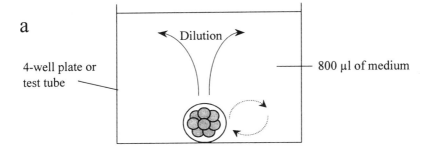

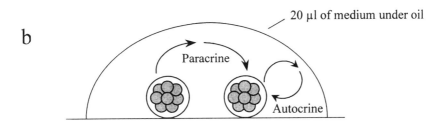

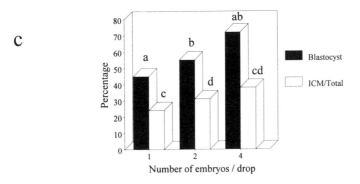

FIGURE 10.2. Effect of incubation volume and embryo grouping on embryo development and differentiation. (a) A single embryo cultured in a four-well plate or test tube, any factor produced by the embryo will become ineffectual due to dilution. (b) Culture of embryos in reduced volumes and/or in groups increases the effective concentration of embryo-derived factors, facilitating their action in either a paracrine or autocrine manner. (c) Effect of embryo grouping on bovine blastocyst development and differentiation. Bovine embryos were cultured either individually or in groups of two or four in 50μl drops of medium.[68] Like pairs are significantly different; $p < 0.05$. From Gardner (58). Reproduced with permission from Martin Dunitz.

relatively large volumes of up to 1 ml of culture medium. It has been shown in both the mouse and cow that increasing the embryo incubation volume ratio specifically stimulates the development of the ICM (Fig. 10.2c). This would explain the increased viability of embryos cultured in reduced volumes in groups (57). Although the beneficial effects of increasing the embryo–incubation volume ratio appear dependent upon the type of macromolecule present (62), the beneficial effect has been found to be evident in medium with or without amino acids (Fig. 10.3). Possible candidates for such autocrine/paracrine factor(s) include platelet-activating factor, insulinlike growth factor II, and FGF-4.

The effects of altering the embryo–incubation volume ratio have been assessed in a limited number of clinical trails. Of the three studies performed with the transfer of cleavage-stage embryos, two found a beneficial effect of group culture as manifest by increased cleavage and pregnancy rates (63, 64). In contrast, Spyropoulou et al. (65) did not observe a benefit of culturing human embryos in groups of three to five followed by transfer on Day 2. In a small study on the effect of culturing human embryos to the blastocyst stage in reduced volumes and/or in groups Rijnders and Jansen (66) did not observe any effect of changing the embryo–incubation volume ratio, however, only six patients were allocated per group and blastocyst cell numbers were not determined. It is therefore hard to reach a meaningful conclusion from this study. Should the human embryo produce specific autocrine or paracrine factors, it is most likely that a benefit would be seen during extended culture to the blastocyst stage when the embryo undergoes a more rapid growth period (67). It would certainly seem prudent to culture human embryos in reduced volumes (50 μL) and in groups (68).

In our experience the move to a reduced oxygen environment (5%) combined with an increase in the embryo–incubation volume ratio resulted in a more stable and improved culture system (Fig. 10.4).

Macromolecules

Embryo culture media historically has been supplemented with protein in the form of either serum, as patient's own or fetal cord, or serum albumin. Although it has been demonstrated that protein is not an absolute requirement for the establishment of a successful pregnancy in human IVF (69), protein is a routine component of embryo culture media. Although the inclusion of protein facilitates ease of gamete and embryo manipulation in vitro, the potential damaging effects of serum and serum albumin now outweigh their benefits; therefore, the time has come to reevaluate their presence in embryo culture systems.

In terms of effect on development per se, then serum albumin has less impact on the embryo's physiology than whole serum. The main problems with serum albumin, or any biological product, is the risk of disease transmission and contamination (70). This alone is reason to consider alternatives. Furthermore, there is considerable variation in the composition of serum albumin from batch to batch (53), making standardization of procedures difficult. The inclusion of whole serum in embryo culture systems, however, whether it be in media or for use in co-

10. Culture Systems and Blastocyst Development 127

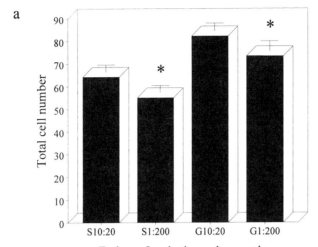

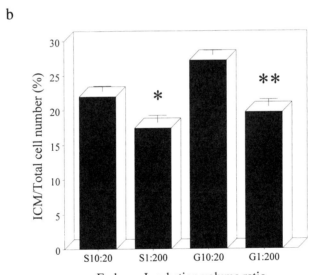

FIGURE 10.3. Effect of embryo:incubation volume ratio and culture medium on mouse embryo development and differentiation. Two-cell mouse embryos from the CF1 strain were cultured in groups of 10 in 20-μl drops (10:20) or individually in 200-μl drops (1:200) of medium. Two types of medium were used: Simple medium (S), which had the same ionic and carbohydrate composition as medium G1.2 but lacked amino acids and EDTA; media containing amino acids (G). In G, embryo were cultured for 24 hours in medium G 1.2 followed by culture for 48 hours in medium G 2.2. (a) Effect on total cell number. (b) Effect on inner cell mass development. *Significantly different from 10:20 in the same medium, $p < 0.05$. **Significantly different from 10:20 in the same medium, $p < 0.01$.

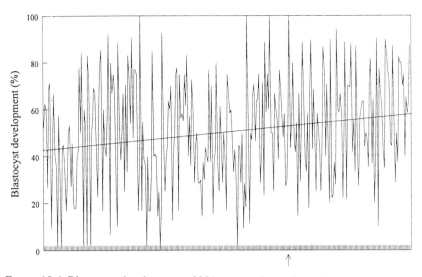

FIGURE 10.4. Blastocyst development of 301 consecutive patients. The x-axis represents the patients in the order in which they attended for infertility treatment. Initial culture conditions were the use of media G 1.2 and G 2.2. Embryos were cultured in groups of up to four in 1 ml of medium in a test-tube in an atmosphere of 5% CO_2 in air (20% O_2). The arrow under the x-axis denotes the time when the culture system was changed. The culture media remained the same, but embryos were cultured in groups of up to four in 50 µl drops in an atmosphere of 6% CO_2 and 5% O_2.

culture, must be challenged. It is important to start out by stressing that mammalian embryos are never exposed to serum in vivo. Oviduct fluid is not a simple serum transudate (71). Serum is instead a pathological fluid and by default is abundant with growth factors such as platelet-derived growth factor and transforming growth factor-α released during platelet aggregation, as well as a host of other growth factors. Serum is poorly defined, and its composition varies from patient to patient, with day of cycle and with nutritional status. The addition of serum to culture medium subsequently makes each medium unique, making comparisons of culture media very difficult, if not impossible. On a practical level, serum also represents a potential source of contamination to both the embryo and laboratory staff who have to prepare it.

Despite this, the addition of serum to culture medium does add a certain degree of protection to the embryo by its ability to minimize transient pH shifts and chelate potential toxins. It is for this ability to confer a degree of robustness to the culture medium that its use has persisted. Data on the development of sheep and cattle blastocysts in the presence of serum, however, have lit a warning beacon regarding the use of serum for extended embryo culture (27,72). Studies on the embryos from other domestic animal species have shown that serum can adversely affect the development of embryos at several levels: precocious blastocoel formation (73,74), sequestration of lipid (74,75), abnormal mitochondrial ultrastructure (74,75), perturbations in metabolism (59), and association with abnormally large offspring in sheep (74).

In attempts to define embryo culture media, Bavister has proposed the use of polyvinyl alcohol (PVA) (76), to replace serum or serum albumin. This approach has worked in the culture of both hamster and cattle embryos; however, the use of such synthetic macromolecules cannot be considered physiological. There are two other issues to consider, however, regarding the use of PVA; first, when embryos are cultured in groups there is a significant effect on blastocyst development and differentiation. To be specific, when embryos are cultured in groups more of them form blastocysts, and there is a significant increase in the development of the inner cell mass; however, the beneficial effects of group culture requires the presence of either albumin or hyaluronan, plausibly to stabilize any paracrine factor produced by the embryo (62). When the culture medium lacks any macromolecule or when PVA is present, there is no observed benefit to culturing embryos in groups. Second, there are some concerns regarding the safety of PVA. A physiological alternative is the glycosaminoglycan hyaluronan, which is present in the cumulus matrix, and whose levels increase significantly in the uterus around the time of implantation (77). Hyaluronan, is a high-molecular mass polysaccharide; therefore, it has the advantage of being nonimmunogenic. It is significant that the human embryo has the receptor for hyaluronan throughout the preimplantation period (78). It has been found that hyaluronan can replace BSA in a mouse embryo culture system, and that its use for embryo transfer results in a significant increase in embryo implantation (79). In the study of Gardner et al. (79) the source of the hyaluronan was the rooster comb. Such studies have subsequently been repeated successfully with hyaluronan from a yeast fermentation procedure. Of perhaps greater significance is the successful use of recombinant human albumin in embryo culture medium (80,81). This albumin, which is, obtained from the genetically engineered bacteria, has the advantage of being physiological, endotoxin and prion free, and does not differ in biological efficacy from batch to batch.

Clinical Experience of Blastocyst Culture and Transfer

The approach of using sequential culture media has been applied in clinical studies at several IVF programs. The use of sequential embryo culture media has been shown to result in blastocyst development of around 50% with a concomitant increase in implantation rates compared to the transfer of cleavage stage embryos (82). Based on further research the original G media (42) were subsequently modified (83). The modifications to the original culture media formulations included reduced glutamine, EDTA, and phosphate levels (medium G 1.2), the inclusion of specific vitamins in medium G2.2, and the use of human serum albumin rather than bovine serum albumin. Using these new media in a prospective randomized clinical trial, it was shown that blastocyst transfer on Day 5 resulted in a significant increase in implantation rate compared to the transfer of embryos on Day 3 in patients with a moderate to good response to gonadotropins (i.e., 10 or more follicles $\geq$ 12 mm in diameter on the day of hCG) (83). This group of patients was chosen due to the fact that at the Colorado Center for Reproductive Medicine (CCRM) they are the source of 90% of the high order multiple gestations. After more than 300 blastocyst transfers, using 10 follicles as the selection criterion for blastocyst culture, an implantation rate of around 50% has been maintained, resulting in a clinical pregnancy rate of 71.5% with a mean of 2.2 blastocysts transferred (Table 10.2) (72). Figure 10.5a shows the relationship between the number of pronucleate embryos and blastocyst development with the number of blastocysts being linearly related ($p < 0.001$) to the number of fertilized oocytes. However, there is no relationship between the number of pronulcear embryos and percentage blastocyst development, which remains on average around 50% (Fig. 10.5b). This means whether a patient has 6 or 26 embryos, the probability that a given embryo will reach the blastocyst stage is 50%. Both Shapiro et al. (84) and Langley et al. (85) have reported that there is a significant linear relationship between the number of cells on Day 3 and subsequent blastocyst development.

In Figure 10.6, the distribution of percentage blastocyst development per patient is shown. Although on average 50% of all embryos will go to the blastocyst stage, there is a considerable variation of development between patients. This should perhaps not be too surprising when one considers that the human is

TABLE 10.2. Outcome of day 5 blastocyst transfers.

No. of patients	301
No. of patients having embryo transfer	296
Mean age (± SEM) in years	33.7 ± 0.2
Age range	20 – 43
FSH (mean ± SEM)	6.8 ± 0.1
Patients with ICSI (%)	37.5
No. of pronulceate embryos (mean ± SEM)	13.8 ± 0.3
Blastocyst development on day 5 (%)	42.7
Blastocyst development on day 6 (%)	7.7
Total blastocyst development (%)	50.5
No. of embryos transferred (mean ± SEM)	2.2 ± 0.04
Patients with embryo freezing (%)[†]	72.4
Mean number of blastocysts frozen embryos (mean ± SEM)	4.2 ± 0.2
Implantation rate (fetal sac) (%)[‡]	51.8
Implantation rate (fetal heart) (%)[‡]	47.9
Clinical pregnancy rate (%)[@]	71.5

[†]Only blastocysts scoring 3BB or higher by the afternoon of Day 6 were cryopreserved.
[‡]Implantation rates are expressed as fetal sac or heart/blastocyst transferred. The calculations included every patient who had an embryo transfer, not just those who subsequently became pregnant.
[@]Includes five patients in the blastocyst culture group who did not have an embryo transferred on Day 5 due to embryonic arrest at the cleavage stages. Clinical pregnancy determined by the presence of a fetal heartbeat. From Gardner et al. (72). Reproduced with permission from the European Society of Human Reproduction and Embryology. Reproduced with permission from Oxford University Press/Human Reproduction.

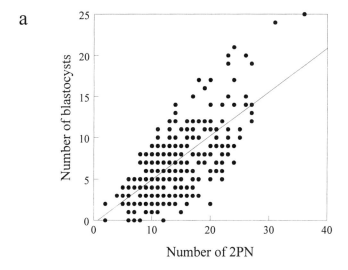

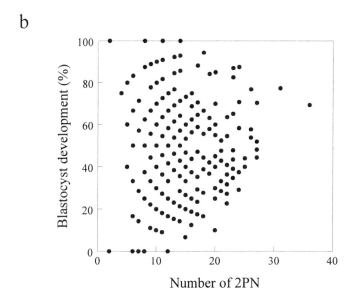

FIGURE 10.5. (a) Relationship between the number of pronulceate embryos and the number of blastocysts formed. There is a significant linear relationship; $r = 0.495$, $p < 0.0001$. (b) Relationship between pronucleate embryo number and percentage blastocyst development. Where two or more patients overlap, only one point is shown on the plot. $n = 301$ patients. From Gardner et al. (72). Reproduced with permission from the European Society of Human Reproduction and Embryology. Reproduced with permission from Oxford University Press/Human Reproduction.

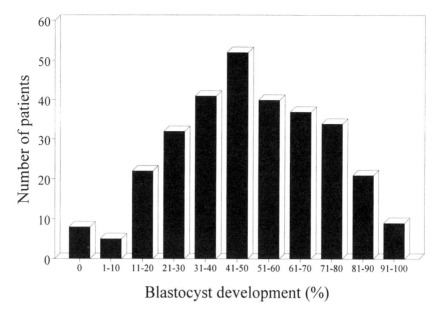

FIGURE 10.6. Distribution of blastocyst development in 301 patients. All embryos were cultured for the first 48 hours in medium G 1.2, and then washed three times in medium G 2.2, followed by culture in medium G 2.2. From Gardner et al. (72). Reproduced with permission from the European Society of Human Reproduction and Embryology. Reproduced with permission from Oxford University Press/Human Reproduction.

the most genetically diverse mammal, and that it is known that genetics have a significant impact on the in vitro development of embryos from other mammals. More than 90% of blastocysts formed using the sequential media G1.2 and G 2.2 were formed on Day 5, with the remainder on Day 6. Eight patients out of the 300 (<3%) did not have any blastocysts (Fig. 10.6). Of these eight patients, two had morulae, which were transferred and resulted in pregnancies. Of the 300 patients, therefore, less than 2% failed to have a transfer. There is also a relationship between the number of blastocysts formed and resultant pregnancy rates (Fig. 10.7). This reflects the ability to select the most viable blastocyst within patients (86). All of these observations have important clinical ramifications because they can help in the decision of whether a patient undergoes blastocyst culture.

Oocyte Donors

Embryo development in culture is determined by the genetics of the parents. It is therefore difficult to establish baseline data on human blastocyst development. This is further compounded by the fact that by default patients with an ART cycle are subfertile, with differing etiologies and typically of advanced reproductive age. With the establishment of oocyte donation as a treatment for some patients, however, a population of oocytes from fertile young women exists that are

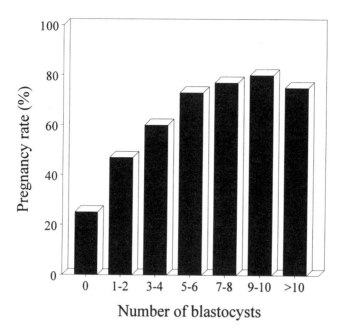

FIGURE 10.7. Relationship between the number of blastocysts and subsequent pregnancy rate. Eight patients had no blastocysts available for transfer. Three of the eight had moruale available for transfer. Of these three patients two conceived. The increase in pregnancy rate with increasing blastocyst number up to five reflects the ability to select blastocysts with the highest developmental potential using the scoring system of Gardner and Schoolcraft (90). From Gardner et al. (72). Reproduced with permission from the European Society of Human Reproduction and Embryology. Reproduced with permission from Oxford University Press/Human Reproduction.

theoretically more competent and have less chromosomal abnormalities. After performing 113 transfers of blastocysts derived from oocyte donation, an implantation rate (fetal heart/blastocyst transferred) of 66% was attained (87), resulting in a clinical pregnancy rate of 88% with a mean of just 2.1 blastocysts transferred. The mean age of the recipients was 41.3. Such high implantation rates are equivalent to those obtained when high-scoring blastocysts are transferred to patients using their own oocytes (86). This observation is consistent with the fact that the embryos from oocyte donors routinely form more blastocysts (60%), and that overall they form more high-scoring blastocysts, therefore allowing for greater selection at transfer.

The Move Toward Single Embryo Transfers

In order to ensure the highest possible pregnancy rates it is imperative to be able to identify the most viable embryo within a given cohort [reviewed by Gardner

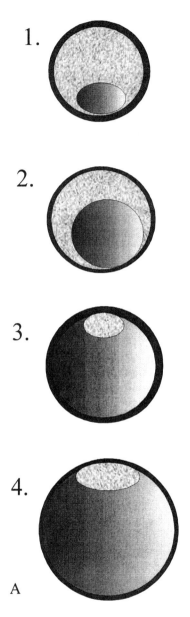

FIGURE 10.8. Scoring system for human blastocysts. (A) Blastocysts are initially given a numerical score from 1 to 6 based upon their degree of expansion and hatching status: (1) early blastocyst; the blastocoel being less than half the volume of the embryo. (2) blastocyst; the blastocoel being greater than half of the volume of the embryo. (3) full blastocyst; the blastocoel completely fills the embryo. (4) expanded blastocyst; the blastocoel volume is now larger than that of the early embryo and the zona is thinning. (5) hatching blastocyst; the trophectoderm has started to herniate though the zona. (6) hatched blastocyst; the blastocyst has completely escaped from the zona. Stages 1–4 are represented schematically to help quantitate the degree of blastocoel expansion. The initial phase of the assessment can be performed on a dissection microscope. The second step in scoring the blastocysts should be performed on an inverted microscope. For blastocysts graded as 3–6 (i.e., full blastocysts onward) the development of the inner cell mass (ICM) and trophectoderm can then be assessed:

ICM Grading—A. Tightly packed, many cells; B. Loosely grouped, several cells; C. Very few cells. *Trophectoderm Grading*—A. Many cells forming a cohesive epithelium; B. Few cells forming a loose epithelium; C. Very few cells. (B) Photomicrograph of a human blastocyst (score 4AA morning of Day 5). The blastocoel cavity is expanding and the zona is thinning (score of 4). The trophectoderm can be seen to be comprised of numerous cells (score of A). Blastocyst diameter is 140 μm. (C) Photomicrograph of the same human blastocyst in (B) taken in a different focal plane. The ICM is visible and can be seen to be comprised of numerous tightly packed cells (score of A). From Gardner and Schoolcraft (90). Reproduced with permission from Parthenon Publishing.

and Leese (88)]. It is possible to use scoring systems to help in the selection of blastocysts for transfer. Dokras et al. (89) developed a scoring system for blastocysts based primarily on the degree of expansion. A blastocyst scoring system based on three parameters (i.e., degree of expansion, development of the ICM, and development of the trophectoderm) was subsequently developed (Fig. 10.8) (90). This scoring system has been used effectively to identify those blastocysts

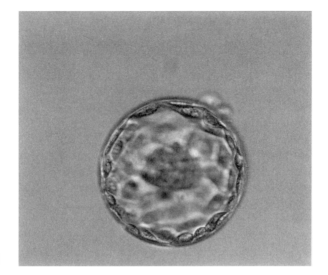

B

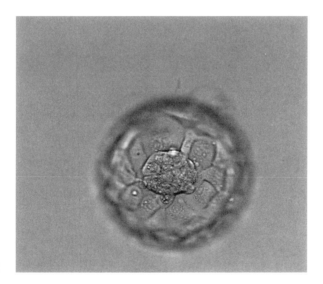

C

FIGURE 10.8. (*Continued*).

with the highest viability within a given cohort (86). When an analysis of patients having just two blastocysts transferred after the scoring system was introduced ($n = 107$ patients), it was observed that when two high-scoring blastocysts ($\geq 3AA$) were transferred, an implantation rate (fetal heart/blastocyst transferred) of 70% was attained (86). When only one high-scoring blastocyst was available for transfer, together with a low-scoring or slower blastocyst, an implantation rate of 54% was observed. If only low-scoring or slow blastocysts were transferred, however, the implantation rate fell to 28%; which can still be considered an acceptable implantation rate, especially when compared with the implantation rates of cleavage stage embryos.

A different approach to assessing viability that has been used with success in animal models is the noninvasive quantification of nutrient consumption and metabolite production by an individual embryo (91–93). Studies on the mouse embryo have revealed that it is possible to identify the most viable blastocysts within a cohort by quantitating their glucose consumption and lactate production (Fig. 10.9) (94). Using the noninvasive technique of ultramicrofluorescence it is possible to select blastocysts for transfer prospectively from a population of morphological similar embryos of the same diameter. Using this approach we have observed that human blastocysts of the same grade exhibit a wide range of metabolic activity, indicating that this approach may be applicable for selecting embryos in a clinical setting (Gardner, Lane, and Schoolcraft; unpublished observations). It is interesting that the nutrient consumption of human blastocysts cultured in sequential media is much higher than those cultured in conventional culture media

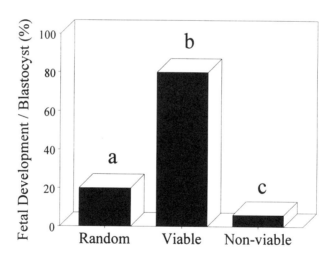

FIGURE 10.9. Fetal development of mouse blastocysts selected for transfer using glycolytic activity as a biochemical marker. "Viable" blastocysts were classified as those with a glycolytic rate in the lowest 15% of the distribution (glycolytic rate <88%), whereas "nonviable" blastocysts were those with a glycolytic rate in the highest 15% of the distribution (glycolytic rate >160%). On each day of the experiment, a selection of blastocysts were transferred at random. Different superscripts indicate significantly different populations ($p < 0.01$). From Lane and Gardner (94). Reproduced with permission from the European Society of Human Reproduction and Embryology. Reproduced with permission from Oxford University Press/Human Reproduction.

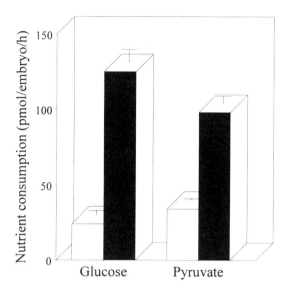

FIGURE 10.10. Nutrient consumption by human blastocysts on Day 5.5 postinsemination. Open bars represent data from Hardy et al. (95), who used medium HLT6 for embryo culture (no amino acids; $n = 25$ embryos). Solid bars represent embryos cultured in medium G 1.2 from the pronucleate stage to 1 P.M. on Day 3 and then cultured in medium G 2.2 ($n = 13$).

(Fig. 10.10), confirming that blastocyst development in culture per se is a poor end point to determine the health of an embryo.

Conclusions

Using sequential media, the human embryo can be cultured to the viable blastocyst stage at acceptable rates, resulting in higher implantation rates that can be attained using the transfer of cleavage-stage embryos. With the development of appropriate scoring systems and new noninvasive methods of quantifying embryo viability, the day of single blastocyst transfer for a significant number of patients is approaching.

The culture system in the clinical laboratory is significantly just one part of the overall treatment cycle. Good oocytes, derived from appropriate stimulation regimes, are able to give rise to good embryos; however, it is not feasible to obtain good embryos from poor oocytes (7). The embryo transfer technique and subsequent luteal support administered have subsequent impact on cycle outcome; therefore, should extended culture not result in the expected blastocyst development and implantation rates, it is important to scrutinize all procedures within an IVF cycle. Blastocyst culture and transfer should therefore not be perceived as a panacea for all of the problems of IVF.

Indeed, should part of an IVF procedure be compromised, then moving to extended culture may actually exacerbate the situation (96).

References

1. Buster JE, Bustillo M, Rodi IA, Cohen SW, Hamilton M, Simon JA, et al. Biologic and morphologic development of donated human ova by nonsurgical uterine lavage. Am J Obstet Gynecol 1985;153:211–17.
2. Scott LA, Smith S. The successful use of pronuclear embryo transfers the day following oocyte retrieval. Hum Reprod 1998;13:1003–13.
3. Edwards RG, Beard HK. Is the success of human IVF more a matter of genetics and evolution than growing blastocysts? Hum Reprod 1999;14:1–4.
4. Gerris J, De Neubourg D, Mangelschots K, Van Royen E, Van de Meerssche M, Valkenburg M. Prevention of twin pregnancy after in-vitro fertilization or intracytoplasmic sperm injection based on strict embryo criteria: a prospective randomized clinical trial. Hum Reprod 1999;14:2581–87.
5. Braude PR, Bolton VN, Moore S. Human gene expression first occurs between the four-and eight-cell stages of preimplantation development. Nature 1988;332:459–61.
6. Taylor DM, Ray PF, Ao A, Winston RM, Handyside AH. Paternal transcripts for glucose-6-phosphate dehydrogenase and adenosine deaminase are first detectable in the human preimplantation embryo at the three- to four-cell stage. Mol Reprod Dev 1997;48:442–48.
7. Gardner DK, Schoolcraft WB. Human embryo viability: what determines developmental potential and can it be assessed? J Assist Reprod Genet 1998;15:455–58.
8. Janny L, Menezo YJ. Evidence for a strong paternal effect on human preimplantation embryo development and blastocyst formation. Mol Reprod Dev 1994;38:36–42.
9. Croxatto HB, Ortiz ME, Diaz S, Hess R, Balmaceda J, Croxatto HD. Studies on the duration of egg transport by the human oviduct. II. Ovum location at various intervals following luteinizing hormone peak. Am J Obstet Gynecol 1978;132:629–34.
10. Gardner DK, Lane M, Calderon I, Leeton J. Environment of the preimplantation human embryo in vivo: metabolite analysis of oviduct and uterine fluids and metabolism of cumulus cells. Fertil Steril 1996;65:349–53.
11. Gardner DK. Changes in requirements and utilization of nutrients during mammalian preimplantation embryo development and their significance in embryo culture. Theriogenology 1998;49:83–102.
12. Marston JH, Penn R, Sivelle PC. Successful autotransfer of tubal eggs in the rhesus monkey (*Macaca mulatta*). J Reprod Fertil 1977;49:175–76.
13. Ertzeid G, Storeng R. Adverse effects of gonadotrophin treatment on pre- and postimplantation development in mice. J Reprod Fertil 1992;96:649–55.
14. Ertzeid G, Storeng R, Lyberg T. Treatment with gonadotropins impaired implantation and fetal development in mice. J Assist Reprod Genet 1993;10:286–91.
15. Van der Auwera I, Pijnenborg R, Koninckx PR. The influence of in vitro culture versus stimulated and untreated oviductal environment on mouse embryo development and implantation. Hum Reprod 1999;14:2570–74.
16. Gardner DK, Schoolcraft WB, McMillan WH. What is the rate limiting factor at implantation: embryo quality or endometrial receptivity? Proc Am Soc Rep Med 2000; 73:P-187.
17. Fanchin R, Righini C, Olivennes F, Taylor S, de Ziegler D, Frydman R. Uterine

contractions at the time of embryo transfer alter pregnancy rates after in-vitro fertilization. Hum Reprod 1998;13:1968–74.
18. Lesny P, Killick SR, Tetlow RL, Robinson J, Maguiness SD. Uterine junctional zone contractions during assisted reproduction cycles. Hum Reprod Update 1998;4: 440–45.
19. Gardner DK, Lane M. Embryo culture systems. In: Trounson A, Gardner DK, eds. Handbook of in vitro fertilization. Boca Raton: CRC Press, 1993:85.
20. Bolton VN, Wren ME, Parsons JH. Pregnancies after in vitro fertilization and transfer of human blastocysts. Fertil Steril 1991;55:830–32.
21. Gardner DK, Lane M. Culture and selection of viable blastocysts: a feasible proposition for human IVF? Hum Reprod Update 1997;3:367–82.
22. Gardner DK, Lane M. Culture of viable human blastocysts in defined sequential serum-free media. Hum Reprod 1998;13(Suppl. 3):148–59.
23. Gardner DK, Lane M. Embryo culture systems. In: Trounson A, Gardner DK, eds. Handbook of in vitro fertilization, 2nd ed. Boca Raton: CRC Press, 1999:205–64.
24. Bavister BD. Culture of preimplantation embryos: facts and artifacts. Hum Reprod Update 1995;1:91–148.
25. Pool TB, Atiee SH, Martin JE. Oocyte and embryo culture: basic concepts and recent advances. In: May JV, ed. Infertility and Reprod. Med. Clinics of North America, Assisted reproduction: laboratory considerations. Philadelphia: WB Saunders Company, 1998:181–203.
26. Bavister BD, McKiernan SH. Regulation of hamster embryo development in vitro by amino acids. In: Bavister BD, ed. Preimplantation embryo development. New York: Springer-Verlag, 1993:57–72.
27. Gardner DK. Mammalian embryo culture in the absence of serum or somatic cell support. Cell Biol Int 1994;18:1163–79.
28. Gardner DK, Lane M. Amino acids and ammonium regulate mouse embryo development in culture. Biol Reprod 1993;4:377–85.
29. Lane M, Gardner DK. Nonessential amino acids and glutamine decrease the time of the first three cleavage divisions and increase compaction of mouse zygotes in vitro. J Assist Reprod Genet 1997;14:398–403.
30. Steeves TE, Gardner DK. Temporal effects of amino acids on bovine embryo development in culture. Biol Reprod 1999;61:731.
31. Miller JGO, Schultz GA. Amino acid content of preimplantation rabbit embryos and fluids of the reproductive tract. Biol Reprod 1987;36:125–29.
32. Moses DF, Matkovic M, Cabrera-Fisher E, Martinez, AG. Amino acid contents of sheep oviductal and uterine fluids. Thereigenology 1977;47:336.
33. Eagle H. Amino acid metabolism in mammalian cell cultures. Science 1959;130: 432–37.
34. Gardner DK, Lane M. The 2-cell block in CF1 mouse embryos is associated with an increase in glycolysis and a decrease in tricarboxylic acid (TCA) cycle activity: alleviation of the 2-cell block is associated with the restoration of in vivo metabolic pathway activities. Biol Reprod 1993;49(Suppl. 1):52.
35. Dawson KM, Collins JL, Baltz JM. Osmolarity-dependent glycine accumulation indicates a role for glycine as an organic osmolyte in early preimplantation mouse embryos. Biol Reprod 1998;59:225.
36. Edwards LE, Williams DA, Gardner DK. Intracellular pH of the preimplantation mouse embryo: amino acids act as buffers of intracellular pH. Hum Reprod 1998;13:3441.

37. Lane M, Gardner DK. Differential regulation of mouse embryo development and viability by amino acids. J Reprod Fertil 1997;109:153–64.
38. Biggers JD, Gardner DK, Leese HJ. Control of carbohydrate metabolism in preimplantation mammalian embryos. In: Rosenblum IY, Heyner S, eds. Growth factors in mammalian development. Boca Raton: CRC Press, 1989:19–32.
39. Leese HJ. Metabolism of the preimplantation mammalian embryo. In: Milligan SR, ed. Oxford reviews of reproductive biology, 13. London: Oxford University Press, 1991:35–72.
40. Rieger D. Relationship between energy metabolism and development of the early embryo. Theriogenology 1992;37:75–93.
41. Gardner DK, Leese HJ. Concentrations of nutrients in mouse oviduct fluid and their effects on embryo development and metabolism in vitro. J Reprod Fert 1990;88:361.
42. Barnes FL, Crombie A, Gardner DK, Kausche A, Lacham-Kaplan O, Suikkari AM, et al. Blastocyst development and pregnancy after in vitro maturation of human primary oocytes, intracytoplasmic sperm injection and assisted hatching. Hum Reprod 1995;10:3243–47.
43. Behr B, Pool TB, Milki AA, Moore D, Gebhardt J, Dasig D. Preliminary clinical experience with human blastocysts development in vitro without co-culture. Hum Reprod 1999;14:454–57.
44. Milki AA, Fisch JD, Behr B. Two-blastocyst transfer has similar pregnancy rates and a decreased multiple gestation rate compared with three-blastocyst transfer. Fertil Steril 1999;72:225–28.
45. Mastroianni L, Jr., Jones R. Oxygen tension in the rabbit fallopian tube. J Reprod Fertil 1965;9:99.
46. Fischer B, Bavister BD. Oxygen tension in the oviduct and uterus of rhesus monkeys, hamsters and rabbits. J Reprod Fertil 1993;99:673.
47. Mass DHA, Storey BT, Mastroianni L, Jr. Oxygen tension in the oviduct of the rhesus monkey (Macaca mulatta). Fertil Steril 1976;27:1312.
48. Quinn P, Harlow GH. The effect of oxygen on the development of preimplantation mouse embryos in vitro. J Exp Zool 1978;206:73.
49. Umaoka Y, Noda Y, Narimoto K, Mori T. Effects of oxygen toxicity on early development of mouse embryos. Mol Reprod Devel 1992;31:28.
50. Gardner DK, Lane M. Alleviation of the "2-cell block" and development to the blastocyst of CF1 mouse embryos: role of amino acids, EDTA and physical parameters. Hum Reprod 1996;11:2703.
51. Li J, Foote RH. Culture of rabbit zygotes into blastocysts in protein-free medium with one to twenty percent oxygen. J Reprod Fertil 1993;98:163.
52. Thompson JGE, Simpson AC, Pugh PA, Donnelly PE, Tervit HR. Effect of oxygen concentration on in vitro development of preimplantation sheep and cattle embryos. J Reprod Fertil 1990;89:573.
53. Batt PA, Gardner DK, Cameron AWN. Oxygen concentration and protein source affect the development of preimplantation goat embryos in vitro. Reprod Fert Devel 1991;3:601–7.
54. Gardner DK, Lane M, Johnson J, Wagley L, Stevens J, Schoolcraft WB. Reduced oxygen tension increases blastocyst development, differentiation and viability. Proc Am Soc Reprod Med 1999;72:30.
55. Wiley LM, Yamami S, Van Muyden D. Effect of potassium concentration, type of protein supplement, and embryo density on mouse preimplantation development in vitro. Fertil Steril 1986;45:111–19.

56. Paria BC, Dey SK. Preimplantation embryo development in vitro: cooperative interactions among embryos and role of growth factors. Proc Natl Acad Sci USA 1990;87:4756–60.
57. Lane M, Gardner DK. Effect of incubation volume and embryo density on the development and viability of mouse embryos in vitro. Hum Reprod 1992;7:558–62.
58. Gardner DK. Improving embryo culture and enhancing pregnancy rate. In: Shoham Z, Howles C, Jacobs H, eds. Female infertility therapy: current practice. London: Martin Dunitz, 1998:283–99.
59. Gardner DK, Lane M, Spitzer A, Batt PA. Enhanced rates of cleavage and development for sheep zygotes cultured to the blastocyst stage in vitro in the absence of serum and somatic cells: amino acids, vitamins and culturing embryos in groups stimulate development. Biol Reprod 1994;50:390–400.
60. Keefer CL, Stice SL, Paprocki AM, Golueke P. In vitro culture of bovine IVM-IVF embryos: cooperative interaction among embryos and the role of growth factors. Theriogenology 1994;41:1323–31.
61. Ahern TJ, Gardner DK. Culturing bovine embryos in groups stimulates blastocyst development and cell allocation to the inner cell mass. Theriogenology 1998;49:194.
62. Gardner DK, Lane MW, Lane M. Development of the inner cell mass in mouse blastocysts is stimulated by reducing the embryo: incubation volume ratio. Hum Reprod 1997;12(Abstr. Book 1):132.
63. Moessner J, Dodson WC. The quality of human embryo growth is improved when embryos are cultured in groups rather than separately. Fertil Steril 1995;64:1034–35.
64. Almagor M, Bejar C, Kafka I, Yaffe H. Pregnancy rates after communal growth of preimplantation human embryos in vitro. Fertil Steril 1996;66:394–97.
65. Spyropoulou I, Karamalegos C, Bolton VN. A prospective randomized study comparing the outcome of in-vitro fertilization and embryo transfer following culture of human embryos individually or in groups before transfer on day 2. Hum Reprod 1999;14:76–79.
66. Rijnders PM, Jansen CAM. Influence of group culture and culture volume on the formation of human blastocysts: a prospective randomized study. Hum Reprod 1999;14:2333–37.
67. Kane MT, Morgan PM, Coonan C. Peptide growth factors and preimplantation development. Hum Reprod Update 1997;3:137–57.
68. Gardner DK, Lane M. Embryo culture. In: Gardner DK, Weissman A, Howles C, Shoham Z, eds. Textbook of assisted reproductive technology: laboratory and clinical rerspectives. London: Martin Dunitz Press, 2001:203–22.
69. Caro CM, Trounson AT. Successful fertilization, embryo development, and pregnancy in human in vitro fertilization (IVF) using a chemically defined culture medium containing no protein. J In Vitro Fert Embryo Transf 1986;3:215.
70. Gray CW, Morgan PM, Kane MT. Purification of an embryotrophic factor from commercial bovine serum albumin and its identification as citrate. J Reprod Fertil 1992;94:471.
71. Leese HJ. The formation and function of oviduct fluid. J Reprod Fertil 1988;82:843–56.
72. Gardner DK, Lane M, Schoolcraft WB. Culture and transfer of viable blastocysts: a feasible proposition for human IVF. Hum Reprod 2000;15(Suppl. 6):9–23.
73. Walker SK, Heard TM, Seamark RF. In vitro culture of sheep embryos without co-culture: success and perspectives. Theriogenology 1992;37:111–26.
74. Thompson JG, Gardner DK, Pugh PA, McMillan J, Tervit RH. Lamb birth weight

following transfer is affected by the culture system used for pre-elongation development of embryos. Biol Reprod 1995;53:1385–91.
75. Dorland M, Gardner DK, Trounson A. Serum in synthetic oviduct fluid causes mitochondrial degeneration in ovine embryos. J Reprod Fertil Abstract Series 1994;13:70.
76. Bavister BD. Substitution of a synthetic polymer for protein in a mammalian gamete culture system. J Exp Zool 1981;217:45–51.
77. Zorn TM, Pinhal MA, Nader HB, Carvalho JJ, Abrahamsohn PA, Dietrich CP. Biosynthesis of glycosaminoglycans in the endometrium during the initial stages of pregnancy of the mouse. Cell Mol Biol 1995;41:97–106.
78. Campbell S, Swann HR, Aplin JD, Seif MW, Kimber SJ, Elstein M. CD44 is expressed throughout pre-implantation human embryo development. Hum Reprod 1995;10:425–30.
79. Gardner DK, Lane M, Rodriguez-Martinez H. Fetal development after transfer is increased by replacing protein with the glycosaminoglycan hyaluronate for embryo culture and transfer in the mouse. Hum Reprod 1999;14:2575.
80. Gardner DK, Lane M. Recombinant human serum albumin and hyaluronan can replace blood-derived albumin in embryo culture media. Proc Am Soc Rep Med 2000;73:86.
81. Hooper K, Lane M, Gardner DK. Toward defined physiological embryo culture media: replacement of BSA with recombinant albumin. Biol Reprod 2000;62(Suppl. 1).
82. Gardner DK, Vella P, Lane M, Wagely L, Schlenker T, Schoolcraft WB. Culture and transfer of human blastocysts increases implantation rates and reduces the need for multiple embryo transfers. Fertil Steril 1998;69:84–88.
83. Gardner DK, Schoolcraft WB, Wagley L, Schlenker T, Stevens J, Hesla J. A prospective randomized trial of blastocyst culture and transfer in in vitro fertilization. Hum Reprod 1998;13:3434–40.
84. Shapiro BS, Harris DC, Richter KS. Predictive value of 72-hour blastomere cell number on blastocyst development and success of subsequent transfer based on the degree of blastocysts development. Fertil Steril 2000;73:582.
85. Langley M, Marek D, Gardner DK, Confer N, Doody KM, Doody KJ. Efficacy of blastocyst transfer in human ART. Hum Reprod 2001 (in press).
86. Gardner DK, Lane M, Stevens J, Schlenker T, Schoolcraft WB. Blastocyst score affects implantation and pregnancy outcome: Towards single blastocyst transfer. Fertil Steril 2000;73:1155–58.
87. Schoolcraft WB, Gardner DK. Blastocyst culture and transfer increases the efficiency of oocyte donation. Fertil Sertil 2000;74:482–86.
88. Gardner DK, Leese HJ. Assessment of embryo metabolism and viability. In: Trounson A, Gardner DK, eds. Handbook of in vitro fertilization, 2nd ed. Boca Raton: CRC Press, 1999:347–72.
89. Dokras A, Sargent IL, Barlow DH. Human blastocyst grading: an indicator of developmental potential? Hum Reprod 1993;8:2119.
90. Gardner DK, Schoolcraft WB. In-vitro culture of human blastocysts. In: Jansen R, Mortimer D, eds. Towards reproductive certainty: infertility and genetics beyond 1999. Carnforth: Parthenon Press; 1999:378–88.
91. Renard JP, Philippon A, Menezo Y. In vitro glucose uptake of glucose by bovine blastocysts. J Reprod Fertil 1980;58:161–64.
92. Gardner DK, Leese HJ. Assessment of embryo viability prior to transfer by the noninvasive measurement of glucose uptake. J Exp Zool 1987;242:103.
93. Gardner DK, Pawelczynski M, Trounson A. Nutrient uptake and utilization can be

used to select viable day 7 bovine blastocysts after cryopreservation. Mol Reprod Dev 1996;44:472.
94. Lane M, Gardner DK. Selection of viable mouse blastocysts prior to transfer using a metabolic criterion. Hum Reprod 1996;11:1975–78.
95. Hardy K, Hooper MA, Handyside AH, Rutherford AJ, Winston RM, Leese HJ. Non-invasive measurement of glucose and pyruvate uptake by individual human oocytes and preimplantation embryos. Hum Reprod 1989;4:188–91.
96. Quinn P, Stone BA, Marrs RP. Suboptimal laboratory conditions can affect pregnancy outcome after embryo transfer on day 1 or 2 after insemination in vitro. Fertil Steril 1990;53:168–70.

11

Apoptosis in the Human Blastocyst: Role of Survival Factors

KATE HARDY AND SOPHIE SPANOS

The developmental potential of human embryos following in vitro fertilization (IVF) is poor. The implantation rate of embryos transferred 2 days after IVF is only around 25% (1), resulting in low pregnancy rates (2). If embryos are cultured in vitro, approximately 50% arrest during the first 6 days (3). The reasons for this high rate of embryo loss during early development are unclear, but they could include suboptimal culture conditions, chromosomal abnormalities, inadequate oocyte maturation, disturbances in embryo–maternal dialogue, or a nonreceptive endometrium.

Both arrested and developing human embryos contain varying proportions of cells with the classic morphological features of apoptosis (4–7), including cytoplasmic, nuclear, and DNA fragmentation. Even though the presence of similar cells in vivo suggests a role for apoptosis in normal development, it could play a significant role in embryonic arrest; however, the causes, roles, and regulation of apoptosis during preimplantation development remain unknown.

It has been proposed that apoptosis is the fate of all cells unless they receive signals to survive (8). These signals include cell–cell contacts, adhesion molecules, extracellular matrix interactions and growth factors. Growth factors are important in the regulation of preimplantation development (9,10), and evidence is accumulating that many may also act as survival factors, playing a role in the regulation of apoptosis (reviewed in 6,7,11).

Apoptosis

Apoptosis is a form of cell death that is under physiological control. It is an essential feature of many normal processes and pathological conditions, and serves a variety of purposes, including tissue homeostasis and remodeling, control of cell number, and the removal of unwanted or damaged cells (12). There has been increasing interest in the importance of apoptosis in reproduction and development. Apoptosis plays a major role in corpus luteum regression, follicle atresia, and endometrium remodeling (reviewed in 13).

Examples of developmental events that require extensive apoptosis include the removal of the tadpole tail during amphibian metamorphosis, and the sculpting of digits in the developing limb bud. During early rodent development, apoptosis plays a crucial role in amniotic cavity formation, soon after implantation (14). It now appears that cell death could play a role during preimplantation development (reviewed in 6,7).

Apoptosis characteristically affects single isolated cells and involves a series of morphologically distinct phases. Chromatin initially condenses on the inner nuclear membrane and condensation of the cytoplasm occurs. The nucleus becomes grossly indented and fragments. The whole cell finally fragments into membrane-bound apoptotic bodies, which are either dispersed in the intercellular tissue spaces and extruded from the tissue, or phagocytozed by neighboring cells. This classical sequence of events has been seen at the ultrastructural level in a wide variety of different cell types (12,15).

In addition to the classic morphological features described here, apoptosis results in biochemical changes in membrane and DNA structure. Early cell surface changes include redistribution of membrane phospholipids within the lipid bilayer, with exposure of phosphatidylserine on the outer leaflet (16). During the later stages of apoptosis, DNA fragmentation is frequently observed where DNA is cleaved between nucleosomes by endonucleases into oligonucleosomal fragments (12).

Two major protein families have been implicated in the regulation and execution of apoptosis: the caspase family of cysteine proteases that mediate proteolytic cleavage of a large number of proteins within the cell leading to the apoptotic morphology described earlier (15) and the Bcl-2 family members that regulate the activity of these effector molecules. The Bcl-2 family is subdivided into pro- (e.g., Bax, Bcl-x_s, Bad, Bak) and antiapoptotic members (e.g., Bcl-2, Bcl-x_L, Mcl-1, Bcl-w). It has been suggested that it is the ratio and ion-channel forming properties of these proteins that determine the fate of the cell (reviewed in 17). The Bcl-2 family of proteins are believed to regulate the release and activation of proapoptotic factors from mitochondria such as cytochrome c and apoptosis-inducing factor (AIF) that lead to the activation of caspases and other downstream execution proteins and, ultimately, cell death.

The cell's decision to undergo apoptosis is governed by the nature of the signals that it receives. These may include intracellular signals (e.g., mitochondrial DNA mutations) or the loss (e.g., serum or growth factor withdrawal) or gain (e.g., FasL/ TNFα; toxin) of an extracellular signal.

Observations of Apoptosis in the Human Preimplantation Embryo

Cells and nuclei with the morphological features of apoptosis (12), including cytoplasmic and nuclear fragmentation, chromatin condensation, DNA fragmentation, and phagocytosis, have been identified during preimplantation development in a range of mammalian species (reviewed in 6) including human (4–7,18–20). Approximately 75% of human blastocysts have one or more apoptotic nuclei.

Chromatin Condensation and Nuclear Fragmentation

Changes in nuclear morphology have been detected in human embryos by labeling DNA with polynucleotide-specific fluorochromes [e.g., propidium iodide, Hoechst or 4',6-diamidino-2-phenylindole (DAPI)]. Nuclei with condensed chromatin have been seen in embryos and blastocysts using fluorescence and confocal microscopy (4,7,20,21). Fragmented nuclei have been observed in cleavage stage embryos (21,22), morulae, and blastocysts (4,7,20). These nuclei appear as discrete clusters of labeled fragments, which are smaller than intact healthy nuclei.

A large proportion of human blastocysts fertilized and cultured in vitro have fragmented nuclei. Retrospective analysis of more than 200 human blastocysts labeled with DNA-specific fluorochromes during a series of studies (reviewed in 6) showed that approximately 75% of blastocysts had one or more dead cells on Day 6. Most of these embryos had fewer than 10 dead cells, although some embryos had significant levels of cell death of more than 15%.

Cell death was present equally in the trophectoderm (TE) and the inner cell mass (ICM), with a dead cell index between 7 and 8% in each lineage. The incidence of cell death appears to be correlated with embryo quality, with the total dead cell index ranging from less than 10% in Day 6 blastocysts of good morphology to 27% in those of poor morphology (4).

DNA Fragmentation

A major hallmark of apoptosis is the degradation of DNA into oligonucleosomal fragments. Because of the small numbers of cells in preimplantation embryos, it is impossible to use electrophoretic techniques to look for DNA laddering typical of apoptotic nuclei; however, the development of TdT-mediated dUTP nick-end labeling (TUNEL) (23) allows the assessment of DNA fragmentation in situ. This technique is based on the fluorescent labeling of the 3'-hydroxyl ends of oligonucleosome fragments resulting from DNA cleavage. It has the additional advantages of allowing both localization and quantification of the percentage of nuclei with DNA fragmentation (23). Positive labeling of fragmented nuclei in mouse (24,25) and human (5) (Spanos and Hardy, unpublished) blastocysts has been demonstrated, providing evidence of DNA fragmentation.

Cytoplasmic Fragmentation

More than 75% of embryos generated during IVF have varying degrees of cytoplasmic fragmentation (7), which is associated with reduced blastocyst formation (7) and implantation (26). Ultrastructural examination of fragmented embryos has shown that these membrane bound fragments contain organelles

(5,27). These fragments resemble apoptotic bodies seen in other cell types. It has been suggested that apoptosis may be involved in early embryonic arrest and that cytoplasmic fragments are equivalent to apoptotic bodies (i.e., the end-product of apoptosis) (5,7). Several studies, however, have failed to demonstrate an association between cytoplasmic fragmentation and DNA fragmentation (28) (Spanos and Karagiannis, unpublished data), indicating that the origin of cytoplasmic fragments remains unclear.

Expression of Cell Death Genes in Embryos

The expression pattern of cell death inducer (e.g., p53, Bax, Bcl-x_s), repressor (e.g., Bcl-2, Bcl-x_L, Bcl-w, Mcl-1), and executor (e.g., caspase-1, -2, -3, -6, -7, -11, -12) genes has been examined during all stages of mouse preimplantation development (29,30). Limited data on human oocytes and preimplantation embryos demonstrates expression of both BAX and BCL-2 mRNA (28,31) (Spanos and Hardy, unpublished) and protein (7).

Timing of Apoptosis in the Human

DNA fragmentation is not seen before compaction in developing embryos with minimal cytoplasmic fragmentation (27) (Spanos and Hardy, unpublished). In a series of 66 normally developing embryos between the four-cell and blastocyst stages, both TUNEL labeling (to detect DNA fragmentation) and DAPI staining (to assess nuclear fragmentation) were used to identify apoptotic nuclei. Nuclear fragmentation was observed rarely before compaction and at increasing levels during blastocyst formation. TUNEL labeling was only seen after compaction, and the proportion of nuclei with DNA fragmentation increased during blastocyst formation to 10% (Spanos and Hardy, unpublished).

Is This an In Vitro Artifact?

Apoptosis in the preimplantation embryo is not an in vitro artifact. It is found in rodent, primate, and human embryos, and blastocysts that have been freshly removed from the reproductive tract (19) (reviewed in 6). More than 80% of mouse blastocysts freshly flushed from the uterus on Days 4 or 5 had one or more fragmented nuclei (6). Pyknotic and fragmented nuclei and cytoplasmic fragmentation have also been described in human embryos in vivo (19,32,33).

Survival Factors and Apoptosis in the Preimplantation Embryo

Growth Factors and Mammalian Preimplantation Development

There is increasing evidence that maternally and embryonically derived growth factors play an important role in preimplantation development (reviewed in

9,10). For example, the preimplantation development of mouse embryos cultured in vitro is retarded when compared with that in vivo (34,35). Moreover, reduced incubation volume or culture of embryos in groups improve preimplantation development (24,36–39), suggesting that there may be autocrine and paracrine pathways operating in vivo that are not present or are diluted in vitro. Furthermore, a range of polypeptide growth factor ligands have been found to be expressed and produced by the reproductive tract and preimplantation embryo, whereas many of their receptors can be detected on the embryo surface (reviewed in 9). Growth factors such as insulin, insulinlike growth factor I (IGF-I), and transforming growth factor α (TGF-α) have generally been shown to promote blastocyst formation and development, and to increase cell number in vitro (36,40–42), in addition to reported effects on protein synthesis (43) and gene expression (44).

Survival Factors and Apoptosis

Most mammalian cells express the cellular machinery necessary to undergo apoptosis. It has been proposed that they only survive if they are signaled to do so (8). Possible signals could take the form of diffusible "survival" factors produced by other cells. Several types of cells deprived of serum or extracellular signaling molecules die (8). Furthermore, culture of cells in staurosporine, a protein kinase inhibitor presumed to inhibit intracellular signaling pathways, induces apoptosis (45). A number of studies have demonstrated that

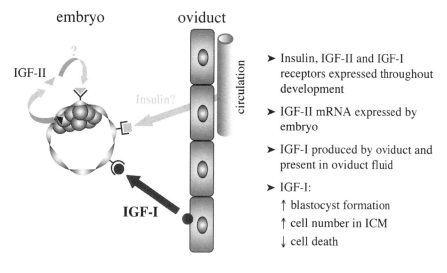

FIGURE 11.1. Possible endocrine, paracrine, and autocrine actions of insulin, IGF-I, and IGF-II during human preimplantation development. Observed receptors, ligands, and their interactions are shown in black (42,45), and proposed ones in gray.

growth factors play a key role in regulating apoptosis during preimplantation embryogenesis (reviewed in 6,7,11).

Mouse embryos cultured in vitro had threefold higher levels of apoptosis than embryos in vivo (24) providing evidence that the maternal reproductive tract produces survival factors. Furthermore, embryos cultured singly had a significantly higher incidence of cell death than that observed in embryos cultured in groups (24,38), suggesting that embryos themselves produce survival factors that act in a paracrine manner.

Supplementation of the culture medium with certain exogenous growth factors (e.g., TGF-α) reduces the incidence of apoptosis, indicating that TGF-α acts as a survival factor during mouse preimplantation development (24). This hypothesis was strengthened by the observation that levels of cell death were higher in the ICM of blastocysts from TGF-α deficient mice compared with wild type mice (46).

Members of the IGF family also appear to regulate apoptosis. Herrler et al. (47) induced apoptosis in rabbit embryos by subjecting them to ultraviolet irradiation, which could be reduced by addition of IGF-I or insulin. Brison (11) also observed a significant reduction in apoptosis in mouse embryos in the presence of IGF-I or insulin.

IGF-I, Human Preimplantation Development, and Apoptosis

The IGF family plays an important role in growth and development. In particular, it is becoming clear that the interaction between IGF-I and the type I receptor (IGF-IR) plays an important role in both stimulation and initiation of the cell cycle and in the regulation of apoptosis. IGF-I is a single-chain polypeptide that is produced by most tissues and is present in high concentrations in circulating serum in association with IGF-binding proteins, which play a regulatory role. IGF-I is thought to have an endocrine mode of action mediating the mitogenic effects of growth hormone, as well as local paracrine or autocrine roles. IGF-IR is similar to the insulin receptor and is a transmembrane tyrosine-specific protein kinase. Upon ligand binding the receptor autophosphorylates tyrosine residues and also phosphorylates cytoplasmic substrates involved in a number of cytoplasmic and nuclear signaling pathways (48).

IGF-I promotes preimplantation embryo development and increases cell number and metabolism in many species, including mouse (38,41), rabbit (47), cow (49,50), pig (51), and human (42). Lighten et al. showed that IGF-I is produced by the maternal tract (42) and that human embryos express IGF-IRs throughout preimplantation development (42,52) but do not express the IGF-I ligand (52) (Fig. 11.1). Furthermore, they showed that addition of IGF-I to culture medium significantly increased the proportion of embryos developing to the blastocyst stage by 25% (42) (Spanos and Hardy, unpublished) and that these blastocysts had a significant (59%) increase in the number of ICM cells (42) (Fig. 11.1).

IGF-I has been shown to be an important inhibitor of cell death in many cell types (reviewed in 48,53). In order to determine whether IGF-I was acting as a mitogenic or an antiapoptotic factor during human preimplantation development the incidence of apoptosis and cell division in embryos cultured in the presence and absence of 1.7 nM IGF-I was examined. Two techniques were used to quantify apoptosis and cell division: TUNEL to identify DNA fragmentation, in conjunction with DAPI staining to examine nuclear morphology and identify fragmenting and mitotic nuclei. IGF-I was shown to reduce significantly the percentage of apoptotic nuclei in human blastocysts by approximately 50%, from ~15 to ~7% (Spanos and Hardy, unpublished data) (Fig. 11.1).

Possible Actions of IGF-I

IGF-I is a powerful inhibitor of apoptosis via an IGF-I receptor mediated cell survival pathway in a wide range of cells (reviewed in 48,53). Reduction in the number of IGF-IRs causes extensive apoptosis whereas overexpression of IGF-IRs protects cells from apoptosis in vivo (54). It is interesting that a direct correlation between expression of IGF-I ligand and receptor and developmental potential to the blastocyst stage in mouse preimplantation embryos has been observed (55).

There are a number of hypotheses for the mechanisms by which the IGF-I survival pathway achieves the inhibition of apoptosis (e.g., transcriptional activation of BCL-2, inhibition of caspases, upregulation of DNA repair enzymes). IGF-I is known to bind to its receptor IGF-IR with highest affinity and survival

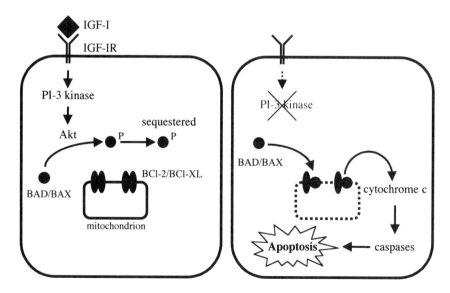

FIGURE 11.2. Possible pathway for the antiapoptotic action of IGF-I in the human preimplantation embryo.

factor inhibition of apoptosis has been shown to occur through activation of the phosphatidylinositide-3'-OH kinase (PI3K) and its downstream target Akt (a serine-threonine kinase). Akt may downregulate cell death by regulating expression or activity of BCL-2 family members or caspases; or by regulating aspects of metabolic homeostasis; or by phosphorylating components of the cell death machinery (56). One current model is that Akt phosphorylates BAD, sequestering it and preventing it from dimerizing with antiapoptotic BCL-2 members in the mitochondrial membrane, thus inactivating its ability to cause apoptosis (Fig. 11.2). Growth factor withdrawal inactivates the kinase pathway, the phosphorylation state of Bad shifts to the dephosphorylated form, leaving BAD free to heterodimerise with BCL-2 and BCL-xL. This leads to the release of cytochrome c from the mitochondria, resulting in activation of effector caspases to cleave a variety of cellular substrates with the final production of the apoptotic phenotype (Fig. 11.2). This is one model for how survival factors could act in the preimplantation embryo, and it is likely that different apoptotic triggers, and even different survival factors, could activate different apoptotic pathways.

Conclusions

During normal human preimplantation development in vitro, nuclei with morphological features of apoptosis are observed following compaction, with increasing incidence at the blastocyst stage. The observation of increased levels of apoptosis in mouse blastocysts in vitro suggests that the maternal reproductive tract is producing survival factors (which could include peptide growth factors) which act on the embryo. Reduction of levels of apoptosis during group culture of embryos provides strong evidence that embryos themselves produce survival factors which act in an autocrine/paracrine manner. Finally, the antiapoptotic action of TGF-α, insulin, and IGF-I in mouse embryos, and of IGF-I in rabbit and human embryos, provides candidates for these putative survival factors.

These observations, however, should be regarded with caution with regard to clinical IVF. Apoptosis is observed in vivo and therefore must play a crucial regulatory role in early development, which is as yet unknown. In vivo, embryos are exposed to a large number of growth factors and their binding proteins. Thus, even though growth factor supplementation of culture medium appears to be beneficial by increasing embryo and cell survival, it is now important to confirm that these survival factors are not overriding natural selection mechanisms and causing developmental abnormalities.

References

1. Dawson KJ, Conaghan J, Ostera GR, Winston RM, Hardy K. Delaying transfer to the third day post-insemination, to select non-arrested embryos, increases development to the fetal heart stage. Hum Reprod 1995;10:177–82.

2. Human fertilisation and embryology authority, eighth annual report, Paxton House. London: HFEA, 1999.
3. Hardy K. Development of human blastocysts in vitro. In: Bavister BD, ed. Preimplantation embryo development. New York: Springer-Verlag, 1993:184–99.
4. Hardy K, Handyside AH, Winston RM. The human blastocyst: cell number, death and allocation during late preimplantation development in vitro. Development 1989;107:597–604.
5. Jurisicova A, Varmuza S, Casper RF. Programmed cell death and human embryo fragmentation. Mol Hum Reprod 1996;2:93–98.
6. Hardy K. Cell death in the mammalian blastocyst. Mol Hum Reprod 1997;3:919–25.
7. Hardy K. Apoptosis in the human embryo. Rev Reprod 1999;4:125–34.
8. Raff MC. Social controls on cell survival and cell death. Nature 1992;356:397–400.
9. Kane MT, Morgan PM, Coonan C. Peptide growth factors and preimplantation development. Hum Reprod Update 1997;3:137–57.
10. Kaye PL. Preimplantation growth factor physiology. Rev Reprod 1997;2:121–27.
11. Brison DR. Apoptosis in mammalian preimplantation embryos: regulation by survival factors. Hum Fertil 2000;3:36–47.
12. Wyllie AH, Kerr JF, Currie AR. Cell death: the significance of apoptosis. Int Rev Cytol 1980;68:251–306.
13. Tilly JL, Strauss JF, Tenniswood M, eds. Cell death in reproductive physiology. New York: Springer-Verlag, 1997.
14. Coucouvanis E, Martin GR. Signals for death and survival: a two-step mechanism for cavitation in the vertebrate embryo. Cell 1995;83:279–87.
15. Wyllie AH. Apoptosis: an overview. Br Med Bull 1997;53:451–65.
16. Martin SJ, Reutelingsperger CP, McGahon AJ, Rader JA, van Schie RC, LaFace DM, et al. Early redistribution of plasma membrane phosphatidylserine is a general feature of apoptosis regardless of the initiating stimulus: inhibition by overexpression of Bcl-2 and Abl. J Exp Med 1995;182:1545–56.
17. Tsujimoto Y, Shimizu S. Bcl-2 family: life-or-death switch. FEBS Lett 2000;466:6–10.
18. Mohr LR, Trounson AO. Comparative ultrastructure of hatched human, mouse and bovine blastocysts. J Reprod Fertil 1982;66:499–504.
19. Hertig AT, Rock J, Adams EC, Mulligan WJ. On the preimplantation stages of the human ovum: a description of four normal and four abnormal specimens ranging from the second to fifth day of development. Contrib Embryol 1954;35:199–220.
20. Hardy K, Warner A, Winston RM, Becker DL. Expression of intercellular junctions during preimplantation development of the human embryo. Mol Hum Reprod 1996;2:621–32.
21. Levy R, Benchaib M, Cordonier H, Souchier C, Guerin JF. Annexin V labelling and terminal transferase-mediated DNA end labelling (TUNEL) assay in human arrested embryos. Mol Hum Reprod 1998;4:775–83.
22. Hardy K, Winston RM, Handyside AH. Binucleate blastomeres in preimplantation human embryos in vitro: failure of cytokinesis during early cleavage. J Reprod Fertil 1993;98:549–58.
23. Gavrieli Y, Sherman Y, Ben-Sasson SA. Identification of programmed cell death in situ via specific labeling of nuclear DNA fragmentation. J Cell Biol 1992;119:493–501.
24. Brison DR, Schultz RM. Apoptosis during mouse blastocyst formation: evidence for a role for survival factors including transforming growth factor alpha. Biol Reprod 1997;56:1088–96.

25. Moley KH, Chi MM, Knudson CM, Korsmeyer SJ, Mueckler MM. Hyperglycemia induces apoptosis in pre-implantation embryos through cell death effector pathways. Nat Med 1998;4:1421–24.
26. Giorgetti C, Terriou P, Auquier P, Hans E, Spach JL, Salzmann J, et al. Embryo score to predict implantation after in vitro fertilization: based on 957 single embryo transfers. Hum Reprod 1995;10:2427–31.
27. Yang HW, Hwang KJ, Kwon HC, Kim HS, Choi KW, Oh KS. Detection of reactive oxygen species (ROS) and apoptosis in human fragmented embryos. Hum Reprod 1998;13:998–1002.
28. Antczak M, Van Blerkom J. Temporal and spatial aspects of fragmentation in early human embryos: possible effects on developmental competence and association with the differential elimination of regulatory proteins from polarized domains. Hum Reprod 1999;14:429–47.
29. Jurisicova A, Latham KE, Casper RF, Casper RF, Varmuza SL. Expression and regulation of genes associated with cell death during murine preimplantation embryo development. Mol Reprod Dev 1998;51:243–53.
30. Exley GE, Tang C, McElhinny AS, Warner CM. Expression of caspase and BCL-2 apoptotic family members in mouse preimplantation embryos. Biol Reprod 1999;61:231–39.
31. Warner CM, Cao W, Exley GE, McElhinny AS, Alikani M, Cohen J, et al. Genetic regulation of egg and embryo survival. Hum Reprod 1998;13(Suppl. 3):178–90; discussion 191–96.
32. Pereda J, Croxatto HB. Ultrastructure of a seven-cell human embryo. Biol Reprod 1978;18:481–89.
33. Buster JE, Bustillo M, Rodi IA, Cohen SW, Hamilton M, Simon JA, et al. Biologic and morphologic development of donated human ova recovered by nonsurgical uterine lavage. Am J Obstet Gynecol 1985;153:211–17.
34. Bowman P, McLaren A. Cleavage rate of mouse embryos in vivo and in vitro. J Embryol Exp Morphol 1970;24:203–7.
35. Harlow GM, Quinn P. Development of preimplantation mouse embryos in vivo and in vitro. Aust J Biol Sci 1982;35:187–93.
36. Paria BC, Dey SK. Preimplantation embryo development in vitro: cooperative interactions among embryos and role of growth factors. Proc Natl Acad Sci USA 1990;87:4756–60.
37. Lane M, Gardner DK. Effect of incubation volume and embryo density on the development and viability of mouse embryos in vitro. Hum Reprod 1992;7:558–62.
38. O'Neill C. Autocrine mediators are required to act on the embryo by the 2-cell stage to promote normal development and survival of mouse preimplantation embryos in vitro. Biol Reprod 1998;58:1303–9.
39. Stoddart NR, Wild AE, Fleming TP. Stimulation of development in vitro by platelet-activating factor receptor ligands released by mouse preimplantation embryos. J Reprod Fertil 1996;108:47–53.
40. Harvey MB, Kaye PL. Insulin increases the cell number of the inner cell mass and stimulates morphological development of mouse blastocysts in vitro. Development 1990;110:963–67.
41. Harvey MB, Kaye PL. Insulin-like growth factor-1 stimulates growth of mouse preimplantation embryos in vitro. Mol Reprod Dev 1992;31:195–99.
42. Lighten AD, Moore GE, Winston RM, Hardy K. Routine addition of human insulin-

like growth factor-I ligand could benefit clinical in-vitro fertilization culture. Hum Reprod 1998;13:3144–50.
43. Harvey MB, Kaye PL. Insulin stimulates protein synthesis in compacted mouse embryos. Endocrinology 1988;122:1182–84.
44. Babalola GO, Schultz RM. Modulation of gene expression in the preimplantation mouse embryo by TGF-alpha and TGF-beta. Mol Reprod Dev 1995;41:133–39.
45. Weil M, Jacobson MD, Coles HS, Davies TJ, Gardner RL, Raff KD, et al. Constitutive expression of the machinery for programmed cell death. J Cell Biol 1996;133:1053–59.
46. Brison DR, Schultz RM. Increased incidence of apoptosis in transforming growth factor alpha-deficient mouse blastocysts. Biol Reprod 1998;59:136–44.
47. Herrler A, Krusche CA, Beier HM. Insulin and insulin-like growth factor-I promote rabbit blastocyst development and prevent apoptosis. Biol Reprod 1998;59:1302–10.
48. O'Connor R. Survival factors and apoptosis. Adv Biochem Eng Biotechnol 1998;62:137–66.
49. Palma GA, Muller M, Brem G. Effect of insulin-like growth factor I (IGF-I) at high concentrations on blastocyst development of bovine embryos produced in vitro. J Reprod Fertil 1997;110:347–53.
50. Matsui M, Takahashi Y, Hishinuma M, Kanagawa H. Insulin and insulin-like growth factor-I (IGF-I) stimulate the development of bovine embryos fertilized in vitro. J Vet Med Sci 1995;57:1109–11.
51. Xia P, Tekpetey FR, Armstrong DT. Effect of IGF-I on pig oocyte maturation, fertilization, and early embryonic development in vitro, and on granulosa and cumulus cell biosynthetic activity. Mol Reprod Dev 1994;38:373–79.
52. Lighten AD, Hardy K, Winston RM, Moore GE. Expression of mRNA for the insulin-like growth factors and their receptors in human preimplantation embryos. Mol Reprod Dev 1997;47:134–39.
53. Rubin R, Baserga R. Insulin-like growth factor-I receptor. Its role in cell proliferation, apoptosis, and tumorigenicity. Lab Invest 1995;73:311–31.
54. Resnicoff M, Abraham D, Yutanawiboonchai W, Rotman HL, Kajstura J, Rubin R, et al. The insulin-like growth factor I receptor protects tumor cells from apoptosis in vivo. Cancer Res 1995;55:2463–69.
55. Kowalik A, Liu HC, He ZY, Mele C, Barmat L, Rosenwaks Z. Expression of the insulin-like growth factor-1 gene and its receptor in preimplantation mouse embryos; is it a marker of embryo viability? Mol Hum Reprod 1999;5:861–65.
56. Datta SR, Brunet A, Greenberg ME. Cellular survival: a play in three Akts. Genes Dev 1999;13:2905–27.

12
Predictors of Viability of the Human Blastocyst

NATALIE A. CEKLENIAK, KATHARINE V. JACKSON, AND CATHERINE RACOWSKY

The challenge to reduce the incidence of high-order multiple gestations resulting from assisted reproduction technology has revived interest in the transfer of blastocysts, as orginally attempted by Bolton et al. (1). Higher implantation rates following blastocyst transfer enable transfer of fewer embryos while maintaining high pregnancy rates; however, suboptimal extended culture systems and intrinsic embryo quality greatly influence development of a cleavage stage embryo to the blastocyst stage. In fact, a cohort of embryos may have no survival on Day 5. The dilemma, therefore, concerns which patients and which embryos are suited to blastocyst transfer.

Morphology of Day 3 embryos has been shown to have some predictive value for successful implantation (2). Parameters such as the number of eight-cell embryos on Day 3 (3), the proportion and distribution of cytoplasmic fragments (4), and the precision of membrane definition between blastomeres (5) are markers for cleavage-stage embryos with superior developmental potential. Racowsky et al. (3) proposed a selection process where only patients with at least three eight-cell embryos on Day 3 were considered good candidates for transfer of a viable blastocyst. The accuracy of this assessment, however, is limited by the fact that the embryo is relying partly on the maternal genome. With embryonic activation at the eight-cell stage (6), extended culture to identify chromosomally normal embryos seems intuitive.

A study by Asakura et al. (7) reported that all (100%) arrested cleavage-stage embryos exhibited aneuploidy. It has been proposed that prolonging embryo culture allows chromosomally normal embryos to develop to the blastocyst stage; however, they also described a 21.2% incidence of aneuploidy among blastocysts. This finding suggests that markers are necessary to identify blastocysts with a normal chromosomal complement. Morphologic criteria to identify a blastocyst with developmental competence is difficult due to the complexity of the embryo at this advanced stage. These factors have made selecting the most viable blastocysts for transfer a unique challenge.

Pregnancy rates with initial attempts using blastocysts for transfer were disappointing (1); however, implementation of sequential media for extended culture has resulted in similar pregnancy rates after transfer on Day 3 or Day 5, with fewer embryos being transferred on Day 5 (8). This protocol has the obvious advantage of decreasing the incidence of multiple gestations, but has potential disadvantages as well. When applying blastocyst transfer to an unselected population, transfer cancellation rates reach 6.7% (9). This may be considered diagnostic of poor cycle outcome regardless of transfer day. It might also indicate the need for improved extended culture conditions that would support development of the embryo to Day 5. The complete effect of extended culture on embryo development is not fully understood. Which requirements are met in our current culture system and which essential components are missing? It seems plausible that a viable embryo on Day 3, although meeting "criterion" reflecting a capacity for blastulation, may either arrest, or develop into a nonviable blastocyst, due to inadequacies of the in vitro culture system.

An increased incidence of monozygotic twinning has been noted with blastocyst transfer (10). This precarious placentation may increase the obstetrical morbidity with Day 5 transfer when compared with dizygotic twinning resulting from Day 3 transfer. It has been suggested that hardening of the zona pellucida may contribute to this observation (11). Patients at low risk for a high-order multiple pregnancy and having very few embryos typically have the same number of embryos transferred, regardless of day of transfer. Such patients, therefore, may not benefit from blastocyst transfer, and may actually be disadvantaged by potential negative effects of extended culture. Last, extended culture systems demand an enormous amount of additional work from the embryology team and laboratory. Identification of both cycle and embryo predictors of blastocyst viability should accordingly allow appropriate, prospective patient selection for blastocyst transfer.

This chapter will address the results of a retrospective analysis that examined various potential cycle and embryo predictors of blastocyst viability. In addition to investigating patient and cycle variables, individual embryo characteristics were assessed in two types of cycles, as classed by their outcomes: unsuccessful cycles (i.e., a negative pregnancy test or a chemical pregnancy) and successful cycles in which the number of fetal hearts equaled the number of blastocysts transferred. This approach allowed definitive identification of morphological features of both Day 3 and Day 5 embryos that are associated with fetal development following blastocyst transfer.

Cycle Predictors of Blastocyst Viability

Although there are several potential cycle predictors of blastocyst viability, we have chosen to target the number of eight-cell embryos on Day 3, the type of artificial reproductive technology (ART) cycle [standard in vitro fertilization (IVF) insemination vs. intracytoplasmic sperm injection (ICSI)], and patient age.

The Number of Eight-Cell Embryos on Day 3

The number of eight-cell embryos was chosen as a potential predictor of blastocyst viability based on data showing higher Day 3 pregnancy rates when at least one eight-cell embryo was available in the cohort (12). In addition, a positive correlation has been observed between the number of eight-cell embryos on Day 3 and blastocyst formation rate on Day 5 (13). Retrospective analysis to compare outcomes of Day 3 and Day 5 transfers was performed after stratification of either Day 3 or Day 5 transfers into three groups according to the number of eight-cell embryos on Day 3 (0, 1 or 2, 3 or more eight-cell embryos). Patients undergoing Day 5 transfers had at least eight zygotes at the fertilization check. The sole inclusion of a minimum of eight zygotes was based on an average blastocyst formation rate of 30–40%, thereby maximizing the probability of having at least two blastocysts available for transfer on Day 3.

When no eight-cell embryos were available on Day 3, no pregnancies occurred following transfer on Day 5, despite the same incidence of blastocyst formation compared with cycles having as many as five eight-cell embryos (Fig. 12.1); however, significantly more ongoing pregnancies were established in patients with no eight-cell embryos who had a Day 3 transfer (33.3%; $p < 0.01$), although implantation rates were not significantly different. Blastocyst formation clearly does not necessarily equate with blastocyst developmental competency in a subquality embryo cohort (i.e., no eight-cell embryos on Day 3) in our clinic. When one or two eight-cell embryos were available on Day 3, ongoing pregnancy rates, implantation rates, and the incidence of gestations with more than 2 fetal hearts were not significantly different between Day 3 and Day 5 transfers. In contrast, when there were at least three

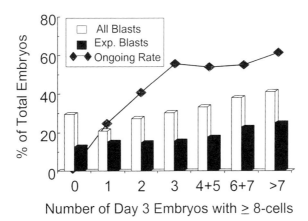

FIGURE 12.1. Relationships among the number of embryos with at least eight-cells on Day 3, blastocyst formation rate and ongoing pregnancy rate. Formation of all blastocysts, and expanded blastocysts, was significantly related to the number of embryos with at least eight-cells on Day 3 ($p < 0.001$ for both).

eight-cell embryos present in the cohort, Day 5 transfers resulted in a significantly increased implantation rate (35.9% vs. 24.2%; $p < 0.003$), but decreased incidence of gestations with more than 2 fetal hearts (4.3% vs. 17.7%; $p < 0.03$) compared with Day 3 transfers. These observations together indicate that blastocysts in these superior embryo cohorts have greater developmental potential.

ICSI Adversely Impacts on Blastocyst Viability

Several previous studies have shown decreased blastocyst formation rates following ICSI as compared with after standard insemination with IVF (14,15). Furthermore, at least one study has reported reduced clinical pregnancy rates after Day 2 or 3 transfers following ICSI (16). These observations together suggest that ICSI may adversely impact on blastocyst viability. We therefore compared blastocyst formation rates, implantation rates, and ongoing pregnancy rates following Day 5 transfer of IVF ($n = 173$) and ICSI ($n = 59$) cycles. Following ICSI, significantly fewer blastocysts formed (4.6 ± 3.8 vs. 5.4 ± 3.2, mean $\pm$ SD; $p < 0.05$), and implantation rates were significantly lower (30.9% vs. 44.2%; $p < 0.04$) when compared with IVF. Ongoing pregnancy rates per embryo transfer were lower in ICSI cycles, although the difference did not reach significance (39.0% vs. 52.0%; $p = 0.08$). These results together indicate that blastocyst development of embryos derived from ICSI is impaired compared with those from standard IVF. Whether this is due to the micromanipulation procedure per se, or from the bias of patient selection for ICSI is unknown. In support of the latter, however, previous reports (13;17; Chap. 4) have shown a reduced blastocyst formation rate without ICSI intervention in male factor patients, in the absence of any female factors.

Patient Age Impacts Pregnancy After Blastocyst Transfer

Maternal age-related aneuploidy is well documented. It has been proposed that extended culture selectively screens out the aneuploid embryos so that only euploid embryos progress to the blastocyst stage (13). Blastocyst culture, therefore, should benefit all patients including those of advanced maternal age. Retrospective analysis of our Day 5 transfers, when stratified by patient age, revealed no significant impact of age on ongoing pregnancy rates ($p = 0.220$), but did show an age-related decline in implantation rate ($p < 0.002$). One study has reported that one fifth of human morulae and blastocysts grown in vitro exhibit aneuploidy (7). The benefit of blastocyst transfer in decreasing the high-order multiple pregnancy rates for patients over 39 years is therefore questioned. Indeed, comparison of outcomes from our Day 3 and Day 5 transfers in this patient population showed similar ongoing pregnancy rates (25.0% vs. 33.3%), with no increase in high-order multiple rates following Day 3 transfer.

Embryo Predictors of Blastocyst Viability

Previous attempts to relate morphological characteristics of cleavage-stage embryos to developmental potential have shown limited predictive value (18). Such analyses have been confounded by the inability to track a particular embryo in the transferred cohort to a developing fetus. In order to be able to make definitive statements regarding the relationships between embryo morphology and blastocyst viability, it is essential to know the developmental fates of all embryos transferred. This is only possible for cycles in which either no fetus developed (negative pregnancy tests or "chemical" pregnancies) or the number of embryos transferred equals the number of fetuses (excluding monozygotic twins). Spontaneous abortions should be excluded in order to avoid a possible confounding influence of uterine factors. We have conducted such an analysis of our Day 5 data. To avoid any other confounders, ICSI cycles and all cycles with fewer than three eight-cell embryos on Day 3 were excluded.

Conventional Day 3 Morphological Characteristics

A total of 117 embryos from 71 unsuccessful cycles were compared with 68 embryos from 35 successful cycles. Stratification of embryos according to cell number on Day 3 showed that blastocyst viability increased proportionally with increasing cleavage stage from less than six-cells to eight-cells (8.3% to 37.7%). Because no further increase in viability was observed when the blastocysts were derived from embryos having more than eight-cells on Day 3 (36.4%), faster-cleaving embryos beyond the eight-cell stage may not exhibit developmental superiority. Analysis of the impact of cleavage stage fragmentation on blastocyst viability revealed a significantly higher implantation rate of blastocysts arising from embryos with less than 10 fragments ($p < 0.003$), compared with those with a greater degree of fragmentation. It is interesting that implantation rates were the same for blastocysts derived from cleavage-stage embryos with no fragmentation (40.7%), as compared with those with up to 10 fragments (43.0%). This observation, although inconsistent with a previous study indicating that embryos with no fragmentation implant at the highest rate (4), supports the possibility that a low incidence of fragmentation may provide some corrective mechanism to achieve developmental competency (19). Blastomere asymmetry on Day 3 was not associated with increased implantation rates after blastocyst transfer.

Unconventional Day 3 Morphological Characteristics

As we have improved our scoring system for Day 3 embryos, we have introduced an additional scoring parameter, referred to as reduced membrane definition (RMD; 5). This phenomenon, appearing as a reduction in definition of blastomere membranes, presumably reflects early tight junction formation in preparation of morula development, (reviewed in 20, and Chap. 8). Although there was a trend toward an increased incidence of RMD in embryos that gave rise to successful cycles, this was not statistically significant (30.9% vs. 22.2%; $p = 0.19$). In contrast, embryos resulting in successful cycles were significantly more likely to exhibit a homogeneous, granular cytoplasm throughout their blastomeres on Day 3 (11.8% vs. 5.8%; $p < 0.05$). In support of this observation, Veeck (21) noted that clinical pregnancy rates were not affected, even with moderate to severe cytoplasmic granularity.

Blastocyst Morphology

Current literature emphasizes the benefits of transferring fully expanded blastocysts to maximize implantation rates following extended culture. This paradigm has been achieved by selectively transferring expanded blastocysts, when available, on Day 5 (8), or occasionally, by obtaining fully expanded blastocysts by extending culture to either Day 6 or Day 7 (13,22). It remains unproven, however, that the most developmentally advanced blastocyst in a cohort (i.e., the one at the fully expanded stage) exhibits the greatest developmental potential. We have addressed this question by analyzing our data set involving cycles in which either no fetus developed (i.e., negative pregnancy tests or "chemical" pregnancies) or the successful cycles in which the number of embryos transferred equals the number of fetuses (excluding monozygotic twins). The successful cycles were further stratified for analysis into those in which all embryos transferred were either at the same developmental stage (i.e., morula, early, expanding, or expanded blastocyst) or at different developmental stages (referred to later as "mixed" transfers).

Consistent with previous observations (23,24), our data revealed that transfer of only morulae on Day 5 resulted in a significantly decreased implantation rate (27.3%) as compared with transfer of expanding blastocysts only (60.9%; $p < 0.05$) or expanded blastocysts (44.4%; $p < 0.05$). Of perhaps greater interest, however, is our observation that implantation rates were significantly higher when mixed transfers involved only early blastocysts combined with expanding blastocysts, as compared with mixed transfers involving at least one fully expanded blastocyst (59.1% vs. 44.4%; $p < 0.05$, Fig. 12.2). These data together argue against the premise that transfer of fully expanded blastocysts maximizes implantation rates. Even though it is possible that these most developmentally advanced blastocysts have the greatest developmental potential, asynchrony of the embryo with the uterine environment, or suboptimal culture conditions may compromise expression of this potential.

Conclusions

The preceding discussion documents cycle and embryo characteristics that appear to be associated with blastocyst viability. Standard insemination with

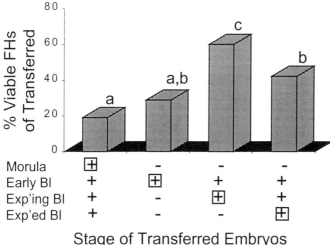

FIGURE 12.2. Stage of transferred embryos on Day 5 and blastocyst viability. Cycles were grouped according to the stages of transferred embryos (+). Groups with different letters exhibited implantation rates that were significantly different. Implantation rates were significantly higher when mixed transfers involved only early blastocysts combined with expanding blastocysts, as compared with mixed transfers involving at least one fully expanded blastocyst ($p < 0.05$).

IVF, patient age under 40 years, and a minimum of three embryos with at least eight-cells on Day 3 all provide positive predictors of blastocyst viability. Regarding embryo characteristics on Day 3, neither blastomere asymmetry nor reduced membrane definition was correlated with implantation following transfer on Day 5. It is surprising that minimal fragmentation and the presence of cytoplasmic granularity, each previously considered negatively associated with embryo viability, were independently and positively associated with increased blastocyst implantation and may actually reflect more robust embryos with a greater likelihood of successful fetal formation. As such, these observations highlight the wealth of information harbored by cleavage-stage embryos and serve to foster further work to define more precise predictors of blastocyst viability. Such research will undoubtedly explore noninvasive biochemical markers associated with developmental competency, as well as expansion of morphologic studies.

References

1. Bolton VN, Wren ME, Parsons JH. Pregnancies after in vitro fertilization and transfer of human blastocysts. Fertil Steril 1991;55:830–32.
2. Schulman A, Ben–Nun I, Ghetler Y, Kaneti H, Shilon M, Beyth Y. Relationship

between embryo morphology and implantation rate after in vitro fertilization treatment in conception cycles. Fertil Steril 1993;60(1):123–26.
3. Racowsky C, Jackson KV, Cekleniak NA, Fox JH, Hornstein MD, Ginsburg ES. The number of eight-cell embryos is a key determinant for selecting day 3 or day 5 transfer. Fertil Steril 2000;73(3):558–64.
4. Alikani M, Cohen J, Tomkin G, Garrisi J, Mack C, Scott RT. Human embryo fragmentation in vitro and its implications for pregnancy and implantation. Fertil Steril 1999;71(5):836–42.
5. Cekleniak NA, Jackson KV, Nurredin A, Shen S, de los Santos MJ, Pillar M, et al. Reduced membrane definition of blastomeres on day 3 identifies embryos resulting in higher ongoing pregnancy rates after transfer on day 5 (abstract P-051). Am Soc Reprod Med 1999;72(3)(Suppl. 1).
6. Braude PR, Bolton V, Moore S. Human gene expression first occurs between the four and eight cell stages of preimplantation development. Nature 1988;332:459–61.
7. Asakura H, Stehlik EF, Wise L, Winchester-Peden K, Stehlik JC, Katayama KP. Correlation between preimplantation genetic diagnosis (PGD) of human embryos by multicolor flourescent in situ hybridization (FISH) and blastocyst development in vitro (abstract 483). J Soc Gynecol Investig 2000;7(Suppl. 1).
8. Gardner DK, Schoolcraft WB, Wagley L, Schlenker T, Stevens J, Hesla J. A prospective randomized trial of blastocyst culture and transfer in in-vitro fertilization. Hum Reprod 1998;13(12):3434–40.
9. Del Marek MA, Langley M, Gardner DK, Confer N, Doody KM, Doody KJ. Introduction of blastocyst culture and transfer for all patients in an in vitro fertilization program. Fertil Steril 1999;72(6):1035–40.
10. Behr B, Fisch JD, Racowsky C, Miller K, Pool TB, Milki AA. Blastocyst-ET and monozygotic twinning. J Assist Reprod Genet 2000;17:349–51.
11. Cohen J, Elsner C, Kort H, Malter H, Massey J, Mayer MP, et al. Impairment of the hatching process following IVF in the human and improvemnet of implantation by assisting hatching using micromanipulation. Hum Reprod 1990;5:7–13.
12. Carrillo AJ, Lane B, Pridham DD, Risch P, Pool TB, Silverman IH, et al. Improved clinical outcomes for in vitro fertilization with delay of embryo transfer from 48 to 72 hours after oocyte retrieval: use of glucose- and phosphate-free media. Fertil Steril 1998;69:329–34.
13. Jones GM, Trounson AO, Lolatgis N, Wood C. Factors affecting the success of human blastocyst development and pregnancy following in vitro fertilization and embryo transfer. Fertil Steril 1998;70(6):1022–29.
14. Shoukir Y, Chardonnens D, Campana A, Sakkas D. Blastocyst development from supernumerary embryos after intracytoplasmic sperm injection: a paternal influence? Hum Reprod 1998;13(6):1632–37.
15. Dumoulin JC, Coonen E, Bras M, Van Wissen LC, Ignoul-Vanvuchele R, Bergers-Jansen JM, Derhaag JG, et al. Comparison of in-vitro development of embryos originating from either conventional in-vitro fertilization or intracytoplasmic sperm injection. Hum Reprod 2000;15(2):402–9.
16. Bar-Hava I, Ashkenazi J, Shelef M, Schwartz A, Brenguaz M, Feldber Orvieto R, et al. Morphology and clinical outcomes of embryos after in vitro fertilization are superior to those after intracytoplasmic sperm injection. Fertil Steril 1997;68(4):653–57.
17. Janny L, Menezo YJ. Evidence for a strong paternal effect on human preimplantation embryo development and blastocyst formation. Mol Reprod Dev 1994;38(1):36–42.

18. Bolton VN, Hawes SM, Taylor CT, Parsons JH. Development of spare human preimplantation embryos in vitro; an analysis of the correlations among gross morphology, cleavage rates, and development to the blastocyst. J In Vitro Fert Embryo Transf 1989;6:30–35.
19. Ziebe S, Petersen K, Lindenberg S, Andersen AG, Gabrielsen A, Andersen AN. Embryo morphology or cleavage stage: how to select the best embryos for transfer after in-vitro fertilization. Hum Reprod 1997;12(7):1545–49.
20. Ducibella T, Albertini DF, Anderson E, Biggers JD. The preimplantation mammalian embryo: characterization of intercellular junctions and their appearance during development. Dev Biol 1975;45:231–50.
21. Veeck LL. An atlas of human gametes and conceptuses. New York: Parthenon Publishing, 1999:64.
22. Shoukir Y, Chardonnens D, Campana A, Bischof P, Sakkas D. The rate of development and time of transfer play different roles in influencing the viability of human blastocysts. Hum Reprod 1998;13(13):676–81.
23. Scholtes MCW, Zeilmaker GH. Blastocyst transfer in day-5 embryo transfer depends primarily on the number of oocytes retrieved and not on age. Fertil Steril 1998;69(1): 78–83.
24. Huisman GJ, Fauser BCJM, Eijkemans MJC, Pieters MHEC. Implantation rates after in vitro fertilization and transfer of a maximum of two embryos that have undergone three to five days in culture. Fertil Steril 2000;73(1):117–22.

Part IV

Blastocyst Transfer
and Fate

13

Which Patients Should Have Blastocyst Transfer?

KEVIN DOODY

The successful attainment of pregnancy via in vitro fertilization (IVF) is dependent on successful embryo culture. The traditional application of IVF relies on short-term (2–3-day) culture of preimplantation embryos prior to transfer. The primary rationale for short-term culture is the belief that the culture conditions available generally fail to support embryo development adequately for the full period of preimplantation development. This belief is hardly surprising in that many embryology laboratories continue to use media that were developed many years ago for somatic cell culture. It has been well documented that these simple salt solutions, and even more complex nutrient media such as Ham's F-10, fail to support viable embryonic development to the blastocyst stage even when supplemented by albumin or whole serum (1).

The widespread growth of IVF in the 1980s prompted the development of culture media designed specifically for the human embryo. These media include B2 (a complex solution containing amino acids, vitamins, and nucleic acid precursors, as well as albumin) developed by Menezo and colleagues (2), as well as human tubal fluid medium (HTF) developed by Quinn and his coworkers (3). HTF is a simple balanced salt solution designed with a higher K^+ content designed to mimic that reported for the tubal lumen in vivo. Despite being designed specifically for human embryo culture, this medium did not prove to be adequate to support consistent development beyond the cleavage stage.

One approach to human embryo culture has been the technique of co-culture in the presence of somatic cells. A variety of cell types have been used from different sources including human, bovine and monkey (4,5). Co-culture may condition the culture environment, either by removing embryotoxic substances or by adding cytokines/growth factors (4,5). The use of co-culture techniques to extend the duration of in vitro development has been reported. The experience with co-culture has led to mixed results unfortunately. Because of theoretical risks associated with co-culture (transmission of infectious disease) and the increased time and expense involved, the widespread adoption of this technique for human IVF remains unlikely.

Sequential culture media has also been designed to promote embryo growth past the first 48 hours of development through Day 5 or 6 of development (1,6). These culture systems have been employed by human IVF programs to culture embryos to the blastocyst prior to transfer successfully (7). Initial studies implementing this type of culture system have demonstrated that extended embryo culture techniques can be used for selected patients who respond well to gonadotropins, and that the resulting implantation and pregnancy rates are high. The high implantation rates of transferred blastocysts have been attributed primarily to an enhanced ability to select healthy embryos. Embryos that are unable to sustain growth and development for 5–6 days in the laboratory are likely to be abnormal. Those that do develop are more likely to be healthy. One highly touted advantage of extended embryo culture is the ability to maintain high pregnancy rates while transferring fewer embryos, thus minimizing the risk of high-order multiple pregnancy. It seems clear that if an IVF program is able to implement a successful program of blastocyst culture, this technique should be performed in all patients who produce several rapidly developing cleavage-stage embryos. The only alternative to blastocyst culture in these patients would be the transfer of three or more cleavage-stage embryos. Although this might achieve a comparable pregnancy rate, the risk of triplet or other high-order gestations would certainly be increased.

Extended laboratory culture of embryos has additional potential benefits beyond the enhanced ability to select the healthiest embryos. An improved embryonic environment has been cited frequently as an additional possible benefit. In the natural state, early embryonic development to the morula stage occurs within the oviduct. The endometrial cavity is very different from the oviduct in terms of composition of its luminal fluid (8). It seems very likely that culture conditions that could closely mimic the environment of the fallopian tube might provide a more optimal environment for growth and development of the cleavage stage embryo and morula. In fact, sequential culture media has been designed to satisfy the known changing metabolic requirements of the developing embryo (6). Although further research will likely identify growth factors or other components of oviductal fluid that enhance embryonic development, currently available media may already be superior to the uterine environment for promotion of early embryo development. If that is the case, currently available blastocyst culture systems would benefit all patients undergoing IVF, not simply those with high numbers of follicles, eggs, or cleavage stage embryos.

Finally, blastocyst culture provides the laboratory and clinician with valuable information on patients who fail to conceive. Failure of embryonic development past the cleavage stage, retarded development or morphologic abnormalities may disclose or provide useful hints as to the cause of failed conception (9). This information can be used clinically to counsel patients regarding future treatment options. In this regard, blastocyst culture may be even more valuable in older or poor responder patients than they are in young high responders.

Some programs have been reluctant to perform blastocyst transfer for fear that the currently available culture systems and techniques may decrease the potential development of some embryos. The concern exists that an impairment of embryonic development, though counterbalanced in high responders by enhanced embryo selection, will result in lower rates of implantation and pregnancy in poor or medium responders where an enhanced capacity to select embryos may be limited or absent. In addition, one would postulate that if embryonic development is impaired, than fewer embryos would be cryopreserved and fewer pregnancies would ultimately result following thaw even in good responders.

Stategies for Patient Selection for Blastocyst Transfer

1. Good-prognosis patients as determined by preretrieval parameters (e.g., 10 or more follicles).

2. Good-prognosis patients as determined by retrieval parameters (e.g., 10 or more eggs).

3. Good-prognosis patients as determined by postinsemination parameters (e.g., seven or eight or more 2PN).

4. Good-prognosis patients as determined by cleavage-stage status (three or more eight-cell embryos on Day 3).

5. Combination criteria (e.g., eight or more 2PN *and* three or more eight-cell embryos on Day 3).

6. Poor-prognosis patients as defined by age, elevated FSH, or prior IVF failure.

7. All patients: Good and poor prognosis.

Blastocyst Transfer in Good-Prognosis Patients as Determined by Preretrieval Parameters

Advantages

1. Enhanced selection of embryos for transfer and cryopreservation.

2. Higher implantation rates can result in high-pregnancy rates with low risk of high-order multiple pregnancy.

3. Environment of cleavage-stage embryos, morulae in laboratory may enhance embryonic development.

170   K. Doody

4. Patient counseling done prior to egg retrieval.

5. Laboratory preparation in advance.

6. Poor blastulation rate may identify occult poor prognosis factor.

Disadvantages

1. Higher risk of no transfer/cycle cancellation than cleavage stage transfers.

2. Potentially reduced embryos for cryopreservation.

3. Poor culture system may decrease embryonic potential.

4. Good follicle numbers do not always correlate with MII egg numbers.

5. Low fertilization rate may result in lack of enhanced selection capacity.

Blastocyst Transfer in Good-Prognosis Patients as Determined by Retrieval Parameters

Advantages

1. Enhanced selection of embryos for transfer and cryopreservation.

2. Higher implantation rates can result in high-pregnancy rates with low risk of high-order multiple pregnancy.

3. Environment of cleavage-stage embryos, morulae in laboratory may enhance embryonic development.

4. Poor blastulation rate may identify occult poor prognosis factor.

5. Less risk of low number of embryos as compared with preretrieval selection.

Disadvantages

1. Higher risk of no transfer/cycle cancellation than cleavage-stage transfers.

2. Potentially reduced embryos for cryopreservation.

3. Poor culture system may decrease embryonic potential.

4. Patient counseling in advance is more difficult.

5. Lab preparation in advance is limited.

6. Low fertilization rate may result in lack of reduced selection capacity.

7. No benefit for poor prognosis patients.

Blastocyst Transfer in Good-Prognosis Patients as Determined by Postinsemination Parameters

Advantages

1. Enhanced selection of embryos for transfer and cryopreservation.

2. Higher implantation rates can result in high-pregnancy rates with low risk of high-order multiple pregnancy.

3. Environment of cleavage-stage embryos, morulae in laboratory may enhance embryonic development.

4. Poor blastulation rate may identify occult poor prognosis factor.

5. Less risk of low number of embryos as compared with selection by follicle or egg number.

Disadvantages

1. Higher risk of no transfer/cycle cancellation than cleavage stage transfers.

2. Potentially reduced embryos for cryopreservation.

3. Poor culture system may decrease embryonic potential.

4. Patient counseling in advance is more difficult.

5. Lab preparation in advance is limited.

6. No benefit for poor prognosis patients.

7. Low cleavage rate may result in lack of reduced selection capacity.

Blastocyst Transfer in Good-Prognosis Patients as Determined by Cleavage-Stage Parameters

Advantages

1. Enhanced selection of embryos for transfer and cryopreservation.

2. Higher implantation rates can result in high-pregnancy rates with low risk of high-order multiple pregnancy.

3. Environment of cleavage-stage embryos, morulae in laboratory may enhance embryonic development.

4. Poor blastulation rate may identify occult poor prognosis factor.

5. Less risk of low number of embryos as compared with selection by follicle, egg, or 2PN number.

Disadvantages

1. Higher risk of no transfer/cycle cancellation than cleavage-stage transfers.

2. Potentially reduced embryos for cryopreservation.

3. Poor culture system may decrease embryonic potential.

4. Patient counseling in advance is increasingly more difficult.

5. Lab preparation in advance is increasingly limited.

6. No benefit for poor prognosis patients.

Blastocyst Transfer in Good-Prognosis Patients Using Combination Criteria (e.g., Eight or More 2PN *and* Three or More Eight-Cell Embryos on Day 3)

Advantages

1. Enhanced selection of embryos for transfer and cryopreservation.

2. Higher implantation rates can result in high-pregnancy rates with low risk of multiple pregnancy.

3. Environment of cleavage-stage embryos, morulae in laboratory may enhance embryonic development.

4. Poor blastulation rate may identify occult poor prognosis factor.

5. Minimal risk of no transfer/cycle cancellation compared with cleavage-stage transfers.

Disadvantages

1. Potentially reduced embryos for cryopreservation.

2. Poor culture system may decrease embryonic potential.

3. Patient counseling in advance is increasingly more difficult.

4. Lab preparation in advance is increasingly limited.

5. No benefit for poor prognosis patients.

6. No benefit for moderate prognosis patients with regard to risk of multiple pregnancy.

Blastocyst Transfer in Poor-Prognosis Patients as Defined by Age, Elevated FSH, Prior IVF Failure, Preretrieval, Retrieval, Postinsemination, or Cleavage-Stage Parameters

Advantages

1. Environment of cleavage-stage embryos, morulae in laboratory may enhance embryonic development.

2. Poor blastulation rate may indicate additional poor prognosis factor.

Disadvantages

1. Higher risk of no transfer/cycle cancellation than cleavage stage transfers.

2. Potentially reduced embryos for cryopreservation.

3. Poor culture system may decrease already limited embryonic potential.

4. Patient counseling in advance is limited in poor prognosis patients identified postretrieval.

5. Lab preparation in advance may be limited.

Blastocyst Transfer in All Patients: Good and Poor Prognosis

Advantages

1. Environment of cleavage-stage embryos, morulae in laboratory may enhance embryonic development.

2. Poor blastulation rate may indicate additional poor prognosis factor.

3. Enhanced selection of embryos for transfer and cryopreservation in good prognosis patients.

4. Higher implantation rates in good prognosis patients can result in high pregnancy rates with low risk of high-order multiple pregnancy.

5. Patient counseling done prior to procedure.

6. Lab preparation in advance.

7. In conjunction with strict adherence to cycle starts and stimulation protocols, can enhance efficiency of IVF team.

Disadvantages

1. Higher risk of no transfer/cycle cancellation than cleavage-stage transfers.

2. Potentially reduced embryos for cryopreservation.

3. Poor culture system may decrease embryonic potential resulting in lower pregnancy rates, especially in poor prognosis subgroups.

Advantages of Nonselective Blastocyst Culture: What Are the Data?

1. In the first clinical application of extended co-culture of embryos on Vero cells, Menezo reported a 56% blastocyst formation rate and a 44%

pregnancy rate in a series of 62 patients with repeated IVF failures (4). In our program, an increased efficiency of IVF in nonselected patients that has been demonstrated suggests that overall embryonic development is enhanced with currently available culture systems. A calculation of cycle efficiency using our data (Tables 13.1 to 13.3) is performed using the following formula (11): [(mean number of embryos transferred × mean implantation rate) + (mean number of embryos cryopreserved × mean implantation rate)] × (1- cancellation rate). This yields an efficiency of Day 3 transfers of 0.83 and of Day 5/6 transfers of 0.99.

2. Poor blastulation rate in one cycle predicts poor blastulation rate in a second cycle even in "good-prognosis" patients (Table 13.4).

3. Higher implantation rates with maintenance of high pregnancy rates and reduced risk of high-order multiple pregnancy in good prognosis patients have been documented by several groups.

4. Uniform counseling of patients in advance: emperic.

5. Uniform laboratory process: emperic.

6. Extended embryo culture together with strict adherence to stimulation protocols can minimize weekend procedures and improve efficiency of IVF team.

Disadvantages of Nonselective Blastocyst Culture: What Are the Data?

1. Higher risk of no transfer/cycle cancellation than cleavage-stage transfers is seen (Table 13.1). Overall increased cancellation will necessarily be an effect of an enhanced ability to select out nonviable embryos. This should not be regarded as a true disadvantage as long as pregnancy rates per retrieval are not diminished. Patients feel no less sorrow if they are allowed to have false hope for an additional 9 days until a blood test confirms embryo nonviability. If it is the goal of the physician and lab to mislead the patient and give unrealistic expectations, nonviable embryos could still be transferred if no healthy embryos are available. Although we feel that patients should not be misled, our policy has been to give embryos the benefit of the doubt, and we will transfer if embryos have exhibited any developmental changes suggesting compaction or blastocoele formation, even if these changes are atypical in nature. This policy has resulted in a minimal increase in actual cancellation of transfers, but still allows acquisition of information that is useful in counseling patients after failed cycles.

TABLE 13.1. Evaluation of embryo transfer cancellations between Day 3 and Day 5: C.A.R. (1997–1998).

	Age <35		Age 35–39		Age >39		Total	
	Day 3	Day 5	Day 3	Day 5	Day 3	Day 5	Day 3	Day 5
No. of retrievals	242	164	165	124	70	25	477	313
No. of cancelled transfers	7	9	7	10	0	2	14	21*
No. of total transfers	235	155	158	114	70	23	463	292

Source: Data from Marek et al. (9).
*$p < 0.05$ (vs. Day 3 total).

2. Potentially reduced embryos for cryopreservation has not been demonstrated in our program (Table 13.2). In addition, the implantation and pregnancy rates following thaw have been considerably improved following embryo thaw at the blastocyst stage (Table 13.3). These findings likely reflect improved environmental conditions for the embryo as well as cryopreservation of supernumerary embryos that might have resulted in a high-order multiple pregnancy if transferred at the cleavage stage according to common protocols in which three or more embryos are transferred.

3. Poor culture systems may reduce the embryonic potential resulting in lower pregnancy rates, especially in poor prognosis groups where embryo selection cannot counterbalance reduced embryo viability. Although this is a significant concern for programs that have not implemented successful blastocyst culture systems, only one study to date has purported to identify a poor prognosis group that has been adversely affected by extended embryo culture (12). In that study, blastocyst cultures in patients meeting the criteria of having at least eight fertilized eggs, with no embryos reaching the eight-cell stage by Day 3 of culture, were compared with historical controls with traditional 3-day culture. The ongoing pregnancy rate was significantly lower in the extended culture group (Tables 13.5 and 13.6) than were the controls. On the other hand, our data demonstrates that Day 3 embryos with retarded development do produce viable blastocysts, albeit at a reduced rate (Table 13.7). The rate of formation of blastocyst from cleavage-stage embryos with retarded development may vary depending on the culture conditions. The rate of progression of embryos in a Vero cell co-culture system (13) is shown in Table 13.8. Data from our program indicates that blastocysts resulting from initially slowly cleaving embryos are capable of implantation with reasonable pregnancy rates (Tables 13.9 and 13.10). These results do not support the selection of patients for early transfer based on low numbers

TABLE 13.2. Comparison of embryo transfer results on Day 3 vs. Day 5 for specific age groups: C.A.R. (1/1997–6/1999).

	Age <35		Age 35–39		Age >39		All ages	
	Day 3	Day 5/6	Day 3	Day 5/6	Day 3	Day 5/6	Day 3	Day 5/6
Mean patient age (years)	31.4 ±0.18	31.1 ±0.16	36.9 ±0.11	37.3 ±0.11	42.3 ±0.19	41.7 ±0.24	34.9 ±0.21	34.1 ±0.19
No. of transfers	235	272	158	173	70	35	463	480
Total no. of oocytes	3354	3850	1765	2076	539	346	5658	6272
Total no. of 2PN zygotes	1740	2159	890	1166	276	213	2906	3538
Mean no. of embryos transferred	2.95 ±0.05	2.22 ±0.04**	3.11 ±0.08	2.46 ±0.06**	3.06 ±0.16	2.77 ±0.15	3.02 ±0.04	2.35 ±0.03**
Mean no. of embryos for cryopreservation	2.15 ±0.24	2.05 ±0.18	1.27 ±0.21	1.13 ±0.17	0.14 ±0.09	0.60 ±0.39	1.54 ±0.14	1.61 ±0.12
No. of clinical sacs: (1/2/3/4)	57/49/15/1	80/54/9/0	36/16/10/1	53/16/9/0	7/3/2/0	8/3/0/0	100/68/27/2	141/73/18/0
Implantation rate (%)	29.5	35.6*	20.7	26.4†	8.9	14.4	23.3	30.3**
Pregnancies (+hCG) (%)	57.0	61.8	44.3	54.3	22.9	37.1	47.	57.3
Ongoing Pregnancy (%)	46.4	45.2	32.9	37.6	14.3	31.4	36.9	41.5

Source: Data from Marek et al. (9).
*Excludes all donor cycles.
*$p < 0.05$ (vs. Day 3 total).
**$p < 0.001$ (vs. Day 3 total).
†$p = 0.054$ (vs. Day 3 total).

TABLE 13.3. Frozen embryo transfer Day 3 vs. Day 5: C.A.R. (1/1997–6/1999).

	Day 3	Day 5
Mean patient age (year)	34.7 ± 0.45	35.9 ± 0.61
No. of transfers	119	72
Mean no. of embryo transferred	3.07 ± 0.10	2.35 ± 0.08**
No. of clinical sacs: (1/2/3/4)	20/7/1/0	22/6/1/0
Implantation rate (%)	10.1	21.9**
Pregnancies (+hCG) per ET (%)	30.2	54.2**
Ongoing pregnancy per ET (%)	18.5	33.3*

Source: Data from Langley et al. (10).
*$p < 0.05$ (vs. Day 3 total).
**$p < 0.01$ (vs. Day 3 total).

Table 13.4. Predictive value of poor blastulation in good-prognosis patients (seven or more 2PN): C.A.R. (1/1998–2/2000).

Patient	Cycle #1			Cycle #2			ΔBlast rate
	Total 2PN	Total blast	Blast rate	Total 2PN	Total blast	Blast rate	
1	14	2	0.14	14	0	0.00	−0.14
2	12	1	0.08	9	2	0.22	0.14
3	8	1	0.13	9	6*	0.67	0.54
4	7	1	0.14	8	3	0.38	0.23
5	7	1	0.14	8	2	0.25	0.11
6	7	1	0.14	9	7*	0.78	0.63
7	13	2	0.15	11	4	0.36	0.21
All Patients	68	9	0.13	68	24**	0.35	0.22

*$p < 0.05$ (vs. total blast cycle #1 using Fisher's exact test).
**$p < 0.01$ (vs. total blast cycle #1 using Fisher's exact test).

TABLE 13.5. Blastocyst transfer in good-prognosis patients (eight or more zygotes).

	Day of ET	Number of eight-cell embryos on Day 3		
		0	1 – 2	≥3
No. of retrievals/	3	27/27	77/77	117
transfers	5	14/11	51/47	83
No. of ongoing	3	9 (33.3)	28 (36.4)	60 (51.3)
pregnancies (% of ETs)	5	0	19 (40.4)	42 (50.6)

Source: Data from Racowsky et al. (12).

Table 13.6. Blastocyst transfer risk of multiple pregnancy.

Number of eight-cell embryos on Day 3	Day of embryo transfer	Number of transfers	Number of patients with fetal hearts	Number of fetal hearts (%)		
				1	2	3
0	3	27	9	8 (88.9)	1 (11.1)	0
	5	11	0	0	0	0
1–2	3	77	33	15 (45.4)	15 (45.4)	3 (9.1)
	5	47	19	12 (63.1)	7 (36.8)	0
≥3	3	117	62	31 (50.0)	20 (32.3)	11 (17.7)
	5	83	46	28 (60.9)	16 (34.8)	2 (4.3)

Source: Data from Racowsky et al. (12).

180   K. Doody

TABLE 13.7. Blastocyst development from Day 3 multicell embryos: C.A.R. (1/1998–6/1999).*

Age	Day 3 cell stage:	Two cell	Three cell	Four cell	Five cell	Six cell	Seven cell	Eight cell	Nine cell	10+ cell
<35	Total number embryos	91	132	497	385	501	454	806	80	124
	Blast day 5 (%)	5/5.5	7/5.3	108/21.7	110/28.6	232/46.3	255/56.2	581/72.1	50/62.5	86/69.4
	Blast day 6 (%)	2/2.2	12/9.1	61/12.3	46/12.0	62/12.4	54/11.9	64/7.9	12/15.0	6/4.8
	Total blast (day 5 + 6) (%)	7/7.7	19/14.4	169/34.0	156/40.5	294/58.7	309/68.1	645/80.0	62/77.5	92/74.2
35–39	Total number embryos	47	65	262	156	180	167	277	18	29
	Blast day 5 (%)	1/2.1	1/1.5	30/11.5	47/30.1	68/37.8	88/52.7	180/65.0	14/77.8	20/69.0
	Blast day 6 (%)	0/0	2/3.1	33/12.6	11/7.1	19/10.6	16/9.6	22/7.9	0/0	2/6.9
	Total blast (day 5 + 6) (%)	1/2.1	3/4.6	63/24.1	58/37.2	87/48.3	104/62.3	202/72.9	14/77.8	22/75.9
>39	Total number embryos	12	12	51	25	36	24	63	3	6
	Blast day 5 (%)	0/0	0/0	7/13.7	6/24.0	11/30.6	12/50.0	42/66.7	3/100	2/33.3
	Blast day 6 (%)	0/0	0/0	7/13.7	3/12.0	2/5.6	3/12.5	1/1.6	0/0	1/16.7
	Total Blast (day 5 + 6) (%)	0/0	0/0	14/27.5	9/36.0	13/36.1	15/62.5	43/68.3	3/100	3/50.0
All ages	Total number embryos	150	209	810	566	717	645	1146	101	159
	Blast day 5 (%)	6/4.0	8/3.8	145/17.9	163/28.8	311/43.4	355/55.0	803/70.1	67/66.3	108/67.9
	Blast day 6 (%)	2/1.3	14/6.7	101/12.5	60/10.6	83/11.6*	73/11.3	87/7.6	12/11.9	9/5.7
	Total blast (day 5 + 6) (%)	8/5.3	22/10.5	246/30.4	223/39.4	394/55.0	428/66.4	890/77.7	79/78.2	117/13.6

*Includes donor statistics in age <35 category.

TABLE 13.8. Blastocyst development from Day 3 cleavage embryos co-cultured with Vero cells.

Cell number	Number of embryos	Number of blasts	Blast/embryo
2	40	0	0
3	42	1	.024
4	103	4	.039
5	99	17	.172
6	137	44	.321
7	128	63	.492
8	245	184	.751
9–12	23	20	.870

Source: Data from Sharpio et al. (13).

TABLE 13.9. Transfer of blastocysts from embryos of known cell number on Day 3: C.A.R. (1/1998–6/1999).

Day 3 cell stage ET	Patients (n)	Ongoing pregnancy	Average number transferred	Implantation rate
1–2	1	0	2.0	0%
3–4	23	4 (17.4%)	1.9	9.3%
5–6	34	11 (32.4%)	1.6	32.7%
7–8	140	69 (49.3%)	2.1	38.8%
9–10	2	1 (50%)	1.5	66.6%

Source: Data from Langley et al. (10).
*Excludes all donor cycles.

TABLE 13.10. Blastocyst transfer in good- and poor-prognosis patients in which no eight-cell embryos were present on Day 3: C.A.R. (1/1998–2/2000).

Results	≥8 2PN	<8 2PN
Mean patient age (±SEM)	33.1 ± 0.97	34.7 ± 0.40
No. retrievals	30	113
No. embryo transfers	29	101
Pregnancies (+hCG)/ongoing	15/11	44/31
Biochemical/miscarriage/ectopic	3/1/0	6/6/1
Pregnancy/ongoing rate per transfer	51.7%/37.9%	43.5%/30.7%
Total embryos/mean transferred	73/2.52	231/2.29
No. 2PN/mean number 2PN	286/9.53	436/3.86
No. blastocyst/per 2PN	111*/38.8%	115/26.4%
No. clinical sacs (1/2/3)	8/3/1	27/8/2
Implantation rate	23.3%	21.2%

Source: Data from Langley et al. (10).
*$p < 0.001$ (vs. <8 2PN category using χ^2 Test).

of rapidly cleaving embryos in our program. In fact, we have been unable to define any subgroup of patients based on clinical or laboratory parameters that appears to have a reduced likelihood of pregnancy per retrieval than our historical controls undergoing traditional three day culture.

Conclusions

Extended embryo culture is technically feasible in nonselected IVF patients using commercially available sequential media together with defined clinical and laboratory protocols.

Advantages of application of this technique to all IVF patients are likely to continue to expand along with improvements in media and culture systems. These advantages include: 1) maintenance of high pregnancy rates with a reduced risk of multiple pregnancy in "good-prognosis" patients, 2) improvements in cryopreservation outcomes, 3) enhanced embryo viability secondary to environmental conditions, and 4) identification of patients with occult poor prognosis factors.

Disadvantages with extended embryo culture will be encountered in programs where suboptimal culture systems result in decreased embryo viability. Although enhanced embryo selection will, to a degree, mask impairments of embryo potential, significant problems would likely be encountered in these programs. This includes decreased embryos for cryopreservation and poor outcome in "poor-prognosis" patients where the advantage of enhanced embryo selection is not present. Although selective application of blastocyst culture is a legitimate short-term approach in these programs, the full advantages of blastocyst culture will not be realized until applied to all patients.

References

1. Gardner DK, Lane M. Culture of viable human blastocysts in defined sequential serum-free media. Hum Reprod 1998;13(Suppl. 3):148–59.
2. Menezo Y, Testart J, Perrone D. Serum is not necessary in human in vitro fertilization, early embryo culture, and transfer. Fertil Steril 1984;42:750–55.
3. Quinn P, Kerin JF, Warnes GM. Improved pregnancy rate in human in vitro fertilization with the use of a medium based on the composition of human tubal fluid. Fertil Steril 1985;44:493–98.
4. Menezo Y, Hazout A, Dumont M, Herbaut N, Nicollet B. Coculture of embryos on Vero cells and transfer of blastocysts in humans. Hum Reprod 1992;7(Suppl. 1): 101–6.
5. Bongso A, Fong CY. The effect of coculture on human zygote development. Curr Opin Obstet Gynecol 1993;5:585–93.
6. Gardner DK, Lane M. Culture and selection of viable blastocysts: a feasible proposition for human IVF? Hum Reprod Update 1997;3:367–82.
7. Gardner DK, Schoolcraft WB, Wagley L, Schlenker T, Stevens J, Hesla J. A

prospective randomized trial of blastocyst culture and transfer in in-vitro fertilization. Hum Reprod 1998;13:3434–40.
8. Gardner DK, Lane M, Calderon I, Leeton J. Environment of the preimplantation human embryo in vivo: metabolite analysis of oviduct and uterine fluids and metabolism of cumulus cells. Fertil Steril 1996;65:349–53.
9. Marek D, Langley M, Gardner DK, Confer N, Doody KM, Doody KJ. Introduction of blastocyst culture and transfer for all patients in an in vitro fertilization program. Fertil Steril 1999;72:1035–40.
10. Langley M, Marek D, Gardner DK, Confer N, Doody KM, Doody KJ. Efficacy of blastocyst transfer in human ART. Hum Reprod 2001 (in press).
11. Gardner DK, Lane M, Schoolcraft WB. Culture and transfer of viable blastocysts: a feasible proposition for human IVF. Hum Reprod 2000;15(Suppl. 6):9–23.
12. Racowsky C, Jackson KV, Cekleniak NA, Fox JH, Hornstein MD, Ginsburg ES. The number of eight-cell embryos is a key determinant for selecting day 3 or day 5 transfer. Fertil Steril 2000;73:558–64.
13. Shapiro BS, Harris DC, Richter KS. Predictive value of 72-hour blastomere cell number on blastocyst development and success of subsequent transfer based on the degree of blastocyst development. Fertil Steril 2000;73:582–86.

14

Embryo Transfer and Luteal Phase Support

WILLIAM B. SCHOOLCRAFT

The main variables affecting pregnancy and implantation rates are uterine receptivity, embryo quality, and transfer efficiency. Much less effort has historically been placed on assessing or maximizing embryo transfer procedures compared with the other aspects of in vitro fertilization. Embryo transfer is usually performed blindly with no attempt to document the variables that might adversely impact pregnancy rates. Physicians too frequently underestimate the importance of the embryo transfer technique and are often unwilling to modify their own personal habits or catheter choices.

Variables Affecting Embryo Transfer Success

The ultimate goal of a successful embryo transfer is to deliver the embryos atraumatically to the uterine fundus in a location where implantation is maximized. A trial transfer in a cycle proceeding in vitro fertilization (IVF) for the purpose of measuring the uterine cavity depth and direction appears to be of value. Mansour (1) evaluated 335 patients randomized to a precycle trial transfer or no trial transfer. Embryo transfer was found to be difficult in 50 (29.8%) cases where no trial transfer was performed, compared with no difficult embryo transfers in the trial transfer group. For the trial transfer group, the pregnancy and implantation rates were 22.8% and 7.2%, respectively, compared with a 13.1% pregnancy rate and 4.3% implantation in the no trial transfer group.

Embryos may occasionally fail to make it into the uterine cavity. Poindexter (2) found that 4 of 46 patients (8.7%) had embryos in the cervix or on the speculum after an apparently routine embryo transfer. Embryos may also be retained in the catheter. Plugging of the catheter tip with mucus, blood, or endometrial tissue is commonly the cause of this complication. Inadequate transfer volume or improper placement of the embryos in the transfer column can also cause embryo retention.

Visser (3) found that pregnancy rates fell from 20.3% to 3% when retained embryos occurred. Cohen (4) found a significant decrease in implantation rates, but not in pregnancy rates, when one or more embryos were retained.

Mucus plugging of the catheter tip can be a cause of retained embryos, damage to the embryos (especially with assisted hatching), and improper embryo placement. Mansour (1) found that prior aspiration of cervical mucus led to methylene blue in the cervix on 23% of mock embryo transfers. Without aspiration, 57% of patients demonstrated methylene blue in the cervix with a mock transfer.

Cervical mucus was shown by Egbase to be culture positive in 71% of cases (5). This in turn led to a positive culture of the catheter tip in 49% of patients. The clinical pregnancy rate was 29.6% in catheter-tip positive patients versus a 57% pregnancy rate when the catheter tip was culture negative.

MacNamee and colleagues (6) evaluated a vigorous cervical lavage technique prior to embryo transfer to remove all visible mucus. In a retrospective study, patients undergoing vigorous lavage demonstrated a 55.5% pregnancy rate and a 26% implantation rate compared with a 41.7% pregnancy rate and 10.4% implantation in control patients.

The benefit of one catheter type over another is controversial. Wisanto (7) studied three catheter types in 400 patients, retrospectively. The pregnancy rate was: Frydman (32.3%), Wallace (19.2%), and TDT (19.4%). In contrast, Al-Shawaf (8) found no difference between the Frydman (30.7%) and the Wallace (30.3%). Findings were similar in a study from Englert (9).

There has been a worldwide trend toward the use of soft catheters (e.g., Wallace). The possible advantages of this catheter are its ability to follow the contour of the endometrial cavity rather than to penetrate the endometrial surface, less chance of the tip becoming plugged with mucus or endometrial tissue, and less bleeding. A disadvantage of the Wallace catheter is the greater difficulty associated with insertion, particularly in patients with significantly anteverted or retroflexed uteri.

Ultrasound-Guided Embryo Transfer

At the Colorado Center for Reproductive Medicine, we have found that the single greatest aid in utilizing the Wallace catheter successfully is the addition of transabdominal ultrasound guidance. Blind catheter placement has been shown to result in the inadvertent location of the catheter tip outside the endometrial cavity in more than 25% of cases (10).

A full bladder is required for transabdominal ultrasound guidance, and it has the benefit of straightening the cervicouterine axis in cases of significant angulation. With ultrasound guidance, the endocervical and endometrial canals can be followed with the catheter, making any adjustments with the catheter and speculum as necessary to avoid forcing the catheter against the endometrial surface. It also allows the physician to avoid hitting the fundus with the catheter, and enables the clinician to confirm that the catheter tip has passed the internal os prior to injection of the embryos. This results in the atraumatic placement of embryos 1–2 cm from the fundus in the lumen of the cavity without traumatizing the uterus or the embryos.

Our experience utilizing this technique for embryo transfer in combination with blastocyst culture in oocyte donation cycles has demonstrated a greater than 60% implantation rate per embryo. Assuming that uterine receptivity, genetics, and unknown factors account for a portion of the 40% of failures, the efficiency of embryo transfer with soft catheters and ultrasound guidance is quite high indeed.

Luteal Support for In Vitro Fertilization

Current methods of IVF predispose patients to luteal phase defects. GnRH analogs which are routinely used for controlled ovarian hyperstimulation, result in continued suppression of LH in the luteal phase. They may also affect ovarian steroid production directly. The net effect is aberrant progesterone production. Follicular aspiration for oocyte retrieval compounds the problem by aspirating granulosa cells that are the source of progesterone production.

A meta-analysis (11) of luteal phase support for IVF has revealed a significantly higher clinical pregnancy rate and lower miscarriage rate with luteal hCG support. No significant difference was found between hCG and progesterone with regard to the beneficial effects on pregnancy and miscarriage rates. Because of the high incidence of ovarian hyperstimulation syndrome when hCG is used for luteal support, progesterone has become the standard of care in IVF cycles.

Controlled ovarian hyperstimulation cycles are associated with elevated progesterone levels prior to ovulation. Elevated progesterone levels in the early luteal phase are also found. The effect of this premature progesterone production is advanced endometrial hystology with premature appearance of endometrial pinopods. Because of these findings, our protocol at the Colorado Center for Reproductive Medicine for luteal support involves starting progesterone a day later than normal in the luteal phase. We initiate progesterone therapy 2 days after oocyte retrieval and utilize either 50 mg of progesterone intramuscularly or one applicator per day of 8% Crinone vaginal gel. Estradiol 0.2 mg transdermally is initiated nine days after retrieval to guard against possible late luteal drop in estradiol production (12).

For patients undergoing oocyte donation, progesterone in the same formulations is initiated the night prior to the donor's retrieval. For frozen embryo transfer patients utilizing blastocysts, progesterone is initiated such that the blastocysts are thawed and transferred on the sixth day of progesterone administration. Patients with pronuclear-stage embryos start progesterone on Day 1, have their pronuclear embryos thawed on Day 2, and then undergo embryo transfer on the third day of progesterone administration.

In summary, a meta-analysis has confirmed the beneficial effects of luteal phase support during in vitro fertilization cycles. Because of the lower incidence of ovarian hyperstimulation syndrome, progesterone is preferred over hCG and can be administered either intramuscularly or vaginally. Because of the accelerated endometrium of ovarian hyperstimulation cycles, a slight delay in the initiation of exogenous progesterone may be beneficial.

References

1. Mansour R, Aboulghar M, Serour G, Amin Y. Dummy embryo transfer using methylene blue dye. Hum Reprod 1994;9:1257–59.
2. Poindexter A, Thompson D, Gibbons W, Findley W, Dodson M, Young R. Residual embryos in failed embryo transfer. Fertil Steril 1986;46:262–67.
3. Visser D, Fourie S, Kruger H. Multiple attempts at embryo transfer: effects on pregnancy outcome in an in vitro fertilization and embryo transfer program. J Assist Reprod Genet 1993;10:37–43.
4. Cohen J. Syllabus: maximizing the potential of every embryo to minimize multiple embryo transfer. ASRM Annual Meeting, 1998.
5. Egbase P, Al-Sharhan M, Al-Othman S, Al-Muta M, Udo E, Grudzinskas J. Incidence of microbial growth from the tip of the embryo transfer catheter after embryo transfer in relation to clinical pregnancy rate following in vitro fertilization and embryo transfer. Hum Reprod 1996;11:1687–89.
6. McNamee PI, Huang TTF, Carwile AH, Kosasa TS, Vu KK. Significant increase in pregnancy rates achieved by vigorous irrigation of endocervical mucus prior to embryo transfer with the Wallace catheter in an IVF-ET program. Proc Am Soc Rep Med 1988;54:P-322.
7. Wisanto A, Janssens R, Deschacht J, Camus M, Devorey P, Van Steirteghem A. Performance of different embryo transfers in a human in vitro fertilization program. Fertil Steril 1989;52:79–84.
8. Al-Shawaf T, Dave R, Harper J, Linehan D, Riley P, Craft I. Transfer of embryos into the uterus: how much do technical factors affect pregnancy rates? J Assist Reprod Genet 1993;10:31–36.
9. Englert Y, Puissant F, Camus M, Van Houck J, Leroy F. Clinical study on embryo transfer after human in vitro fertilization. J In Vitro Fert Embryo Transfer 1986;3:243–46.
10. Woolcott R, Stanger J. Potentially important variables identified by transvaginal ultrasound-guided embryo transfer. Hum Reprod 1997;12:963–66.
11. Soliman S, Daya S, Collins J, Hughes EG. The role of luteal phase support in infertility treatment: a meta-analysis of randomized trials. Fertil Steril 1994;6:1068–76.
12. Schoolcraft W, Hesla J, Gee M. Experience with Crinone 8% for luteal support in a highly successful IVF program. Hum Reprod 2000;15:1278–83.

15
Cryopreservation of Blastocysts

YVES MENEZO, DENNY SAKKAS, AND ANNA VEIGA

Based on observations collected from IVM-IVF bovine blastocysts, we developed and modified cryopreservation programs for human co-cultured blastocysts. We have used glycerol as cryoprotectant, and sucrose. We were surprised to observe that the in vitro grown blastocysts are rather more sensitive to high concentrations of cryoprotectants. Our current protocol includes cryoprotectant addition in two steps and removal in two steps. The final concentration of glycerol, however, has been decreased to 9% (i.e., 1.125 M).

In our program, from 1989 to 1999, two thirds of patients that have supernumerary embryos had blastocysts frozen. One third of the supernumerary embryos are frozen, and the mean number of embryos frozen per patient is 3.4. On more than 1,000 freezing and thawing cycles, the transfer rate is around 90%, and the recovery rate per embryo 80%. The miscarriage rate is 20%. The take home baby rate per transferred blastocyst is around 13%. If with transfer of fresh blatocysts the sex ratio shifts toward males (60/40). For frozen and thawed (F/T) blastocysts the sex ratio is not statistically different from 0.5.

Co-cultured blastocysts and the ones obtained from sequential media (SM) have not the same cryoresistance. SM blastocysts need serum for cryopreservation and thawing; however, we have switched to a propanediol program with encouraging results.

Introduction

Mammalian embryos have been successfully frozen and thawed since 1972, when Whittingham and co-workers (1) reported the birth of live mice after transfer of frozen–thawed embryos. In the human, the first baby was born in Australia after the replacement of a frozen-thawed embryo (2) in 1984. Cryobiology techniques became an essential part of IVF programs because ovarian stimulation for IVF often leads to the production of a high number of oocytes. Thus, excess embryos have to be cryopreserved. Because embryo replacements are performed very early (Day 2 or 3 following in vitro insemination), freezing at early preimplantation stages, from zygote to the eight-cell stage, was established universally. No major changes have occurred in that field since the standardization of the techniques. The results obtained are still clearly worse than they are with fresh embryos or in comparison with other mammalian species.

In domestic animals, embryos are frozen at the blastocyst stage. Blastocysts are much easier to freeze and thaw. In the human, however, in vitro culture techniques did allow blastocyst formation at high rates. Moreover, the quality of the blastocysts obtained with conventional culture techniques is usually not really fair (3). The co-culture techniques have allowed us to obtain in vitro good blastocysts with reasonable rates (4,5). Blastocysts are easier to freeze for two main reasons: The cytoplasmic volume of the cells is lower, thus the nucleus–cytoplasm ratio is higher, then the higher cell number allows embryo recovery even if some cells have been destroyed during the freezing and thawing procedures. In bovine, blastocysts were usually obtained, after in vivo collection, from superovulated heifers and cows. The appearance of IVM-IVF has provided a new source of blastocysts obtained after long-term culture and/or co-culture in vitro. As the in vivo and in vitro produced embryos appear to exhibit some differences, we have tried to adapt conventional cryopreservation protocols (6). Both bovine and human blastocysts were obtained using the same co-culture technique.

Blastocyst Freezing Protocols

In most of the animal experiments, glycerol is the cryoprotectant; now, ethylene glycol is used in bovine and ovine as well (7). Propanediol is rather used for cleaving stage embryos (see Table 15.1). Glycerol seems to be a good compromise because it is a natural metabolic compound present in all cells. It is probably not the perfect molecule as cryoprotectant. Glycerol was used in the first technique concerning blastocyst freezing, reported in 1985 (8). In a first approach, we tested this protocol, based on bovine data, and then simplified it (9).

For cryoprotectant addition, we first decreased the number of steps from six to two (of 10mM), and we added sucrose in the final step immediately before starting the freezing program. By maintaining the sucrose, we decreased the concentration of glycerol from 10% (1.25M) to 9% (1.125 M). The third protocol of the first series of experiment was the basis of a second modification (started in 1995, see Refs. 10,11) with a drop of glycerol concentration from 10 to 9%. Finally, the thawing protocol was simplified in two steps (Table 15.2). The same experiments were performed in the bovine, with the same co-culture techniques. The programmed freezing curve is $-2°C$ per minute from $22°C$ to $-6.5°C$, then manual seeding after a 30-second delay; after seeding, from $-6.5°C$ to $-37°C$, slow cooling at $-0.3°C$ per minute, then plunging directly into liquid nitrogen.

TABLE 15.1. The two major cryoprotectants used in human IVF embryo cryopreservation.

Croprotectant	Formula	MW	d
Glycerol	$CH_2OH-CHOH-CH_2OH$	92.1	1.47
Propanediol	$CH_3-CHOH-CH_2OH$	76.1	1.04

In all steps of embryo manipulations, the blastocysts were set at room temperature under a stream of gas (5% O_2, 5% CO_2, and 90% N_2). After thawing, the embryos were allowed to recover 3–4 hours in the culture medium before transfer. Embryo quality was assessed at this time. Only the morphologically normal embryos that had reexpanded were replaced in synchronized patients: They were prepared for transfers either in natural cycles or by hormone replacement. Progesterone was administrated for improving the luteal phase. In cows, one blastocyst was transferred in each synchronized recipient.

As we observed a difference in cryoresistance of blastocysts originating from co-culture and sequential media, the propanediol procedure (12) used for early stage embryos was tested.

Results

Lowering the concentration of cryoprotectant improves the recovery after freezing and thawing; sucrose addition is beneficial as well. Increasing serum addition does not seem to be of any benefit: No improvement was observed in

TABLE 15.2. Protocol used for blastocyst freezing (final).

Preparation for Freezing: Two steps
- Solution of 5% (v/v*) glycerol in bicarbonate buffered medium for 10 minutes
- Solution of 9% (v/v**) glycerol in bicarbonate buffered medium containing 0.2 M sucrose, for 10 minutes

Thawing: Two steps
- Solution of 0.5 M sucrose in bicarbonate buffered medium for 10 minutes
- Solution of 0.2 M in bicarbonate buffered medium for 10 minutes

Then passage in culture medium and culture for 2 hours before transfer. If the reexpension seems delayed, add another rinse in culture medium.

*Taking care of the density, a 5% v/v Glycerol solution is 6.25 g/L.
**9% v/v 11.3 g/L.

TABLE 15.3. The two thawing protocols for tranfers of co-cultured frozen blastocysts.*

	Stepwise	Two-step (no glycerol)	
Thawing cycles	563	380	
Transfer cycles	516 (92%)	341 (89.7%)	
No thawed blastocysts	1239	754	
No transferred blastocysts	1033 (83%)	563 (74,6%)	($p < 0.02$)
Clinical pr./transfer	112 (21.7%)	92 (27%)	
Ongoing pr./transfer	98 (19%)	73 (21,4%)	
Cin. impl./tr. embryo	138 (13.4%)	95 (17.%)	
Ongoing impl./tr. embryo	124 (12%)	76 (13.5%)	
Live birth/*frozen* blastocyst	**10%**	**10%**	

*Cryoprotectant addition is realized in two steps: 5% and 9% glycerol (V/V).

bovine when serum supplementation was increased from 20 to 50%. In human, the freezing rate of the supernumerary embryos for the last 4 years was 35%. On a *per patient* basis, the freezing ratio was 61%. A mean number of 3.4 blastocysts was frozen per patient.

The blastocyst recovery rate is a little bit lower with the simplified thawing protocol, but the final yield per frozen embryo is the same at the end. Our freezing activity for 1995-1999 is summarized in Table 15.3. When 100 blastocysts were frozen, we obtained 10 babies at the end of the artificial reproduction technology (ART) process. The overall miscarriage rate (including two ectopic pregnancies) is 20%. The best implantation rates are obtained with the artificial cycles (26.2%). The remaining uterine preparations led to lower implantation rates (12%-16%, see Ref. 10).

The use of sequential media led to high differences in the results: SM blastocyst are not as cryoresistant as the co-culture ones. There is a 50% loss in the implantation rates per transferred embryo (Table 15.4).

The results with the propanediol protocol are encouraging but for a very small population. Six out of six thawed blastocysts recovered. They were transferred in three patients (two per patient). All three patients became pregnant.

In bovine, where the donors are not the recipients, the implantation rate is 27% per blastocyst: This is the double that is observed in the human for overall patients. In the human, where more than one blastocyst is transferred per patient, we can calculate the implantation rates per embryo in the overall population and in the pregnant patients. We can observe (Table 15.5) that, if we consider the overall population, the freezing and thawing processes seem to severely damage one half of the in vitro-grown embryos. This is true for bovine IVM-IVF frozen thawed blastocysts.

Freezing at the blastocyst stage does not modify the sex ratio (Table 15.6). It does not interfere as well with the birthweights (Table 15.7).

TABLE 15.4. Freezing and thawing blastocysts from sequential media versus co-culture.

	Same period of time		Significance*
	Sequential media	Co-culture	
No. of couples	249	127	
	82.3%	93.7%	0.003
No. of transfers	205	119	
No. of thawed embryos	430	220	
	74.2%	83.2%	0.01
No. embryos transferred	319	183	
Pregnancies	25 PR/T = 12/2%	28 PR/T = 23,5%	0.02
Implantations	25 Imp/embryo = 7,8%	28 Imp/emb = 15,3%	0.03
Take home baby rate per frozen embryo			
	21/430 = 5%	24/220 = 10.9%	0.01

*Determined by χ^2.

TABLE 15.5. Comparison of implantation rates after fresh and frozen–thawed blastocyst transfers (ongoing and/or life births).

	Fresh	Frozen–thawed
Human	Overall 547/2580 = 21.2%	200/1596 = 12.5%
	Pregnant 493/865 = 57%	200/428 = 46.7%
Bovine	28/56 = 50%	13/48 = 27%

TABLE 15.6. Blastocyst freezing and sex ratio.

Births	Males	Females	Sex ratio
150	78 (52%)	72 (48%)	1.08 (NS)

TABLE 15.7. Birthweights (kg) after blastocyst freezing (150 babies total).

	Males	Females
FT		
Single	3.33 +/− 0.55	3.42 +/− 0.54
Multiple	2.12 +/− 0.79	2.44 +/− 0.47
Control		
Single	3.31 +/− 0.52	3.33 +/− 0.46
Multiple	2.28 +/− 0.60	2.23 +/− 0.53

Discussion

Due to the long-term maintenance in vitro bovine IVF-IVF blastocyst is a nice tool and model for human IVF embryos. Observations picked up from bovine protocols can be directly transferred for human blastocysts. High concentrations of cryoprotectant seems rather toxic for in vitro–grown blastocysts. This may explain the poor successes obtained with vitrification, but this point is still open in humans.

There appears to be some inherent advantages to using blastocysts for cryopreservation in humans. In terms of cryobiology, the small volume of the blastocyst cell allows a more important recovery rate after the freezing and thawing process than the one observed for earlier stages. Co-culture of preembryo before freezing allows first an increase in final cell number (4–12). It is then clear that prolonged culture times allow a selection of the best embryos. Early preembryos may block due to biochemical or cytogenetic problems (13). These cytogenetic problems are ineluctable and occur in vitro as well in vivo (14). It has also been demonstrated that ICSI embryos have an increased tendency to block before blastocyst formation (15). Our experience is similar, with a loss in blastocyst formation of around 10% on blastocyst formation of the spare embryos: IVF : 594/1424 = 41.8%, ICSI : 190/560 = 33.9%. Freezing zygotes limits the selection of embryos for fresh transfer and even after thawing. This is also exactly the same handicap for cell-stage freezing because it is now clear that most of the preembryos submitted to developmental arrests for biochemical reasons block at the time of genomic activation, which is far before blastocyst formation.

In humans the ongoing implantation rate is around 12.5%, half of what is currently expected for fresh blastocyst transfers. The miscarriage rate (20%) is lower than the 32% reported after transfers of blastocysts grown in simple media (16), but this observation concerning the lowest freezing and thawing ability of the blastocysts grown in simple culture media is also true for the postthaw transfer rates, survival, and implantation rate per blastocyst. The co-culture system may be promoting a better blastocyst quality. An important point needs to be focused: If we observed the implantation rates in overall patients, and in pregnant patients, we can conclude that there is a big embryo wastage due to the inadequate preparation of the endometrium.

If we consider the overall implantation rate per embryo as Ov, and the implantation rate in the pregnant patient is p, then the following formula

$$L = \frac{(P - Ov)}{P} \times 100 \text{ or } (1 - Ov/P) \times 100$$

gives the estimated losses (in percentages) *in vivo* of the fair quality embryos related to inadequacy of the epithelium. There is a huge loss related to an unsuitable environment. We observed this same type of embryonic losses with fresh blastocysts. In any case, the loss related to the freezing procedure can be estimated at one half.

In conclusion, if we have to improve our knowledge in cryobiology, more progress should be made in the knowledge of uterine physiology. It is still not clear whether artificial cycles are better, even if there is a tendency for better results with artificial and/or slightly stimulated cycles (10–17). The endometrium is still a black box. Culture conditions have to be improved as well to improve cryoresistance. Prevention of free radical formation should be emphasized in order to avoid lipid peroxidation. They first distort and fragilize the membranes (through the formation of prostaglandin like Peroxides) (18). Moreover, it is now common knowledge that the oxidation products of membrane polyunsaturated fatty acids have deleterious effects on cell survival (19). The use of growth factors (20) may also be, at least partly, the beginning of an answer.

References

1. Whittingham DG, Leibo SP, Mazur P. Survival of mouse embryos frozen to –196°C and –269°C. Science 1972;178:411–14.
2. Trounson A, Mohr L. Human pregnancy following cryopreservation, thawing and transfer of an eight-cell embryo. Nature (London) 1983;305:707–9.
3. Dokras A, Sargent LL, Ross C, et al. The human blastocyst: morphology and human chorionic gonadotropin secretion in vitro. Hum Reprod 1991;3(Suppl. 1):1143–51.
4. Ménézo YJR, Hazout A, Dumont M, et al. Coculture of embryos on Vero cells and transfer of blastocysts in human. Hum Reprod 1992;7:101–6.
5. Quinn P. Use of coculture with cumulus cells in insemination medium in human in vitro fertilization. J Assist Reprod Genet 1994;11:270–77.
6. Leibo S, Loskutoff NM. Cryobiology of in vitro derived bovine embryos. Theriogenology 1993;39:81–94.
7. Prather RS, Spire MF, Schalles RR. Evaluation of cryopreservation techniques for bovine embryos. Theriogenology 1987;28:195–204.
8. Cohen J, Simons R, Fehilly C, et al. Birth after replacement of hatching blastocyst cryopreserved at expanded blastocyst stage. Lancet 1987;i:647.
9. Ménézo Y, Nicollet B, Herbaut N, André D. Freezing co-cultured human blastocysts. Fertil Steril 1992;58:977–80.
10. Kaufmann RA, Ménézo YJR, Hazout A, Nicollet B, Dumont M, Servy E. Cocultured blastocyst cryopreservation: experience of more than 500 transfer cycles. Feril Steril 1995;64:1125–29.
11. Ménézo Y, Veiga A. Cryopreservation of blastocysts. In: Gomel V, Leung PCK, eds. In vitro fertilization and assisted reproduction. Tenth World Congress of In Vitro Fertilization and Assisted Reproduction, Vancouver (Canada), Monduzzi, 1997:49–53.
12. Lassale B, Testart J, Renard JP. Human embryo features that influence the success of cryopreservation with the use of 1.2 propanediol. Fertil Steril 1985;44:645–51.
13. Vlad M, Walker D, Kennedy RC. Nuclei number in human embryos cocultured with human ampullary cells. Hum Reprod 1996;11:1678–86.
14. Benkhalifa M, Ménézo Y, Janny L, Pouly JL, Qumsiyeh MB. Cytogenetics of uncleaved

oocytes and arrested zygotes in IVF programs. J Assist Reprod Genet 1996;13: 140–46.
15. Shoukir Y, Chardonnens D, Campana A, Sakkas D. Blastocyst development from supernumerary embryos after intracytoplasmic sperm injection: a paternal influence? Hum Reprod 1998;13:1632–37.
16. Hartshorne GM, Elder K, Crow J, et al. The influence of in vitro development upon post-thaw survival and implantation of cryopreserved human blastocysts. Hum Reprod 1991;6:136–41.
17. Schmidt CL, de Ziegler D, Gagliardi CL, et al. Transfer of cryopreserved-thawed embryos: the natural cycle versus controlled preparation of the endometrium with gonadotropin-releasing hormone agonist and exogenous estradiol and progesterone. Fertil Steril 1989;46:268–72.
18. Pryor WA, Stanley JP, Blair E. Autoxidation of polyunsaturated fatty acids: II; a suggested mechanism for the formation of TBA-reactive materials from prostaglandin-like peroxides. Lipids 1976;11:370–79.
19. Begin ME. Effects of polyunsaturated fatty acids and their oxidation products on cell survival. Lipids 1987;45:269–313.
20. Carnegie JA, Morgan JJ, McDiarmid N, Durnford R. Influence of protein supplements on the secretion of leukemia inhibitory factor by mitomycin-pretreated Vero cells: possible application to the in vitro production of bovine blastocysts with high cryotolerance. J Reprod Fertil 1999;117:41-48.

Part V

Implantation

16

Embryo–Maternal Dialogue in the Apposition and Adhesion Phases of Human Implantation

CARLOS SIMÓN, JOSE LOUIS DE PABLO, JULIO C. MARTIN,
MARCOS MESEGUER, ARANCHA GALÁN, AND ANTONIO PELLICER

Embryonic implantation, which is the process by which the human embryo orientates, attaches, and finally invades the underlying maternal endometrial tissue is a highly regulated mechanism. Embryonic implantation requires a receptive endometrium, a competent blastocyst, and a coordinated development and communication between them. Considerable advances have been made in understanding the cell biology of the embryo and the maternal endometrium separately. Nevertheless, communication between them, and the reciprocal effect on each other, constitute an exciting and as yet unsolved paradigm in reproductive medicine. This embryo–maternal dialogue is differentially regulated in an autocrine/paracrine manner during the apposition and adhesion phases. We will show in this chapter the capacity of the human embryo to regulate the endometrial antiadhesion molecule MUC1 to prevent unwanted attachment in the apposition phase and to allow selective attachment in the adhesion phase. In addition, similar coordinated mechanism will be shown for the embryonic regulation of endometrial epithelial cell (EEC) apoptosis in the apposition and adhesion phase of human implantation.

Introduction

Different authors have shown the important role of mucins as barriers present in epithelia to protect from the invasion of microorganism to the underlying tissues. In human EEC the mucin MUC1 has also been pointed out as the main stop signal that embryos must pull up to establish a successful attachment. Mucins are a family of highly glycosylated, high molecular weight (>250 kDa) glycoproteins present on epithelial surfaces, including human EEC (1,2). MUC1 is a large transmembrane mucin that is present in the apical domain of the EEC during the implantation phase (3). In addition, an alternatively spliced product without transmembrane domain, the MUC1/SEC protein, can be expressed in epithelial cells. The expression of the former at the cell surface area inhibits cell–cell adhesion. This antiadhesive property is therefore dependent on the presence of the long ectodomain and is probably the result of steric hindrance of the interactions receptor–ligand of the families of adhesion molecules (e.g., the cadherins) (4,5).

In humans, endometrial MUC1 is hormonally regulated in natural cycles (6,7). There is an increased abundance of MUC1 mRNA from the proliferative to midsecretory phase, followed by a decrease in late secretory phase (7). MUC1 levels increase in glands during the secretory phase (7). Moreover, we have investigated the hormonal regulation of endometrial MUC1 in agonadal women undergoing mock cycles of hormonal replacement therapy (HRT) in an ovum donation program, and we found an increase of mRNA levels in the receptive compared with nonreceptive endometrium. We also analyzed MUC1 in preimplantation blastocysts using RT-nested PCR, and a product corresponding to an amplification of MUC1 cDNA has been showed (8). In parallel we used an in vitro model for the apposition and adhesion phases of human implantation to analyze the distribution and embryonic regulation of MUC1 in EEC (9–11).

Apoptosis, or the highly orchestrated form of programmed cell death, in which cells neatly commit suicide without producing an inflammatory response in the tissue, is becoming a relevant event in the study of reproductive physiology (12). In the uterine tissue, apoptotic cells increase throughout the menstrual cycle. There is a lower number of apoptotic cells in the proliferative phase, and this number increases significantly in the secretory phase, peaking in the menstrual phase (13). It is remarkable that in the endometrium, the epithelium is more affected with apoptotic cells than the stroma (14). In rodents, ultrastructural studies have demonstrated that uterine epithelial cells in the attachment site undergo apoptotic changes (15) and are phagocytozed by the trophoectoderm during epithelial invasion (16). Indeed, TGF-β mediates the autocrine/paracrine regulation of apoptosis induced by the embryo as previously shown in mice (17). In the stromal invasion phase, rat pregnancy is characterized by a progressive continuous induction of apoptosis in the maternal tissues lining the conceptus (18). Our aim was to investigate the effect of single human blastocysts on the regulation of apoptosis in an in vitro model of cultured human endometrial epithelial cells in the apposition and adhesion phases of human implantation.

Materials and Methods

Endometrial Culture

Endometrial samples were minced into small pieces of less than 1 mm, subjected to mild collagenase digestion, and endometrial stromal cells (ESC) and EEC were isolated as previously described (19). Both cell types were cultured, and grown to confluence in steroid-free medium: 75% Dulbecco's Modified Eagle's Medium (Gibco, Grand Island, NY) and 25% MCDB-105 (Sigma, St. Louis, MO) containing antibiotics, supplemented with 10% charcoal-Dextran treated fetal bovine serum (FBS) (Hyclone, Logan, Utah) and 5 µg/ml insulin (Sigma). EEC and ESC were cultured until they formed confluent monolayers with typical whirled and polygonal morphology, respectively. The homogeneity of cultures was determined by morphological characteristics and verified by immunocytochemical localization of cytokeratin, vimentin, and CD68 antigen as markers for epithelial cells, stromal cells, and human macrophages, respectively. As defined by these criteria, ESC monolayers contained less than 2% of EEC and less than 0.1% of macrophages. EEC cultures contained less than 3% of ESC and less than 0.1% of macrophages. After cultures were confluent (1–2 weeks), culture media was supplemented with 5 µg/ml ascorbic acid, 10 µg/ml transferring, and the indicated hormones. Confluent monolayers of EEC and ESC were cultured for 8 days with progesterone (P) (3.18 µg/ml) (Sigma), EGF (20 ng/ml) (Beckton & Dickinson Labware, Bedford, MA), and hrIL-1b (20 pg/ml) (Genzyme Corporation, Cambridge, MA). They were compared with control cells cultured only with P and EGF. Growth medium was renewed every 2 days. Media was collected and cells were removed every 2 days for RNA analysis. The conditioned media was centrifuged and the supernatant stored at –70°C for PRL and PGE2 analysis.

Co-Culture of Human Embryos with EEC for the Study of the Apposition Phase

Forty-eight hours after insemination, single two-to-four-cell embryos were transferred individually into co-culture wells with the confluent AEEC monolayer. Embryos were grown until they reached the eight-cell stage; the culture was then continued in S2 medium up to the blastocyst stage. Embryonic development was checked daily and media changed every 24 hours. On Day 6, blastocysts were transferred back to the mother or frozen. Control wells were developed culturing EEC under the same conditions, but without human embryos.

Human In Vitro Attachment Assay for the Study of the Adhesion Phase

Three-dimensional cultures were prepared for the in vitro embryo attachment assays. Epithelial cells were obtained from endometrial biopsies and processed as before. Epithelial cells grew polarized on 24-well plates coated with extracellular matrigel. Spare blastocysts were cultured on those EEC achieving confluence, and allowed to attach to the epithelial surface. After 48–72 hours cells were washed with phosphate buffered saline (PBS), fixed 30 minutes in 4% paraformaldehyde (PFA) in PBS at 4°C, and washed as before. Attached blastocysts were first localized by phase-contrast microscopy. The labeling experiments were developed later for the corresponding molecule and analyzed by confocal microscopy or flow cytometry.

Flow Cytometry (FCM) and Confocal Microscopy (CM)

For FCM experiments, EEC monolayers were detached using a cell scraper, retrieved with the co-culture medium, centrifuged, and the cell pellet was blocked with 1% BSA in PBS for 120 minutes at 4°C. To study intracytoplasmic epitopes of MUC1, the cell pellet was resuspended in cold 70% ethanol for 20 minutes. After washing with PBS-T, cells were incubated overnight at 4°C with the following antibodies: HMFG-1, BC-2, CT-1, and antihuman cytokeratin CK-5. For the HMFG-1 and BC-2 assays, the EEC suspensions were incubated with an FITC-conjugated goat antimouse IgG as the secondary antibody; for CT-1 assays we used an FITC-conjugated goat antirabbit IgG. Cell suspensions incubated with BC-2 or HMFG-1 were fixed with 1% PFA (1 hour at 4°C). The extracellular domain of MUC1 was labeled using BC-3 as primary antibody. Negative controls were included in each experiment by the omission of the primary antibody. Finally, cells were analyzed using an Epics Elite Flow Cytometer (Coulter Cytometry, Hialeah, FL) (10). Data were expressed as luminosity intensity (FAU: fluorescence arbitrary units). Variability in the intensity of the signal was obtained with FPCV value (full peak coefficient of variation).

To determine Annexin-V^+ cells (apoptotic positive cells) by FCM (20), EEC were mechanically detached by pipetting wells after trypsin/EDTA (1:10) incubation (10 minutes, 37°C). Cells were collected by centrifugation, then washed with PBS, and resuspended in 490 µl of 1:10 diluted binding buffer. After this, cells were stained with 5 µl of Annexin V-FITC and 5 µl of propidium iodide (PI). Cell suspensions were fixed with 4% PFA for 30 minutes at 4°C, resuspended in PBS, and analyzed in the flow cytometer. Live, apoptotic, and necrotic cells were differentiated according to their annexin V and PI fluorescence pattern (live cells: annexin V^-/PI^-; apoptotic cells: annexin V^+/PI^{dim}; necrotic cells: annexin V^+/PI^{bright}).

All FCM determinations were performed in an Epics XL flow cytometer (Beckmann-Coulter) using an argon-ion laser tuned at 488 nm and 15 mW. FITC-fluorescence was collected by 575 DL+ 525BP and PI was collected by 600DL +575BP filters. Data were collected in four-decade logarithmic amplification. Debris was excluded by analysis of scatter properties. At least 10,000 events per sample were stored in list-mode files. Data were expressed as the percentage of stained cells.

Confocal analysis was performed using an NRC 1024 instrument (Bio-Rad, Hempstead, UK). The excitation line used was 488 (FITC). The filter used was: HQ515/10 (FITC). Transmitted light images were acquired for every field.

Northern Blot Analysis

The MUC1 cDNA probe (pMUC7, in pBluescriptSK) was provided by Dr. J. Burchell (ICRF, UK) (6), and corresponds to the variable number tandem repeats (VNTR) region of the MUC1 exon 2. Transformed DH5α *E. coli* cells were used to isolate the plasmid, and a band of 450 bp was isolated after a digestion with EcoRI. The cDNA was ^{32}P-radiolabeled as previously described (21). A cDNA probe for 28S rRNA was provided by Dr. Iris L. Gonzalez (Hahnemann University, Philadelphia).

Endometrial tissue for RNA isolation was collected, weighed, frozen in liquid nitrogen, and stored at -70°C. As control RNA, adenoids were collected and processed as before. Total RNA was extracted from the tissue homogenate and/or EEC following the guanidinium isothiocyanate method (22) using the Trizol reagent. Then, 10 µg of total RNA from EEC and 15 µg from endometrial biopsies were used for the analysis (6,19). The relative intensities of Northern hybridization signals were determined by analysis of autoradiograms after image capture (TDI, Madrid, Spain). MUC1 mRNA levels were normalized to 28S rRNA hybridization signals.

Detection of DNA Strand Breaks by TUNEL

In situ detection of apoptotic cells was performed in EEC plated in chamberslides. EEC monolayers were fixed as before, permeabilized with 0,2% Triton X-100 (5 minutes, 4°C), and washed with PBS. Apoptotic cells were detected using a Cell Death Detection Kit. Incubation with TdT-enzyme and FITC-dUTP was done for 60 minutes at 37°C in the dark. Cells were then counterstained with PI (1µg/mL) or DAPI. Negative controls were made by omitting the TdT enzyme. Slides were viewed under a fluorescence microscope (Nikon, Labophot-2).

For TUNEL studies, EEC were fixed in 4% PFA for 10 minutes, exposed to 0.3% hydrogen peroxide in methanol for 30 minutes, permeabilized in 0.1% Triton X-100 for 10 minutes on ice, washed twice in PBS and then pre-stained in 25 mg/ml of bisbenzimide for 25 minutes at 37°C. Cell cultures were incubated with 50 U/ml of terminal transferase and 15 mM of fluorescein-dUTP for 60 minutes at 37°C, and then exposed to a sheep antifluorescein antibody conjugated to peroxidase for 30 minutes at 37°C. After four washes in PBS, TUNEL staining was developed in a solution of diaminobenzidine and nickel chloride, and the preparations were mounted and observed under combined UV and visible light.

TUNEL on Detached EEC (FCM Analysis)

DNA strand breaks were also assessed by FCM on detached EEC using the following procedure. Detached EEC were collected by centrifugation, fixed with 4% PFA (30 minutes, 4°C) and permeabilized with 0,2% Triton X-100 (5 minutes, 4°C), and washed with PBS. Apoptotic cells were detected using the Cell Death Detection Kit. Cells were resuspended in equilibration buffer (5 minutes, room temperature), incubated with TdT-enzyme and FITC-dUTP for 60 minutes at 37°C in the dark and counterstained with PI. Negative controls were made omitting the TdT enzyme. Cell suspensions were analyzed by FCM.

Results

Hormonal Regulation of Endometrial MUC1 mRNA and Protein

Northern blot of MUC1 mRNA and immunohistochemical studies using different antibodies against different epitopes of MUC1 demonstrate an increase of MUC1 in the receptive compared with nonreceptive endometrium (8). The upregulation of MUC1 during the peri-implantation period in hormone replacement therapy (HRT) cycles is in agreement with the regulation described in natural cycles (6,7).

Embryonic Regulation of Endometrial Epithelial MUC1 mRNA and Protein at the Apposition Phase

EEC cultures were maintained with or without the presence of developing human embryos from the cleavage until blastocyst stage. Northern blot hybridization detected two transcripts in some cases, but the two alleles co-migrated in others. Bands were observed in the range of 4–7 kb. Quantitative

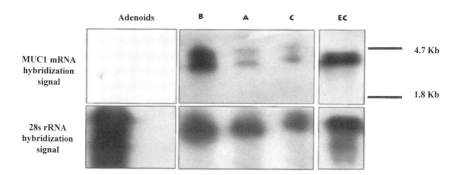

FIGURE 16.1. Northern blot analysis of MUC1 mRNA and the corresponding 28Ss hybridization signal from two or three pooled confluent endometrial epithelial cell cultures wells. This figure shows endometrial epithelial cells isolated from the biopsy (EC), adenoids (lymphoid tissue), EEC cultured with a human blastocyst (B), EEC cultured with arrested blastocysts (A), and EEC cultured without embryo (C).

16. Embryo–Maternal Dialogue in the Apposition and Adhesion Phases 205

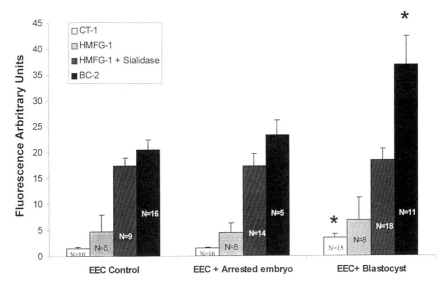

FIGURE 16.2. Data for CTF experiments with each antibody were combined and expressed as the mean ± SEM of the luminous intensity of cells expressed as fluorescence arbitrary units (FAU). Asterisks (*) denote a significant increase ($p < 0.05$) of intensity from cells in contact with blastocyst versus control cells. N indicates the number of wells studied in each category. When the secondary Ab was used alone, no appreciable fluorescence was detected.

densitometric analysis showed more than twofold increase of MUC1 mRNA in EEC cultured in the presence of embryos compared with controls (Fig. 16.1).

To quantify the embryonic regulation of immunoreactive MUC1, FCM analysis was performed on EEC co-cultured with blastocysts, with embryos that arrested during development, or in the absence of embryos (control). Because glycosylation may affect antibody binding to the ectodomain, FCM was performed with two different mAbs (BC-2 and HMFG-1). Sialidase unmasking treatment was also used. In addition, the cytoplasmic C-tail antibody CT-1 was used. Data for the experiments with each antibody were combined and expressed as intensity of stained cells in fluorescence arbitrary units (FAU). Heterogeneity (measured as FPCV) is higher when extracellular epitopes are studied compared with the intracellular epitope detected with CT-1, probably because glycosylation leads to more variation in binding in the former case. The results indicate that human pre-implantation embryos upregulate endometrial epithelial MUC1 compared to controls (Fig. 16.2). This effect is observed with three different antibodies and is statistically significant with BC-2 and CT-1 ($p < 0.05$). Arrested embryos show an endometrial effect that is intermediate between controls and embryos that develop to blastocysts (8).

Embryonic Regulation of Endometrial/Epithelial MUC1 During the Adhesion Phase

Using an in vitro model for embryonic adhesion (see Materials and Methods), the extracellular domain of MUC1 was immunolocalized with BC-3 by confocal microscopy at the implantation sites. Sites were fixed before significant trophoblast migration had occurred from the embryo. Despite the fact that MUC1 was expressed in pre-adhesion blastocysts, we were unable to detect MUC1 in attached embryos. MUC1 was similarly absent from EEC subjacent and adjacent to the attached embryo (8). Expression in EEC gradually increased with distance from the implantation site (8). Strong and uniform staining was observed away from the blastocyst.

Embryonic Induction of EEC Apoptosis Studies During the Apposition Phase

The presence of a human blastocyst induces a reduction of EEC apoptotic cells (35.2%) compared with EEC cultured without blastocyst (48.8%) ($p <$ 0.05). It is interesting that EEC monolayers cultured in the presence of an arrested-embryo also have a decreased number of apoptotic cells (39.2%) compared with EEC without embryos (48.8%), which suggests an anti-apoptotic effect induced by soluble factor(s) secreted by the human embryo even for a few days (Fig. 16.3) (23).

This anti-apoptotic embryonic effect was detected by Annexin-V FITC FCM. Late apoptosis events (i.e., DNA strand breaks) in EEC monolayers were not detected. To understand this discrepancy, TUNEL on detached EEC and measurement of cellular DNA content were performed. TUNEL experiments demonstrated that unlike Annexin-V FCM on detached cells, TUNEL positive cells on detached EEC were low (10%) and showed a similar pattern regardless of the presence or absence of the human embryo. This suggests that cell detachment is a stress situation that might induce apoptosis in those cells not protected by the anti-apoptotic effect exerted by the embryo (as demonstrated by phosphatidylserine externalization). Moreover, the study of the DNA content revealed that EEC cell cycle was normal and DNA was not fragmented nor degraded.

Embryonic Induction of EEC Apoptosis Studies in the Adhesion Phase

Unlike the apposition phase, when a human blastocyst adheres to polarized human EEC we found an induction of apoptosis in EEC beneath and around the embryo attachment site compared with cells away from the blastocyst and control cultures (23, Fig. 16.3). This is an embryonic pro-apoptotic effect because it can be detected late in the apoptotic pathway by TUNEL with

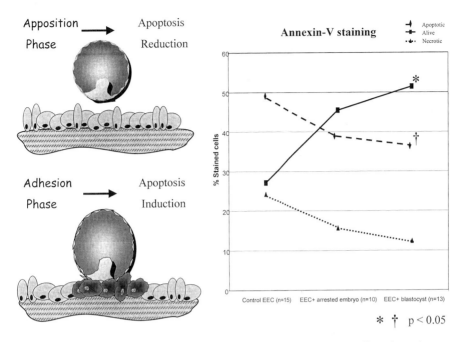

FIGURE 16.3. Annexin-V-FITC and propidium iodide flow cytometry. Bar chart shows the percentage of apoptotic, alive, and necrotic cells in control EEC, EEC with arrested embryos, and EEC with blastocyst. *,†$p < 0.05$ versus control by ANOVA (Bonferroni correction). All data are expressed as the mean ± SEM of four separate experiments.

conventional fluorescence and confocal microscopy. This embryonic pro-apoptotic effect seems to be mediated by a direct contact between the trophoectoderm of the blastocyst and EEC and regulated at least in part by the Fas-Fas ligand system (23).

Conclusions

Blastocyst implantation is a robust phenomenon that has evolved during the course of evolution in eutherian mammals. Apposition and adhesion between the embryonic trophectoderm and EEC plasma membrane and rupture of the endometrial epithelial barrier require a coordinated interaction between blastocyst and maternal endometrium.

MUC1 in the apical luminal glycocalyx is predicted to extend as much as 500 nm above the plasma membrane, and, given its abundance in the receptive phase, it is expected to be encountered by an embryo that approaches the maternal cell surface. It has been proposed that MUC1 acts as an antiadhesion molecule and may inhibit the interaction between embryo and maternal apical epithelium during implantation, thus creating a uterine barrier for implantation. Since EEC tend to show increased MUC1 reactivity in the apposition phase, the healthy embryo may act to reinforce the maternal barrier to premature attachment. Expression of MUC1 in the blastocyst may similarly prevent attachment at an anatomically inappropriate site (e.g., the tubal epithelium). Another interesting and complementary hypothesis is that its presence could provide protection from enzymatic and microbial attack coming from the uterus to the embryo or have suppressive activity from the maternal immune response to the blastocyst. In the adhesion phase, our studies reinforce this hypothesis by addressing the question of how this barrier may eventually be overcome by the embryo. Human blastocyst produce a specific, highly localized downregulation/cleavage of MUC1 at attachment sites (8).

Here we also show that EEC apoptosis occurs in implantation sites both in the mouse (24), rat (15), and hamster (25) as well as in humans. Furthermore, this in vitro work demonstrates for the first time in the human, a coordinated regulation of embryonic induction of EEC apoptosis crucial for the embryo to breach the epithelial barrier. In the apposition phase, the presence of a blastocyst rescues EEC from the apoptotic pathway maintaining more EEC prepared for the initial contact. When the blastocyst adheres to the EEC monolayer, however, it induces a paracrine apoptotic reaction that is maximal in EEC in close contact with the blastocyst.

In conclusion, our data suggest a novel hypothesis of mutual cooperative paracrine signaling between maternal and embryonic cells at implantation, affecting different molecules leading to the loss of an inhibitory barrier to implantation.

References

1. Devine P, Mackenzie IFC. Mucins: structure, function and association with malignancy. Bioassays 1992;14:619–25.
2. Lagow E, DeSouza MM, Carson DD. Mammalian reproductive tract mucins. Hum Reprod Update 1999;5:280–92.
3. Meseguer M, Pellicer A, Simón C. MUC1 and endometrial receptivity. Mol Hum Reprod 1998;4(12):1089–98.
4. Wesseling J, Van der Valk SW, Hilkens J. Epsialin (MUC1) overexpression inhibits integrin-mediated cell adhesion to extracellular matrix components. J Cell Biol 1995;129:255–65.
5. Aplin JD, Hey NA. MUC1, endometrium and embryo implantation. Biochem Soc Trans 1995;23:826–31.
6. Hey NA, Graham RA, Seif MW, Aplin JD. The polymorphic epithelial mucin MUC1 is regulated with maximal expression in the implantation phase. J Clin Endocrinol Metab 1994;78(2):337–42.
7. Aplin JD, Hey NA, Graham RA. Human endometrial MUC1 carries keratan sulphate: characteristic glycoforms in the luminal epithelium at receptivity. Glycobiology 1998;8(3):269–76.

8. Meseguer M, Aplin JD, Caballero-Campo P, O´Connor JE, Martin JC, Remohí J, et al. Hormonal and embryonic regulation of human endometrial MUC-1. Biol Reprod 2001;64:181–92.
9. De los Santos MJ, Mercader A, Francés A, Portoles E, Remohí J, Pellicer A, et al. Immunoreactive human embryonic interleukin-1 system and endometrial factors regulating their secretion during embryonic development. Biol Reprod 1996;54:563–74.
10. Simón C, Gimeno MJ, Mercader A, O'Connor JE, Remohí J, Polan ML, et al. Embryonic regulation of integrins β, α_4 and α_1 in human endometrial epithelial cells in vitro. J Clin Endocrinol Metab 1997;82:2607–16.
11. Simón C, Mercader A, Garcia Velasco J, Remohí J, Pellicer A. Co-culture of human embryos with autologous human endometrial epithelial cells in patients with repeated implantation failures. J Clin Endocrinol Metab 1999;84:2638–46.
12. Tilly JL, Strauss JF III, Tenniswood M, eds. Cell death in reproductive physiology. Serono Symposia USA. New York: Springer-Verlag, 1997.
13. Tao XJ, Tilly KI, Maravei DV Shifren JL, Kajewski S, Reed JC, et al. Differential expression of members of the bcl-2 gene family in proliferative and secretory human endometrium: glandular epithelial cell apoptosis is associated with increased expression of bax. J Clin Endocrinol Metab 1997;82:2739–46.
14. Rango UV, Classen-Linke I, Krusche CA, Beier H. The receptive endometrium is characterized by apoptosis in the glands. Hum Reprod 1998;13:3177–89.
15. Parr EL, Tung HN, Parr MB. Apoptosis as the mode of uterine epithelial cell death during embryo implantation in mice and rats. Biol Reprod 1987;36:211–25.
16. Schlafke S, Enders AC. Cellular basis of interaction between trophoblast and uterus at implantation. Biol Reprod 1975;12:41–65.
17. Kamijo T, Rajabi MR, Mizunuma H, Ibuki Y. Biochemical evidence for autocrine/paracrine regulation of apoptosis in cultured uterine epithelial cells during mouse embryo implantation in vitro. Mol Hum Reprod 1998;4:990–98.
18. Piacentini M, Autuori F. Immunohistochemical localization of tissue transglutaminase and Bcl-2 in rat uterine tissues during embryo implantation and post-partum involution. Differentiation 1994;57:51–56.
19. Simón C, Piquette GN, Francés A, El-Danasouri I, Irwin JC, Polan ML. The effect of interleukin-1 beta on the regulation of IL-1 receptor type I and IL-1 beta m RNA levels and protein expression in cultured human endometrial stromal and glandular cells. J Clin Endocinol Metab 1994;78:675–82.
20. Koopman G, Reutelingsperger CPM, Kuijten GAM, Keehnen RMJ, Pals ST, van Oers MHJ. Annexin V for flow cytometric detection of phosphatidylserine expression on B cells undergoing apoptosis. Blood 1994;84:1415–20.
21. Feinberg AP, Volgstein B. A technique for radiolabeling DNA restriction endonuclease fragments to high specific activity. Anal Biochem 1983;132:6–13.
22. Chomczynski P, Sacchi N. Single-step method for RNA isolation by acid guanidinium thiocyanate-phenol-chloroform extraction. Biochemistry 1987;162:156–59.
23. Galán A, O'Connor JE, Valbuena D, Herrer R, Remohí J, Pampfer S, et al. The human blastocyst regulates endometrial epithelial apoptosis in embryonic adhesion. Biol Reprod 2000;63:430–39.
24. Pampfer S, Donnay I. Apoptosis at the time of embryo implantation in mouse and rat. Cell Death Differ 1999;6:533–45.
25. Parkening TA. An ultrastructural study of implantation in the golden hamster II. Trophoblastic invasion and removal of the uterine epithelium. J Anat 1976;122:211–30.

17
Biomarkers and the Assessment of Uterine Receptivity

BRUCE A. LESSEY

The use of biomarkers is an expanding and challenging area of biomedical research. At the turn of twentieth century, we can look back proudly at the steady advances in the field of medicine. In 1999, the NIH organized a symposium on the use of biomarkers for the diagnosis and treatment of a wide variety of medical conditions (*http://www4.od.nih.gov/biomarkers/index.htm*). It was pointed out during this conference that efficient use and selection of appropriate biomarkers in diagnosis and assessment of any condition or interest requires an extensive infrastructure of investigators, comprised of: (1) an environment in which basic science can proceed to translational research; (2) availability of technological resources; and (3) clinical researchers, biostatisticians, and epidemiologists who design studies to validate the use of biomarkers. As interest in the assessment of the endometrium has grown, many of these concepts involving biomarkers will need to be applied to the data emerging on endometrial markers.

Infertility remains a growing problem for couples who have put off or delayed childbearing. There are indeed increasing numbers of couples who seek help in establishing or maintaining a pregnancy. In 1995, it was estimated that one in six couples were infertile. The number of patients seeking care for infertility that year exceeded 9 million couples (1), up from 2.4 million reported in 1989 (2). A large percentage of this increase is now thought to harbor defects in implantation and a relative or absolute lack of uterine receptivity, and "unexplained" infertility may account for up to 37% of these cases (3). The use of biomarkers offers a means to better understand potentially *occult* defects in endometrial receptivity. This chapter will focus on updating the current information on endometrial biomarkers in implantation research and to discuss how many of the protein entities function to improve embryo quality. Our goal is ultimately to use such markers to understand the implantation process, to appreciate the regulatory components of endometrial receptivity, and to improve opportunities for diagnosis of disorders that affect fertility due to interference with embryo–endometrial interactions.

Embryo–Endometrial Interactions

During the earliest events of implantation process, the ovulated oocyte is picked up by the fimbriated end of the fallopian tube and transported toward the uterus. Sperm and egg meet and fertilization occurs in the tube. Cell divisions ensue as the zygote moves closer to the uterine cavity, reaching blastocyst stage by the time endometrial receptivity is achieved. The endometrium undergoes a series of developmental changes in response to ovarian steroids that result in a defined period of receptivity toward embryo implantation (4,5). The putative "window" of implantation, as first suggested by Finn (6), has been demonstrated in both animal models (7–10) and in humans (11,12).

These early stages of implantation have been documented by Hertig and colleagues in women who were pregnant at the time of secretory phase hysterectomy (13). Of 34 embryos identified in such specimens, all had undergone attachment and ingrowth when taken from women whose surgery was beyond Day 21 of the secretory phase. In hysterectomies obtained prior to Day 20 all embryos were still free within the uterine cavity or fallopian tube. These samples formed the basis for many of the known examples of early implantation sites (Fig. 17.1). The concept of a defined period of receptivity in hu-

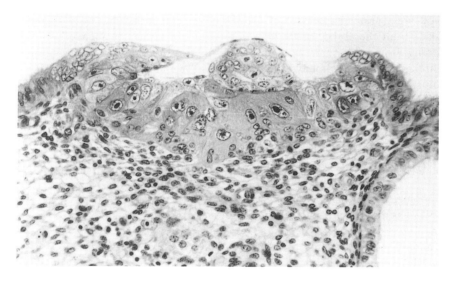

FIGURE 17.1. Photomicrograph of an early implantation site during Stage 5a of implantation. At this stage the maternal vasculature remains intact, but becomes surrounded by the expanding syncytium. This example of a human implantation site was generously provided and photographed from the Carnegie Collection by Dr. Allen Enders and is used with his permission.

mans has subsequently come from studies by Navot and co-workers. These investigators described the early rise in hCG as an indicator of early attachment (14) and from the use of donor embryos replaced into hormonally prepared recipients from different stages of the secretory phase. Their results support the concept of a defined period of uterine receptivity that most likely corresponds to cycle days 20 to 24 (11,15). It is these studies that serve as the underpinnings for the use of biomarkers described below.

The development of uterine receptivity is ultimately driven by ovarian steroids, estrogen and progesterone (16). The endometrium undergoes its developmental changes from a proliferative tissue to a secretory structure through elaboration of a complex series of cytokines, receptors, extracellular matrix molecules, and matrix-degrading enzymes. Induction of signal transduction pathways and cell adhesion molecules prepares the endometrium for what may come. Estradiol is mitogenic toward uterine epitheium and results in a greatly expanded endometrial lining. Estradiol is also important for the induction of estrogen and progesterone receptors (ER and PR) that allows for an adequate secretory response (17,18). Following ovulation, rising progesterone levels transform the straight glandular structures of the endometrium into secretory structures that make the proteins and factors that nurtures the early blastocyst and promote its ability to attach and growth.

There is increasing data to suggest that the progestational effect is not direct; rather, it is orchestrated through paracrine interactions arising in the endometrial stroma. This transformation is accompanied by sequential and well-orchestrated expression of specific genes that both facilitate and sometimes limit the ability of the blastocyst and trophoblast to invade into the uterine lining. Many of the resulting proteins are critical for implantation, although no clear role has been established for many others. Whatever proteins are expressed during the window of implantation serve as potential biomarkers that can be used to understand the implantation process and to help unlock the secrets of its regulation.

Biomarkers of Uterine Receptivity

Endometrial "dating," as first described by Noyes more than 50 years ago, has served as the first meaningful and useful measure of the endometrial capacity for implantation (19). The histologic changes collectively remain the "gold standard" for endometrial assessment despite problems with reproducibility and interpretation. The use endometrial dating resulted in the first recognized defect in the endometrium, termed luteal phase deficiency (LPD) by Georgiana Seegar Jones in the late 1940s (20). The diagnosis of LPD as a heterogeneous condition related to subfertility is thought to be the result of insufficient hormone stimulation or suboptimal endometrial response (21). It is now clear than many of the cases of "LPD" may be artifact of the dating criteria themselves (22). This entity is nevertheless not uncommon and can be found in couples with otherwise unexplained infertility (23), and it can contribute to recurrent pregnancy loss (24,25). Histology correlates poorly with other measures of luteal function [e.g., serum progesterone levels (26) and the usefulness of histologic dating may be limited by the discovery that some uterine receptivity defects exist in the absence of histologic delay] (27,28). The presence of such *occult* defects may account for many cases of truly unexplained infertility or recurrent failure in assisted reproductive technology (ART) cycles (24,29,30). Thus, histology alone does not provide a complete picture of the functional state of the endometrium.

The identification of appropriate biomarkers for the assessment of endometrial function is now underway. Histology-independent measures of the functional state of the endometrium that accurately predicts the potential for successful pregnancy will eventually reduce our reliance on empiric therapies and ameliorate the frustration of patients with "unexplained" infertility or recurrent pregnancy loss. The list of available candidate biomarkers that can be used to assess uterine receptivity is rapidly growing due to the increasing availability of powerful molecular techniques. These include immunohistochemical markers (e.g., the integrins), ultrastructural components (e.g., pinopods), and serum markers (such as glycodelin). Each of the many candidates still need to be closely studied to better define their spatial and temporal distribution within the cycling endometrium. Extensive epidemiologic studies await any candidate biomarker to determine the sensitivity, specificity and predictive value related to its use. It is safe to say that none of the currently available endometrial biomarkers have achieved this level of validation. Selected biomarkers are described in greater detail below.

Ovarian Steroids and Their Receptors

In 1988, we and others described the interesting pattern of distribution for ER and PR in the endometrium of cycling women (18,31). During the mid-secretory phase, in response to rising serum P levels, both ER and PR virtually disappear from the epithelial components of the endometrium, while maintained in the stromal cells of the endometrium. This shift in steroid receptor levels was unexpected at the time, and the significance was not understood. Since then, this same pattern for PR has been observed in several different mammals, including the pig and mouse (32,33), with loss of epithelial PR occurring at the corresponding time of embryo implantation in each species. In women, LPD associated with histologic delay correlated with a delay in PR downregulation and aberrant expression of other endometrial proteins (34). The presence of PR in the presence of elevated secretory phase levels of P is now thought to inhibit the production of other key biomarkers (e.g., endometrial integrins). Elevations in other steroid receptors (e.g., androgen receptors) may have a similar effect (35).

Progesterone (P_4) itself has been employed as an indirect biomarker of adequate luteal function (34). This major steroid hormone of pregnancy is a product first of the corpus luteum following ovulation and later of the placenta. The production of P_4 begins at the time of the LH surge and is primarily responsible for the myriad of progestin-induced proteins that regulate the conversion from a proliferative endometrium to a secretory structure. As a marker, P_4 has been studied extensively, primarily to diagnose LPD, a leading cause of recurrent pregnancy loss and infertility. Unfortunately, a single measurement of P_4 may not accurately reflect the true measure of the cumulative P_4 levels and does not correlate well with endometrial histologic dating (26).

Peptide Hormones

Calcitonin is a peptide hormone, primarily made in the thyroid, that is well known for its endocrine role in calcium homeostasis. Bagchi and colleagues, using the rat model, have demonstrated that this hormone is also made by the endometrial epithelium (36), a finding later described for human endometrium (37). The discovery that endometrium is a source of calcitonin was unexpected and the pattern of calcitionin confined to the window of implantation suggested a role in the process of endometrial–embryonic-interaction. Expression by glandular and luminal epithelium is hormonal dependent (38,39), and it now appears that this hormone functions as a paracrine factor targeting the blastocyst (39). Further studies by this group have also suggested a role in loosening of cell–cell contacts at the luminal surface (work in progress).

Integrins

There are four major classes of cell adhesion molecules, as shown in Figure 17.2. The integrin family is composed of a large family of heterodimeric glycoproteins composed of α and β subunits. The number of subunits now exceed 20 members and associate in predictable patterns to form membrane-bound receptors for the extracellular matrix (ECM). The integrins are perhaps the best characterized of the immunohistochemical biomarkers of uterine receptivity (40). There is now increasing interest in the use of integrins to assess uterine receptivity (41–43) and significant data to suggest their involvement in both fertilization and implantation (44–47).

Every cell in the body maintains patterns of integrin expression, with the exception of red blood cells, and the endometrium is no exception. We and others have described both constitutive and cycle-dependent expression of integrins in normal endometrium (23,40–42,48–51) and noted alterations in endometrial cancer (52). At least three integrins—the $\alpha v \beta 3$ vitronectin receptor, the $\alpha 1 \beta 1$ collagen receptor, and the $\alpha 4 \beta 1$ fibronectin receptor—have been reported to frame the window of implantation in the human, co-expressed on glandular epithelium only during cycle days 20–24 corresponding to the putative window of implantation (53). Apical distribution of luminal $\alpha v \beta 3$ and related $\alpha v \beta 5$ integrins points to these as first in line to interact with the

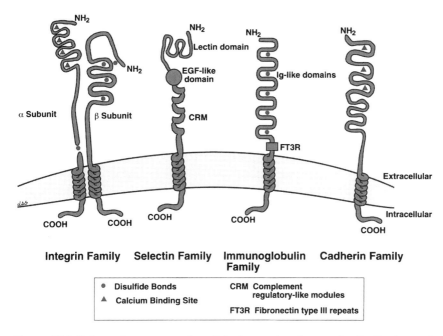

FIGURE 17.2. Schematic representation of the four major classes of cell adhesion molecules including the integrin family, selectin family, immunoglobulin family, and the cadherin family. Note that each of these are membrane-bound receptors that extend to the outside of the cell and signal to the cell through intracytoplasmic tails. Reproduced with permission by Thieme Medical Publishers, NY, from *Seminars in Reproductive Endocrinology*.

incoming embryo at the time of implantation (51,54). The former appears around midsecretory phase of the cycle, whereas αvβ5 increases during the early secretory phase. Both integrins recognize ligands containing the three amino acid sequence arg-gly-asp (RDG). This recognition sequence has been implicated in trophoblast attachment and outgrowth (55,56), and we have shown that neutralization of αvβ3 integrin reduces the number of embryos that will implant in the mouse model (47).

The functional significance of apical integrins at the time of implantation at first suggested a possible role in embryo attachment. Even though this may be true for integrins on the embryonic surface, endometrial integrins are more likely involved in signaling mechanisms that activate cell migration and invasion in response to embryonic fibronectin motifs (57,58). Interactions between integrins and matrix-degrading enzymes, reported in melanoma cells (59), provide a clue that this combination in the receptive endometrium could stimulate the invasive phenotype of the embryo or placental cytotrophoblast (60). Furthermore, degradation products of this digestion may promote cell motility and migration.

Other cell adhesion molecules have been examined in the endometrium at the time of implantation in either epithelial or stromal cells as possible participants in embryo–trophoblast interactions. These include the α6β4 integrin (61) but careful examination of this integrin throughout the cycle shows it to be constitutively present and not a suitable marker of uterine receptivity (62). The hyaluronic acid receptor, CD44 (51,63,64), trophinin (65), and cadherin-11 (66,67) have all been suggested as candidate biomarkers. CD44 is present in various isotypes (68) and is more strongly expressed in the secretory endometrium and decidua. Trophinin is a novel cell adhesion molecule that has been well described in the mouse (65), and has been shown to be present in human endometrium as well. It is expressed on the luminal surface in both rodents and humans and may mediate cell–cell interaction between epithelial cells from maternal and epithelial surfaces. Cadherin-11 is another unique member of the cadherin family of CAMs. It is interesting because it is both an epithelial marker and is expressed in a cycle-dependent manner in the decidua (66). This cadherin is also expressed on the epithelial component of the trophoblast suggesting a role in endometrial–embryonic interaction (67).

Mucins are large glycoproteins that coat the luminal and glandular surfaces. These complex glycopeptides have been suggested to have utility as detectable markers for both LPD and unexplained infertility (69,70). MUC1 is a mucin that has been suggested to present a barrier to implantation when the endometrium is nonreceptive and must be removed at the time of implantation in both rodent (71) and primates (72). In humans, the situation for MUC1 is less clear because it is present throughout the secretory phase in normal cycles (73). An antibody, D9B1 recognizing an oligosaccharide epitope detected reduced expression of this marker in women with unexplained infertility compared to fertile controls (70). MAG is another mucin recognized by mouse ascites fluid that has been studied in women with infertility and also appears to detect those with poor reproductive outcome (74).

Secreted Proteins, Growth Factors, and Cytokines

One of the first and most abundant endometrial products is known as PP14, which is now referred to as glycodelin (75). This protein has been shown to reduce sperm binding to the zona pellucida (76) and was thought to have immune regulatory roles (77). Glycodelin may play a greater role after pregnancy has been established and thus may not be as useful in scrutinizing the initial phases of uterine receptivity during the putative window of implantation (78). Although it can readily be measured by immunohistochemistry, its usefulness has been primarily reserved for serum testing. Glycodelin appears to be reduced in women with luteal phase defect (79) and may be reduced in recurrent pregnancy loss (80).

Several cytokines and growth factors, including leukemia inhibitiory factor (LIF) (81–83), heparin-binding epidermal growth factor (HB-EGF) (84,85), and insulinlike growth factor II (IGF-II) (86), appear in the endometrium at or slightly before the receptive period in women and may be useful as markers of a receptive endometrium. Leukemia inhibitory factor was one of the first cytokines found to be critical for implantation (see 87). LIF was originally shown to induce differentiation of a myeloid leukemia cell line, M1 (88). For those of us who study implantation, interest in this cytokine was significantly increased by the observation that LIF appears in the mouse uterus on Day 4 of pregnancy, corresponding to the day that embryos implant in this species (89). It was observed that female LIF –/– homozygous mice were infertile, whereas the fertility of the males was unaffected. Normal free-floating blastocysts were found within the uteri of the LIF –/– females that failed to implant unless transferred to the uteri of normal female mice (82). Exogenous LIF partially reverses the defect in implantation in the LIF –/– mice. It now appears that LIF is essential for decidualization as attempts to induce decidualization in LIF –/– mice was unsuccessful (83). In humans, LIF is expressed during the window of implantation (88,90) and may be reduced in some women with infertility (84).

In the human HB-EGF is temporally expressed during the time of uterine receptivity (85,86,91). Based on studies, it is tempting to postulate that HB-EGF maintains a role in both adhesion and development in the embryo (92,93). HB-EGF has been shown to improve the development or quality of human embryos in vitro (94,95) and appears to be a paracrine factor in human endometrium regulating other key epithelial gene products (96).

Transcription Factors

Other marker proteins that appear critical to implantation in rodents include the homeobox genes HOXA-10 (97,98) and HOXA-11 (99). These transcription factors now appear to have relevance for human implantation as well (100,101). The HOXA genes are important in segmental development and are both expressed by the endometrium specifically during the midsecretory phase of the menstrual cycles. They are now thought to be master regulatory genes that control other factors important for implantation. Another implantation-critical factor is the enzyme cyclo-oygenase-2, which is a rate-limiting enzyme in prostaglandin synthesis (102). This factor also appears to be a promising as potential biomarkers in the endometrium of primates as well (103,104). Finally, the receptor for the cytokine IL-11 appears to be critical for implantation and decidualization (105). The similarity in phenotype between these gene knock-out mice and the COX-2 and LIF knock-outs emphasize the importance of decidualization, but also suggest that common pathways are being targeted in these gene mutation studies.

Pinopodes

Pinopodes are an ultrastructural feature of receptive endometrium that has been proposed as a reliable marker of receptive endometrium (106). These projections from the apical pole of the luminal surface of the endometrium were first described by Psychoyos (107) and are best viewed by scanning electron microscopy. The pinopodes' principal value resides in the correlation between the appearance of pinopods and the putative window of implantation, their spatial localization to the luminal surface (108), and the in vitro data showing embryo–pinopode interactions (109). Even though these endometrial microprojections have been suggested to function in the absorption of luminal fluid from the uterine cavity (110), another purpose of pinopodes may be to elevate the implantation surface toward the embryo above any antiadhesion molecules (e.g., MUC1) that have been associated with a blockade of implantation (111). Modification of the luminal surface could facilitate the intereaction between embryonic and endometrial adhesion molecules (72,112–114).

Markers of Uterine Receptivity and Infertility

The discovery of biomarkers (e.g., those described earlier) immediately begged the question regarding their patterns of expression in women with suspected defects in uterine receptivity. Graham and colleagues reported early on that women with unexplained infertility had aberrant expression of an epitope defined by an antibody against mucins (71). Patients with LPD were identified as having delayed or absent expression of integrins (49), mucin moieties (70), or PP14 (Glycodelin) (79). Klentzeris proposed the $\alpha 4\beta 1$ integrin as a potential marker for endometrial dysfunction in unexplained infertility (115). We have proposed the $\beta 3$ integrin subunit as a potential marker of such defects in women with subfertility due to various causes, including unexplained infertility (23), endometriosis (27), hydrosalpinges (28), and PCOS (116). It is interesting that this integrin appears to be normally expressed in women taking emergency contraceptives as part of the Yuzpe prototocol (117,118), but is reduced in women on oral contraceptives (119).

The existence of occult uterine receptivity defects has also been advanced by the study of other endometrial marker proteins, including the mucins (69,70), endometrial bleeding associated factor (ebaf) (120), leukemia inhibitor factor (LIF) (83), and HOXA10 (121,122). Ongoing studies include the pattern of expression of these and other markers in women with repetitive failure in ART cycles. Such approaches may provide insights into some of the unexplained implantation failures observed during in vitro fertilization attempts. Pinopods, for example, have been extensively examined to determine the effect of different stimulation protocols, including superovulation (123) or estrogen replacement cycles (124) on endometrial receptivity. Evidence from these and similar studies suggest that the endometrium in ART cycles are altered compared with that observed in natural cycles.

There is now considerable interest in establishing the nature of such defects. A better clarification of their existence, prevalence, and effective means to treat such defects will lead to better diagnosis and treatment of unexplained infertility, recurrent pregnancy loss, and improvement in the selection criteria for in vitro fertilization.

The Next Steps

It now is possible to describe the pattern of expression of numerous factors or indexes in the endometrium of a normal, fertile cycle. We and others are now in position to validate these patterns and define the normative data for old and new biomarkers. With carefully defined subpopulations of infertile women, it may soon be possible to apply one or more of these biomarkers to identify women at risk for implantation failure. This is clearly a challenging next step and will require the help of statisticians, epidemiologists, and clinical investigators. The development of appropriate animal models will allow insights into the functioning of individual biomarkers. Though animal to animal differences exist, the study of the regulation of these biomarkers will provide better strategies for treatment of infertility or methods to effectively disrupt the establishment of uterine receptivity for purposes of contraception. It is an exciting time to be in the field of implantation and embryo–endometrial interactions, and much remains to be learned about the complex interactions that lead to a single, wanted pregnancy for any couple that desires it.

References

1. Abma JC, Chandra A, Mosher WD, Peterson L, Piccinino L. Fertility, family planning, and women's health: new data from the 1995 National Survey of Family Growth. Center for Disease Control and Prevention 1997;19: Series 23.
2. Marchbanks PA, Peterson HB, Rubin GL, Wingo PA. Research on infertility: definition makes a difference. The Cancer and Steroid Hormone Study Group. Am J Epidemiol 1989;130:259–67.
3. Kim HH, Hornstein MD. Unexplained infertility: defining the problem and understanding study design. Infert Reprod Med Clin NA 1997;8:487–99.
4. Anderson TL, Hodgen GD. Uterine receptivity in the primate. Prog Clin Biol Res 1989;294:389–99.
5. Rogers PAW, Murphy CR. Uterine receptivity for implantation: human studies. In: Yoshinaga K, ed. Blastocyst implantation. Boston: Adams Publishing Group, 1989: 231–38.
6. Finn CA, Martin L. The control of implantation. J Reprod Fertil 1974;39:195–206.
7. Shapiro SS, Johnson MH, Jr. Progesterone altered amino acid accumulation by human endometrium in vitro. Biol Reprod 1989;40:555–64.
8. Beier HM. Oviducal and uterine fluids. J Reprod Fertil 1974;37:221–37.
9. Psychoyos A. Hormonal control of ovoimplantation. Vitams Horm 1973;31: 201–56.
10. Hodgen GD. Surrogate embryo transfer combined with estrogen-progesterone therapy in monkeys: implantation, gestation, and delivery without ovaries. JAMA 1983; 250:2167–71.

11. Navot D, Bergh PA, Williams M, et al. An insight into early reproductive processes through the in vivo model of ovum donation. J Clin Endocrinol Metab 1991;72: 408–14.
12. Bergh PA, Navot D. The impact of embryonic development and endometrial maturity on the timing of implantation. Fertil Steril 1992;58:537–42.
13. Hertig AT, Rock J, Adams EC. A description of 34 human ova within the first 17 days of development. Am J Anat 1956;98:435–93.
14. Navot D, Bergh P. Preparation of the human endometrium for implantation. Ann NY Acad Sci 1991;622:212–19.
15. Navot D, Scott RT, Droesch K, Veeck LL, Liu HC, Rosenwaks Z. The window of embryo transfer and the efficiency of human conception in vitro. Fertil Steril 1991;55:114–18.
16. Brenner RM, West NB. Hormonal regulation of the reproductive tract in female mammals. Ann Rev Physiol 1975;37:273–302.
17. Brenner RM, West NB, McClellan MC. Estrogen and progestin receptors in the reproductive tract of male and female primates. Biol Reprod 1990;42:11–19.
18. Lessey BA, Killam AP, Metzger DA, Haney AF, Greene GL, McCarty KS, Jr. Immunohistochemical analysis of human uterine estrogen and progesterone receptors throughout the menstrual cycle. J Clin Endocrinol Metab 1988;67:334–40.
19. Noyes RW, Hertig AI, Rock J. Dating the endometrial biopsy. Fertil Steril 1950; 1:3–25.
20. Jones GS. Some newer aspects of management of infertility. JAMA 1949;141: 1123–29.
21. Fritz M.A, Lessey BA. Defective luteal function. In: Fraser IS, Jansen RPS, Lobo RA, Whitehead MI, eds. Estrogens and progestogens in clinical practice. London: Churchhill Livingstone, 1998:437–94.
22. Lessey BA, Castelbaum AJ, Harris J, Meyer WR, Wolf L, Fritz MA. Use of integrins to date the endometrium. Fertil Steril 2000;73:779–87.
23. Lessey BA, Castelbaum AJ, Sawin SJ, Sun J. Integrins as markers of uterine receptivity in women with primary unexplained infertility. Fertil Steril 1995;63:535–42.
24. Stephenson MD. Frequency of factors associated with habitual abortion in 197 couples. Fertil Steril 1996;66:24–29.
25. Wilcox AJ, Baird DD, Wenberg CR. Time of implantation of the conceptus and loss of pregnancy. N Engl J Med 1999;340:1796–99.
26. Batista MC, Cartledge TP, Merino MJ, et al. Midluteal phase endometrial biopsy does not accurately predict luteal function. Fertil Steril 1993;59:294–300.
27. Lessey BA, Castelbaum AJ, Sawin SJ, et al. Aberrant integrin expression in the endometrium of women with endometriosis. J Clin Endocrinol Metab 1994;79:643–49.
28. Meyer WR, Castelbaum AJ, Somkuti S, et al. Hydrosalpinges adversely affect markers of endometrial receptivity. Hum Reprod 1997;12:1393–98.
29. Somkuti S, Appenzeller MF, Lessey BA. Advances in the assessment of endometrial function. Infert Reprod Med Clin NA 1995;6:303–28.
30. Yaron Y, Botchan A, Amit A, Peyser MR, David MP, Lessing JB. Endometrial receptivity in the light of modern assisted reproductive technologies. Fertil Steril 1994;62: 225–32.
31. Garcia E, Bouchard P, De Brux J, et al. Use of immunoctyochemistry of progesterone and estrogen receptors for endometrial dating. J Clin Endocrinol Metab 1988;67: 80–87.
32. Geisert RD, Pratt TN, Bazer FW, Mayes JS, Watson GH. Immunocytochemical local-

ization and changes in endometrial progestin receptor protein during the porcine oestrous cycle and early pregnancy. Reprod Fertil Dev 1994;6:749–60.
33. Tan J, Paria BC, Dey SK, Das SK. Differential uterine expression of estrogen and progesterone receptors correlates with uterine preparation for implantation and decidualization in the mouse. Endocrinology 1999;140:5310–21.
34. Lessey BA, Yeh IT, Castelbaum AJ, et al. Endometrial progesterone receptors and markers of uterine receptivity in the window of implantation. Fertil Steril 1996;65: 477–83.
35. Lovely LP, Appa Rao KBC, Gui Y, Lessey BA. Characterization of the androgen receptor in a well-differentiated endometrial adenocarcinoma cell line (Ishikawa). J Steroid Biochem Mol Biol 2000;74:235–41.
36. Zhu LJ, Cullinan-Bove K, Polihronis M, Bagchi MK, Bagchi IC. Calcitonin is a progesterone-regulated marker that forecasts the receptive state of endometrium during implantation. Endocrinology 1998;139:3923–34.
37. Kumar S, Zhu LJ, Polihronis M, et al. Progesterone induces calcitonin gene expression in human endometrium within the putative window of implantation. J Clin Endocrinol Metab 1998;83:4443–50.
38. Zhu LJ, Bagchi MK, Bagchi IC. Attenuation of calcitonin gene expression in pregnant rat uterus leads to a block in embryonic implantation. Endocrinology 1998;139: 330–39.
39. Wang J, Rout UK, Bagchi IC, Armant DR. Expression of calcitonin receptors in mouse preimplantation embryos and their function in the regulation of blastocyst differentiation by calcitonin. Development 1998;125:4293–302.
40. Lessey BA. Endometrial integrins and the establishment of uterine receptivity. Hum Reprod 1998;13(Suppl. 3):247–58.
41. Lessey BA. Integrins and uterine receptivity. In: Carson DD, ed. Embryo implantation: molecular, cellular and clinical aspects. New York: Springer-Verlag, 1999:210–22.
42. Creus M, Balasch J, Ordi J, et al. Integrin expression in normal and out-of-phase endometria. Hum Reprod 1998;13:3460–68.
43. Hii LPP, Rogers PAW. Endometrial vascular and glandular expression of integrin $\alpha_v\beta_3$ in women with and without endometriosis. Hum Reprod 1998;13:1030–35.
44. Giudice LC. Potential biochemical markers of uterine receptivity. Hum Reprod 1999;14(Suppl. 2):3–16.
45. Bronson RA, Fusi FM. Integrins and human reproduction. Mol Hum Reprod 1996;2:153–68.
46. Sueoka K, Shiokawa S, Miyazaki T, Kuji N, Tanaka M, Yoshimura Y. Integrins and reproductive physiology: expression and modulation in fertilization, embryogensis, and implantation. Fertil Steril 1997;67:799–811.
47. Illera MJ, Cullinan E, Gui Y, Yuan L, Beyler SA, Lessey BA. Blockade of the $\alpha n\beta 3$ integrin adversely affects implantation in the mouse. Biol Reprod 2000;62:1285–90.
48. Lessey BA, Damjanovich L, Coutifaris C, Castelbaum A, Albelda SM, Buck CA. Integrin adhesion molecules in the human endometrium. Correlation with the normal and abnormal menstrual cycle. J Clin Invest 1992;90:188–95.
49. Tabibzadeh S. Patterns of expression of integrin molecules in human endometrium throughout the menstrual cycle. Hum Reprod 1992;7:876–82.
50. Lessey BA, Castelbaum AJ, Buck CA, Lei Y, Yowell CW, Sun J. Further characterization of endometrial integrins during the menstrual cycle and in pregnancy. Fertil Steril 1994;62:497–506.

51. Albers A, Thie M, Hohn HP, Denker HW. Differential expression and localization of integrins and CD44 in the membrane domains of human uterine epithelial cells during the menstrual cycle. Acta Anat (Basel) 1995;153:12–19.
52. Lessey BA, Albelda S, Buck CA, et al. Distribution of integrin cell adhesion molecules in endometrial cancer. Am J Pathol 1995;146:717–26.
53. Lessey BA, Ilesanmi AO, Sun J, Lessey MA, Harris J, Chwalisz K. Luminal and glandular endometrial epithelium express integrins differentially throughout the menstrual cycle: implications for implantation, contraception, and infertility. Am J Reprod Immunol 1996;35:195–204.
54. Aplin JD, Spanswick C, Behzad F, Kimber SJ, Vicovac L. Integrins $\beta 5$, $\beta 3$, αv are apically distributed in endometrial epithelium. Mol Hum Reprod 1996;2:527–34.
55. Armant DR, Kaplan HA, Mover H, Lennarz WJ. The effect of hexapeptides on attachment and outgrowth of mouse blastocysts cultured in vitro: evidence for the involvement of the cell recognition tripeptide Arg-Gly-Asp. Proc Natl Acad Sci USA 1986;83:6751–55.
56. Yelian FD, Yang Y, Hirata JD, Schultz JF, Armant DR. Molecular interactions between fibronectin and integrins during mouse blastocyst outgrowth. Mol Reprod Dev 1995;41:435–48.
57. Turpeenniemi-Hujanen T, Feinberg RF, Kauppila A, Puistola U. Extracellular matrix interactions in early human embryos: implications for normal implantation events. Fertil Steril 1995;64:132–38.
58. Shiokawa S, Yoshimura Y, Sawa H, et al. Functional role of Arg-Gly-Asp (RGD)-binding sites on β_1 integrin in embryo implantation using mouse blastocysts and human decidua. Biol Reprod 1999;60:1468–74.
59. Brooks PC, Strömblad S, Sanders LC, et al. Localization of matrix metalloproteinase MMP-2 to the surface of invasive cells by interaction with integrin $\alpha v \beta 3$. Cell 1996;85:683–93.
60. Murray MJ, Lessey BA. Embryo implantation and tumor metastasis: common pathways of invasion and angiogenesis. Semin Reprod Endocrinol 1999;17:275–90.
61. Lanteri E, Pistritto M, Bartoloni G, Cordaro S, Stivala F, Montoneri C. Expression of $\alpha 6$ and $\beta 4$ integrin subunits on human endometrium throughout the menstrual cycle and during early pregnancy. Fertil Steril 1998;69:37–40.
62. Murray MJ, Zhang JN, Lessey BA. Expression of $\alpha 6$ and $\beta 4$ integrin subunits throughout the menstrual cycle: no correlation with uterine receptivity. Fertil Steril 1999;72:522–26.
63. Yaegashi N, Fujita N, Yajima A, Nakamura M. Menstrual cycle dependent expression of CD44 in normal human endometrium. Hum Pathol 1995;26:862–65.
64. Saegusa M, Hashimura M, Okayasu I. CD44 expression in normal, hyperplastic, and malignant endometrium. J Pathol 1998;184:297–306.
65. Fukuda MN, Sato T, Nakayama J, et al. Trophinin and tastin, a novel cell adhesion molecule complex with potential involvement in embryo implantation. Genes Dev 1995;9:1199–210.
66. MacCalman CD, Furth EE, Omigbodun A, Bronner M, Coutifaris C, Strauss JF III. Regulated expression of cadherin-11 in human epithelial cells: a role for cadherin-11 in trophoblast-endometrium interactions? Dev Dyn 1996;206:201–11.
67. Getsios S, Chen GTC, Stephenson MD, Leclerc P, Blaschuk OW, MacCalman CD. Regulated expression of cadherin-6 and cadherin-11 in the glandular epithelial and stromal cells of the human endometrium. Dev Dyn 1998;211:238–47.

68. Behzad F, Seif MW, Campbell S, Aplin JD. Expression of two isoforms of CD44 in human endometrium. Biol Reprod 1994;51:739–47.
69. Seif MW, Aplin JD, Buckley CH. Luteal phase defect: the possibility of an immunohistochemical diagnosis. Fertil Steril 1989;51:273–79.
70. Graham RA, Seif MW, Aplin JD, et al. An endometrial factor in unexplained infertility. Br Med J 1990;300:1428–31.
71. Carson DD, Rohde LH, Surveyor G. Cell surface glycoconjugates as modulators of embryo attachment to uterine epithelial cells. Int J Biochem 1994;26:1269–77.
72. Hild-Petito S, Fazleabas AT, Julian J, Carson DD. Mucin (Muc-1) expression is differentially regulated in uterine luminal and glandular epithelia of the baboon (*Papio anubis*). Biol Reprod 1996;54:939–47.
73. Aplin JD, Seif MW, Graham RA, Hey NA, Behzad F, Campbell S. The endometrial cell surface and implantation: expression of the polymorphic mucin MUC-1 and adhesion molecules during the endometrial cycle. Ann NY Acad Sci 1994;734:103–21.
74. Kliman HJ, Feinberg RF, Schwartz LB, Feinman MA, Lavi E, Meaddough EL. A mucin-like glycoprotein identified by MAG (mouse ascites Golgi) antibodies: menstrual cycle-dependent localization in human endometrium. Am J Pathol 1995;146:166–81.
75. Rutanen EM, Seppala M. Insulin-like growth factor binding protein-1 in female reproductive functions. Int J Gynaecol Obstet 1992;39:3–9.
76. Oehninger S, Coddington CC, Hodgen GD, Seppala M. Factors affecting fertilization: endometrial placental protein 14 reduces the capacity of human spermatozoa to bind to the human zona pellucida. Fertil Steril 1995;63:377–83.
77. Clark GF, Oehninger S, Patankar MS, et al. A role for glycoconjugates in human development: the human feto-embryonic defense system hypothesis. Hum Reprod 1996;11:467–73.
78. Westergaard LG, Wiberg N, Yding C, et al. Circulating concentrations of placenta protein 14 during the natural menstrual cycle in women significantly reflect endometrial receptivity to implantation and pregnancy during successive assisted reproduction cycles. Hum Reprod 1998;13:2612–19.
79. Klentzeris LD, Bulmer JN, Seppälä M, Li TC, Warren MA, Cooke ID. Placental protein 14 in cycles with normal and retarded endometrial differentiation. Hum Reprod 1994;9:394–98.
80. Tulppala M, Julkunen M, Tiitinen A, Stenman U-H, Seppälä M. Habitual abortion is accompanied by low serum levels of placental protein 14 in the luteal phase of the fertile cycle. Fertil Steril 1995;63:792–95.
81. Bhatt H, Brunet LJ, Stewart CL. Uterine expression of leukemia inhibitory factor coincides with the onset of blastocyst implantation. Proc Natl Acad Sci USA 1991;88:11408–12.
82. Stewart CL, Kaspar P, Brunet LJ, et al. Blastocyst implantation depends on maternal expression of leukaemia inhibitory factor. Nature 1992;359:76–79.
83. Cullinan EB, Abbondanzo SJ, Anderson PS, Pollard JW, Lessey BA, Stewart CL. Leukemia inhibitory factor (LIF) and LIF receptor expression in human endometrium suggests a potential autocrine paracrine function in regulating embryo implantation. Proc Natl Acad Sci USA 1996;93:3115–20.
84. Das SK, Wang X-N, Paria BC, et al. Heparin-binding EGF-like growth factor gene is induced in the mouse uterus temporally by the blastocyst solely at the site of its

apposition: a possible ligand for interaction with blastocyst EGF-receptor in implantation. Development 1994;120:1071–83.
85. Yoo HJ, Barlow DH, Mardon HJ. Temporal and spatial regulation of expression of heparin-binding epidermal growth factor-like growth factor in the human endometrium: a possible role in blastocyst implantation. Dev Genet 1997;21:102–8.
86. Giudice LC. Endometrial growth factors and proteins. Semin Reprod Endocrinol 1995;13:93–101.
87. Stewart CL. The role of leukemia inhibitory factor (LIF) and other cytokines in regulating implantation in mammals. Ann NY Acad Sci 1994;734:157–65.
88. Hilton DJ, Gough NM. Leukemia inhibitory factor: a biological perspective. J Cell Biochem 1991;46:21–26.
89. Kojima K, Kanzaki H, Iwai M, et al. Expression of leukemia inhibitory factor in human endometrium and placenta. Biol Reprod 1994;50:882–87.
90. Birdsall MA, Hopkisson JF, Grant KE, Barlow DH, Mardon HJ. Expression of heparin-binding epidermal growth factor messenger RNA in the human endometrium. Mol Hum Reprod 1996;2:31–34.
91. Leach RE, Khalifa R, Ramirez ND, et al. Multiple roles for heparin-binding epidermal growth factor-like growth factor are suggested by its cell-specific expression during the human endometrial cycle and early placentation. J Clin Endocrinol Metab 1999;84:3355–63.
92. Raab G, Kover K, Paria BC, Dey SK, Ezzell RM, Klagsbrun M. Mouse preimplantation blastocysts adhere to cells expressing the transmembrane form of heparin-binding EGF-like growth factor. Development 1996;122:637–45.
93. Tamada H, Higashiyama C, Takano H, Kawate N, Inaba T, Sawada T. The effects of heparin-binding epidermal growth factor-like growth factor on preimplantation-embryo development and implantation in the rat. Life Sci 1999;64:1967–73.
94. Martin KL, Barlow DH, Sargent IL. Heparin-binding epidermal growth factor significantly improves human blastocyst development and hatching in serum-free medium. Hum Reprod 1998;13:1645–52.
95. Sargent IL, Martin KL, Barlow DH. The use of recombinant growth factors to promote human embryo development in serum-free medium. Hum Reprod 1998;13(Suppl. 4):239–48.
96. Lessey BA, Gui Y, Yuan L, Appa Rao KBC, Mulholland J. Endometrial heparin binding epidermal growth factor (HB-EGF): A paracrine signal for uterine receptivity? J Clin Endocrinol Metab 2001 (submitted).
97. Benson GV, Lim HJ, Paria BC, Satokata I, Dey SK, Maas RL. Mechanisms of reduced fertility in *Hoxa-10* mutant mice: uterine homeosis and loss of maternal *Hoxa-10* expression. Development 1996;122:2687–96.
98. Satokata I, Benson G, Maas R. Sexually dimorphic sterility phenotypes in Hoxa-10 deficient mice. Nature 1995;374:460–63.
99. Taylor HS, Vanden Heuvel GB, Igarashi P. A conserved Hox Axis in the mouse and human female reproductive system: late establishment and persistent adult expression of the Hoxa cluster genes. Biol Reprod 1997;57:1338–45.
100. Taylor HS, Arici A, Olive D, Igarashi P. HOXA10 is expressed in response to sex steroids at the time of implantation in the human endometrium. J Clin Invest 1998;101:1379–84.
101. Taylor HS, Igarashi P, Olive DL, Arici A. Sex steroids mediate HOXA11 expression

in the human peri-implantation endometrium. J Clin Endocrinol Metab 1999;84: 1129–35.
102. Chakraborty I, Das SK, Wang J, Dey SK. Developmental expression of the cyclo-oxygenase-1 and cyclo-oxygenase-2 genesin the peri-implantation mouse uterus and their differential regulation by the blastocyst and ovarian steroids. J Mol Endocrinol 1996;16:107–22.
103. Jones RL, Kelly RW, Critchley HOD. Chemokine and cyclooxygenase-2 expression in human endometrium coincides with leukocyte accumulation. Hum Reprod 1997;12:1300–6.
104. Kim JJ, Wang J, Bambra C, Das SK, Dey SK, Fazleabas AT. Expression of cyclooxygenase-1 and-2 in the Baboon endometrium during the menstrual cycle and pregnancy. Endocrinology 1999;140:2672–78.
105. Robb L, Li RL, Hartley L, Nandurkar HH, Koentgen F, Begley CG. Infertility in female mice lacking the receptor for interleukin 11 is due to a defective uterine response to implantation. Nature Med 1998;4:303–8.
106. Psychoyos A, Nikas G. Uterine pinopodes as markers of uterine receptivity. Assist Reprod Rev 1994;4:26–32.
107. Psychoyos A, Mandon P. Etude de la surface de l'epithelium uterin au microscope electronique a balayage. CR Hebd Seances Acad Sci Paris 1971;272:2723–29.
108. Martel D, Frydman R, Sarantis L, Roche D, Psychoyos A. Scanning electron microscopy of the uterine luminal epithelium as a marker of the implantation window. In: Yoshinaga K, ed. Blastocyst implantation. Boston: Adams Publishing Group, 1993: 225–30.
109. Bentin-Ley U, Sjögren A, Nilsson L, Hamberger L, Larsen JF, Horn T. Presence of uterine pinopodes at the embryo-endometrial interface during human implantation in vitro. Hum Reprod 1999;14:515–20.
110. Anderson TL. Biomolecular markers for the window of uterine receptivity. In: Yoshinaga K, ed. Blastocyst implantation. Boston: Adams Publishing Group, 1993: 219–24.
111. Carson DD, Tang J-P, Julian J. Heparan sulfate proteoglycan (perlecan) expression by mouse embryos during acquisition of attachment competence. Dev Biol 1993;155: 97–106.
112. Campbell S, Swann HR, Seif MW, Kimber SJ, Aplin JD. Cell adhesion molecules on the oocyte and preimplantation human embryo. Hum Reprod 1995;10:1571–78.
113. Sutherland AE, Calarco PG, Damsky CH. Expression and function of cell surface extracellular matrix receptors in mouse blastocyst attachment and outgrowth. J Cell Biol 1988;106:1331–48.
114. Sutherland AE, Calarco PG, Damsky CH. Developmental regulation of integrin expression at the time of implantation in the mouse embryo. Development 1993; 119:1175–86.
115. Klentzeris LD, Bulmer JN, Trejdosiewicz LK, Morrison L, Cooke ID. Beta-1 integrin cell adhesion molecules in the endometrium of fertile and infertile women. Hum Reprod 1993;8:1223–30.
116. Appa Rao KBC, Lovely LP, Gui Y, Lessey BA. Over expression of endometrial androgen receptors in women with polycystic ovarian syndrome: an underlying cause of poor reproductive function? Biol Reprod 2001 (submitted).
117. Taskin O, Brown RW, Young DC, Poindexter AN, Wiehle RD. High doses of oral

contraceptives do not alter endometrial α1 and αvβ3 integrins in the late implantation window. Fertil Steril 1994;61:850–55.
118. Raymond EG, Lovely LP, Chen-Mok M, Seppälä M, Kurman RJ, Lessey BA. Effect of the Yuzpe regimen of emergency contraception on markers of endometrial receptivity. Hum Reprod 2000;15:2351–55.
119. Somkuti SG, Sun JH, Yowell CW, Fritz MA, Lessey BA. The effect of oral contraceptive pills on markers of endometrial receptivity. Fertil Steril 1996;65:484–88.
120. Tabibzadeh S, Shea W, Lessey BA, Satyaswaroop PG. Aberrant expression of ebaf in endometria of patients with infertility. Mol Hum Reprod 1998;4:595–602.
121. Taylor HS, Bagot C, Kardana A, Olive D, Arici A. HOX gene expression is altered in the endometrium of women with endometriosis. Hum Reprod 1999;14:1328–31.
122. Gui Y-T, Zhang J, Yuan L, Lessey BA. Regulation of Hoxa-10 and its expression in normal and abnormal endometrium. Mol Hum Reprod 1999;5: 866–73.
123. Kolb BA, Paulson RJ. The luteal phase of cycles utilizing controlled ovarian hyperstimulation and the possible impact of this hyperstimulation on embryo implantation. Am J Obstet Gynecol 1997;176:1262–67.
124. Nikas G, Drakakis P, Loutradis D, et al. Uterine pinopodes as markers of the "nidation window" in cycling women receiving exogenous oestradiol and progesterone. Hum Reprod 1995;10:1208–13.

18

Endometrial Pinopodes: Relevance for Human Blastocyst Implantation

URSULA BENTIN-LEY AND GEORGE NIKAS

Implantation failure after assisted reproductive technology (ART) is still a major problem. Even after blastocyst transfer, implantation rates do not exceed 50% (1,2), most likely due to suboptimal endometrial preparation for implantation (3,4).

Psychoyos (5,6) formulated the theory of an implantation or nidation window, a transient period during which the endometrium is receptive and implantation can initiate. A lot of effort has been invested into a clear definition of endometrial receptivity, using both morphological markers (7–11) and molecular markers (12–22), but the ethical constraints for use of human material mean that only indirect evidence has been provided by investigations of the human endometrium during the midluteal phase, whereas direct information on human blastocyst–endometrial interactions in vivo are missing. This chapter will concentrate on morphological markers of endometrial receptivity, as observed by scanning electron microscopy (SEM), and their relevance for blastocyst–endometrial interactions in vitro.

Scanning Electron Microscopy of the Endometrial Surface Epithelium

SEM studies in human and animals show presence of two different cell types in the luminal epithelium: ciliated cells and secretory cells presenting microvilli at the apical plasma membrane. Whereas the morphology of ciliated cells is relatively constant, the secretory cells undergo pronounced hormone-dependent morphological changes during the menstrual cycle.

Animal Studies

Studies by Psychoyos (23) in the rat model has shown that after 3 days of progesterone priming in spayed animals, the endometrium is in a neutral phase that allows ovum survival but not ovum implantation. Addition of a small dose of estrogen induces formation of a receptive endometrium within 24 hours that lasts for a short period of 12 hours, the so-called implantation window. After this short receptive period, the endometrium enters a refractory state during which the endometrium is hostile to the embryo.

During the receptive phase, the apical plasma membranes of the epithelial cells lining the uterine cavity loose their microvilli and develope large and smooth apical protrusions resembling sponges (24). Intrauterine tracer studies have shown that these structures are involved in apical-to-basal transport of fluid and macromolecules (25). Several studies indicate that pinopodes are a specific marker of endometrial receptivity in the rat (26–28). Pinopode formation and disappearance is dependent on both estrogen and progesterone (29). Furthermore, high levels of estrogen interfere with normal pinopode formation.

Human Studies

Pinopode formation has also been observed in the human endometrium (30,31). Under the influence of estrogen during the proliferative phase, cells vary greatly in size and shape (11). Bulging of the apical plasma membrane is minimal, cell borders are barely marked, and the microvilli are short and slender. Cell bulging increases 2 days postovulation. On Day 3 the microvilli are long, thick, and upright, having reached their maximum of development. On the fourth postovulatory day, the tips of microvilli appear swollen. Day 5, a pronounced and general bulging appears, the microvilli decrease both in number and length, fuse or disappear. Smooth and slender projections arise from the entire cell apex. These are developing pinopodes. Day 6 postovulation, the microvilli are virtually absent and the naked membranes protrude and fold maximally (fully developed pinopodes). Day 7 the protrusions decrease in size and small stubby microvilli reappear on the wrinkled membranes (regressing pinopodes). Day 8, the pinopodes have almost disappeared and the microvilli develop further. The "implantation window" is estimated to be between Day 5 and Day 7 postovulation.

Sequential biopsies from patients undergoing hormone-controlled cycles (HC) with exogenous estrogen and progesterone confirm that pinopodes only are present in a short period of 48 hours (8). Furthermore, even though the duration of pinopode formation is constant in all patients, the interpatient variation of onset of pinopode formation varies up to 5 days, from Day 6 to Day 10 of progesterone treatment. There is no correlation between serum steroid hormone levels on the day of biopsy and pinopode expression. In normally menstruating fertile women, fully developed pinopodes are found on Day 6, 7, and 8 postovulation (11). Other clinical studies show a positive correlation of the number of pinopodes present in sequential endometrial biopsies and pregnancy after embryo transfer (ET) (32) and absence of pinopodes in recipients with repeated implantation failure after ET (Nikas

18. Endometrial Pinopodes: Relevance for Human Blastocyst Implantation   229

et al., unpublished). Representative SEM micrographs of the endometrial surface before and during pinopode formation are shown in Figure 18.1.

Biopsies from oocyte donors undergoing controlled ovarian hyperstimulation (COH) (11) also show presence of fully developed pinopodes in only a

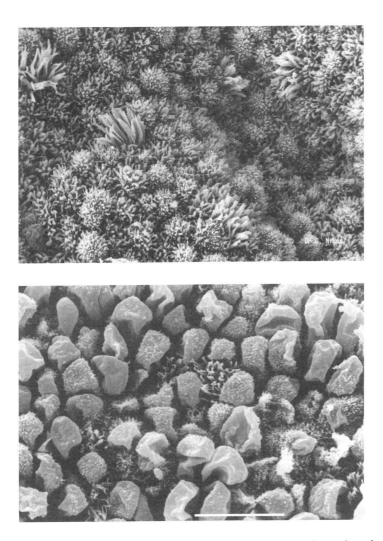

FIGURE 18.1. Representative SEM micrographs of midsecretory endometrium. In the upper photo, the secretory cells appear bulging, with their apices covered with dense microvilli. Note that in some cells, the tips of the microvilli appear swollen. Some ciliated cells are also present. This is a typical picture of a Day 18 endometrium. In the lower photo, the secretory cells bear smooth and folded membrane projections that are devoid of microvilli. These are fully developed pinopodes, typical of a Day 20 endometrium. Note that pinopodes may protrude beyond the length of the cilia. The bar represents 10 µm, and applies to the magnification of the images (×3250).

single biopsy in each patient, confirming the short lifespan of maximally 48 hours in pinopode formation, also in the COH cycles. It is interesting that pinopode formation seems to be accelerated 1–2 days (11,33), apparently due to premature progesterone rise at the day following hCG. In a preliminary study (34), administration of a small dose of antiprogestin (2.5 mg of RU486) shortly after ovum pick-up and the following day was shown to normalize the timing of pinopode formation.

Experience from ovum donation programs show that women undergoing HC cycles and ET have higher chances of conception compared with women undergoing COH (3,35). This may be due to a better priming of the endometrium, avoiding high estradiol levels (4). The retardation of pinopode formation in HC cycles, however, compared with both COH- and normal menstrual cycles, suggests that the opening and closure of the implantation window is relatively retarded. The extra time might allow more embryos to develop to the hatched blastocyst stage before closure of the implantation window, and by that means increase conception rates.

Presence of Endometrial Pinopodes During Human Blastocyst–Endometrial Interactions In Vitro

For investigations on human blastocyst–endometrial interactions, a three-dimensional human endometrial cell culture system has been developed (36) in which endometrial epithelial and stromal cells are co-cultured, separated by a thin layer of artificial basal membrane (Matrigel®). Comparative studies of immediately fixed biopsies and cultured epithelial cells from the same patients show that the cultured cells preserve their ultrastructure corresponding to the day of biopsy (37).

For these studies, human surplus embryos from in vitro fertilization (IVF) treatments are cultured to the expanded or hatched blastocyst stage, and then applied onto the endometrial cell culture. Forty-eight hours following attachment, three cultures were fixed and prepared for SEM (38). Furthermore, seven attachment sites were cut into 3-µm serial sections for light microscopy (LM) and subsequent transmission electron microscopy (TEM).

SEM of Embryo Attachment Sites

Cultured cells demonstrated a confluent epithelial surface that was slightly folded into ridges. Most cell surfaces seemed flattened, but interspersed clusters of cells with pinopodes were present. Some pinopodes presented a smooth naked surface (developing pinopodes), others a folded naked surface (fully developed pinopodes). Endometrial cells without pinopode formation, presenting dense short microvilli or cilia, separated the pinopode accumulations that covered roughly 5%–10% of the surface.

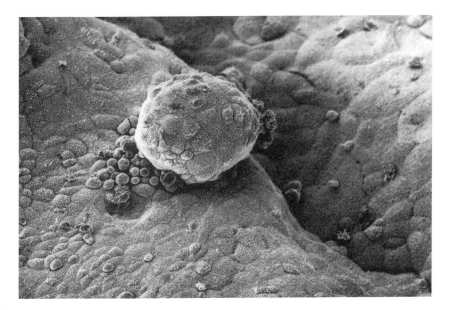

FIGURE 18.2. SEM of embryo–endometrial interface. The majority of endometrial epithelial cells display flattened apical plasma membranes with microvilli present; however, the blastocyst attaches to a cluster of pinopode presenting cells with naked bulging apical plasma membranes. The bar represents 90 μm and applies to the magnification of the images (×225).

All three blastocysts were fully hatched and attached to the endometrial surface. The blastocysts were not evenly rounded; rather, they were more or less oblong and flattened. Dense short microvilli covered the surface of the trophectodermal cells. All three blastocysts were attached to areas where epithelial cells displayed pinopodes (Fig. 18.2). It is remarkable that cells in neighbor areas were devoid of pinopodes, showing microvilli or cilia at the apical surface. Many pinopodes were fully developed or developing right at the embryo–endometrial interface and were contacting the surface of the trophectodermal cells.

LM and TEM of Embryo Attachment Sites

LM and TEM also showed sections with pinopodes in attachment areas. Trophoblastic cells, however, did not interact directly with apical plasma membranes of endometrial epithelial cells (Bentin-Ley et al., unpublished). Transmission electron microscopy of early blastocyst attachment revealed that the first morphological sign of attachment, defined as *junction formation*, was found at the apical-to-lateral border of endometrial epithelial cells. Pinopode presenting apical plasma membranes were located closely to trophoblastic apical plasma membranes, but direct participation in trophoblast–endometrial interactions were not observed.

Discussion

The upcoming and lifespan of pinopodes (8) is tightly regulated. Furthermore, pinopode formation is hormone dependent. The correlation of pinopode expression to embryo implantation after ET suggests that pinopodes are good indicators of endometrial receptivity. The preference of human blastocyst to attach to pinopode-presenting cells further supports this hypothesis.

Given the importance of implantation in ART, pinopode detection appears to be a promising clinical tool for assessing endometrial function and optimizing embryo transfer on an individual basis. Preliminary trials using SEM on endometrial biopsies taken in mock HC cycles appear to improve pregnancy rates following transfer of donated embryos (39). Larger studies are needed to establish the clinical value of this procedure.

The pilot study by Paulson et al. (34), who used RU486 to postpone pinopode formation for about 2 days, is very interesting for standard IVF cycles. In theory, a delayed opening of the implantation window in IVF cycles would allow sufficient time for the blastocyst to develop to a stage capable of commencing implantation; however, this preliminary report was not followed by any clinical trials. In the rat, displacement of receptivity with the use of RU486 was successfully reported by Sarantis et al. (28). Beier et al. (40) used antiprogestins to achieve a transposition of the implantation window in the rabbit. These reports encourage the hope that a similar postponement of receptivity could be possible in the human; however, clinical trials would be complicated by ethical constraints, and by the difficulty to define the exact dose of antiprogestin that would produce a temporary arrest of endometrial maturation without disrupting tissue integrity.

It remains to be elucidated whether apical plasma membranes on pinopodes present specific receptors for trophoblast attachment. Immunohistochemical studies have in fact shown that luminal endometrial cells do present the interleukin-1 receptor type 1 (IL-1R t1) and the integrin subunit β_3, which are supposed to participate in embryo–endometrial interactions during attachment (12–18). Both the IL-1R t1 and the IL-1 receptor antagonist are actually expressed as patches (13), whereas this pattern is not found for integrin subunit β_3 distribution (Lessey, personal communication). So far, however, observations on co-expression of pinopodes and possible trophoblast receptors have not been published.

Serial sections of human blastocyst attachment sites in vitro also showed presence of pinopodes at the trophoblast–endometrial interface; however, pinopode presenting apical plasma membranes were not directly involved in blastocyst attachment to the endometrium. This suggests that pinopode formation is only a part of the cellular and molecular changes in the endometrial epithelium that allows blastocyst attachment and penetration.

Acknowledgments. These studies have been supported by Snedkermester Sophus Jacobsen og hustru Astrid Jacobsens Foundation, The Michaelsen Foundation and the Danish Research Counsil (no. 28809).

References

1. Gardner DK, Schoolcraft WB, Wagley L, Schlenker T, Stevens J, Hesla J. A prospective randomized trial of blastocyst culture and transfer in in-vitro fertilization. Hum Reprod 1998;13(12):3434–40.
2. Schoolcraft WB, Gardner DK, Lane M, Schlenker T, Hamilton F, Meldrum DR. Blastocyst culture and transfer: analysis of results and parameters affecting outcome in two in vitro fertilization programs. Fertil Steril 1999;72(4):604–9.
3. Edwards RG, Morcos S, MacNamee M, Balmaceda JP, Walters DE, Asch R. High fecundity of amerorrhoic women in embryo-transfer programmes. Lancet 1991;338: 292–94.
4. Simón C, Cano F, Valbuena D, et al. Clinical evidence for a detrimental effect on uterine receptivity of high serum estradiol levels in high and normal responder patients. Hum Reprod 1995;10:2432–37.
5. Psychoyos A. Hormonal control of uterine receptivity for nidation. J Reprod Fertil 1976;25(Suppl. 1):17–28.
6. Psychoyos A. Uterine receptivity for nidation. Ann NY Acad Sci 1986;476:36–42.
7. Psychoyos A, Nikas G. Uterine pinopodes as markers of uterine receptivity. Assist Reprod Rev 1994;4:26–32.
8. Nikas G, Drakakis P, Loutradis D, et al. Uterine pinopodes as markers of the nidation window in cycling women receiving exogenous oestradiol and pogesterone. Hum Reprod 1995;10:1208–13.
9. Nikas G. Cell surface morphological events relevant to human implantation. Hum Reprod 1999;14(Suppl. 2):37–44.
10. Nikas G. Pinopodes as markers of endometrial receptivity in clinical practice. Hum Reprod 1999;14(Suppl. 2):99–106.
11. Nikas G, Develioglu OH, Toner JP, Jones HW, Jr. Endometrial pinopodes indicate a shift in the window of receptivity in IVF cycles. Hum Reprod 1999;14:787–92.
12. Simón C, Piquette GN, Frances A, et al. Localization of interleukin-1 type I receptor and interleukin-1β in human endometrium throughout the menstrual cycle. J Clin Endocrinol Metab 1993;77:549–55.
13. Simón C, Frances A, Lee BY, et al. Immunohistochemical localisation, identification and regulation of the interleukin-1 receptor antagonist in the human endometrium. Hum Reprod 1995;10:2472–77.
14. Simón C, Gimeno MJ, Mercader A, et al. Embryonic regulation of integrine β3, α4 and α1 in human endometrial epithelial cells *in vitro*. J Clin Endocrinol Metab 1997;82: 2607–16.
15. Lessey BA, Damjanovich L, Coutifaris C, et al. Integrin adhesion molecules in the human endometrium. Correlation with the normal and abnormal menstrual cycle. J Clin Invest 1992;90:188–95.
16. Lessey BA, Yeh I, Castelbaum AJ, et al. Endometrial progesterone receptors and markers of uterine receptivity in the window of implantation. Fertil Steril 1996;65: 477–83.
17. Lessey BA. Integrins and the endometrium: new markers of uterine receptivity. Ann NY Acad Sci 1997;828:111–22.

18. Meyer WR, Castelbaum AJ, Somkuti S, et al. Hydrosalpinges adversely affect markers of endometrial receptivity. Hum Reprod 1997;12:1393–98.
19. Giudice LC. Multifaceted roles for IGFBP-1 in human endometrium during implantation and pregnancy. Ann NY Acad Sci 1997;828:146–56.
20. Giudice LC. Potential biochemical markers of uterine receptivity. Hum Reprod 1999;14(Suppl. 2):3–16.
21. Aplin JD. MUC-1 in glycosylation in endometrium: possible roles of the apical glycocalyx at implantation. Hum Reprod 1999;14(Suppl. 2):17–25.
22. Smith SK, Charnock-Jones DS, Sharkey AM. The role of leukaemia inhibitory factor and interleukin-6 in human reproduction. Hum Reprod 1998;13(Suppl. 3):237–43.
23. Psychoyos A. Recent research on egg implantation. In: Wolstenholme W, O'Connor M, eds. Ciba Foundation study group on egg implantation. London: Churchill, 1966: 4–28.
24. Potts M, Psychoyos A. Evolution de l'ultrastructure des relations ovoendométriales sous l'influence de l'oestrogene, chez la Ratte en retard expérimental de nidation. CR Acad Sci Paris 1967;264:370–73.
25. Enders AC, Nelson DM. Pinocytotic activity of the uterus of the rat. Am J Anat 1973;138:277–300.
26. Psychoyos A, Mandon P. Scanning electron microscopy of the surface of the rat uterine epithelium during delayed implantation. J Reprod Fertil 1971;26:137–38.
27. Psychoyos A, Mandon P. Etude de la surface de l'épithélium utérin au microscope électronique à balayage. Observation chez la ratte au 4ème et 5ème jours de la gestation. CR Acad Sci Paris 1971;272:2723–29.
28. Sarantis L, Roche D, Psychoyos A. Displacement of receptiviry for nidation in the rat by the progesterone antagonist RU 486: a scanning electron microscopy study. Hum Reprod 1988;3:251–55.
29. Martel D, Monier MN, Roche D, et al. Hormonal dependence of pinopode formation at the uterine luminal surface. Hum Reprod 1991;6:597–603.
30. Nilsson O. Correlation of structure for function of the luminal cell surface in the uterine epithelium of mouse and man. Z Zellforsch microsk Anat 1962;56:803–8.
31. Martel D, Malet C, Gautray JP, et al. Surface changes of the luminal uterine epithelium during the human menstrual cycle: a scanning electron microscopic study. In: de Brux J, Gautrey JP, eds. The endometrium: hormonal impacts. New York: Plenum, 1981: 15–29.
32. Nikas G, Reddy N, Winston RML. Implantation correlates highly with the expression of uterine pinopodes in ovum recipients uner HRT: a preliminary study (Abstr. FR 21). Ninth World Congress in Human Reproduction, Philadelphia, May 29–June 1, 1996.
33. Kolb BA, Najmabadi S, Paulson RJ. Ultrastructural characteristics of the luteal phase endometrium in patients undergoing controlled ovarian hyperstimulation. Fertil Steril 1997;67:625–30.
34. Paulson RJ, Sauer MV, Lobo RA. Potential enhancement of endometrial receptivity in cycles using controlled ovarian hyperstimulation with antiprogestins; a hypothesis. Fertil Steril 1997;67:321–25.
35. Paulson RJ, Sauer MV, Lobo RA. Factors affecting embryo implantation after human in vitro fertilization: a hypothesis. Am J Obstet Gynecol 1990;163:2020–23.
36. Bentin-Ley U, Petersen B, Lindenberg S, et al. Isolation and culture of human endometrial cells in a three dimensional cell culture system. J Reprod Fert 1994;101:327–32.
37. Bentin-Ley U, Lindenberg S, Horn T, et al. Ultrastructure of endometrial epithelial cells

in a three-dimensional cell culture system for human implantation studies. J Assist Reprod Gen 1995;12:632–38.
38. Bentin-Ley U, Sjögren A, Nilsson L, et al. Presence of uterine pinopodes at the embryo–endometrial interface during human implantation in vitro. Hum Reprod 1999;14:515–20.
39. Nikas G, Garcia-Velasco J, Pellicer A, Simon C. Assessment of uterine receptivity and timing of embryo transfer using the detection of pinopodes (abstr.). Hum Reprod 1997;12(Suppl.):O-069.
40. Beier HM, Hegele-Hartung C, Mootz U, Beier-Hellwig K. Modification of endometrial cell biology using progesterone antagonists to manipulate the implantation window. Hum Reprod 1994;9(Suppl. 1):98–115.

19
The Future: Toward Single Embryo Transfer

LARS HAMBERGER, PETER SVALANDER, AND MATTS WIKLAND

In the beginning of the in vitro fertilization (IVF) era only the natural cycle was utilized. Since the introduction of controlled ovarian hyperstimulation (COH) in the beginning of the 1980s (1) more and more aggressive gonadotrophic stimulations, in combination with either GnRH agonists or antagonists, have become the vast predominating treatment regimens. When more than one oocyte was available for fertilization and development in vitro, the temptation became too great to replace more than one embryo to improve the pregnancy outcome. It has taken more than 15 years of follow up of children born after IVF to understand fully that multiple pregnancy is a risk factor for the children, even if the result is "only twins." Data from the literature concerning natural conceived twins or twins born after gonadotrophic stimulation combined with intrauterine insemination (IUI) were clearly indicating higher risks for the offspring. Multiple pregnancy is thus a serious risk factor. In a Swedish IVF-material gathered between 1982 and 1995 (2) the outcome of children has been studied by use of register data collected by the Swedish Government. Just to mention one factor from this material, a fourfold increase in cerebral palsy (CP) was registered among the multiples.

Patients and Doctors

The subfertile couple may suffer from a primary or secondary infertility; they may or may not have children with other partners in the past, and the work up of a patient prior to treatment does not always tell with certainty which one in the couple is "responsible" for the reproductive problem. It may well be an advantage not to stress this issue in the clinical situation because subfertility and its consequences are the couples problem. The man or the woman in the couple is clearly pointed out only in cases where donor gametes have to be utilized. It is important to stress these questions because many IVF units seem to have forgotten the psychosocial aspect of the infertility work up and treatment. The couple seeks help from our profession to try to improve quality of

Question   Why utilize ART?

Answer   To improve the couples quality of life

	singleton	twins	triplets	higher order
	+ +	– / –	–	– –

FIGURE 19.1. Quality of life for the family as related to multiple pregnancy.

life for the family (Fig. 19.1). Singletons or twins, at least if healthy, seem to meet with the couples hope and expectations, whereas high-order multiple pregnancies always create unwanted, and (not to the professional staff) unexpected, complications.

Comparison of results between different IVF centers is often unfair because important facts may be (deliberately) missing. Take home baby rate per transfer, which is commonly reported, is a relatively uninteresting measure, if figures on multiple pregnancy rate, prematurity rate, perinatal mortality, health of the children, and the like, are not given. The fight for enough patients to the program has sometimes driven our profession to unethical decisions. It should also be pointed out that it is not small IVF units that set the standard; rather, big centers with large programs and high impact factors do. A higher degree of facts reporting from these centers is therefore needed.

Hormonal Stimulation

The natural cycle was gradually replaced by gonadotrophin-stimulated cycles 20 years ago. GnRH agonists were introduced to avoid premature LH surges. This resulted in more convenient working hours as well as in an even higher number of mature oocytes, which then resulted in a higher number of embryos. Replacement of more embryos increased the pregnancy rate with the previously mentioned complications. Downregulation with GnRH agonists for prolonged periods of time (3–5 weeks) prior to stimulation with gonadotrophins probably helped the syncronization of the follicle cohorts and further suppressed circulating cytokines released by those such as active endometriosis.

The introduction of the GnRH antagonists gives a shorter protocol with less adverse effects for the patients, but it also limits some of the possibilities for the most aggressive ovarian stimulation regimes and reduces the number of oocytes.

Lowering of the length of gonadotrophin treatment and a reduction of the dose are other promising modifications of the simulation. Harvesting of immature oocytes and in vitro maturation (IVM) prior to fertilization is a relatively new exciting possibility (3,4).

Replacement

The replacement policy today has two problems: (1) how many embryos should be replaced? and (2) at what developmental stage should it (they) be replaced?

In northern Europe a maximum of two embryos per transfer is already general practice. Published guidelines from The American Society for Reproductive Medicine (ASRM) are more "liberal" in their recommendations, with an allowance of three embryo replacements in wide patients groups, and even four embryo replacements in certain groups. Compared with the Nordic countries in 1999 the United States still have 10 times more high-order multiple births.

In the beginning of year 2000 the Royal College of Obstetricians and Gynecologists (RCOG) published more restrictive guidelines for replacement of embryos, which partly agree to the Nordic guidelines. In the Nordic countries an increasing percentage of the transfers are now elective single embryo transfers (ESET) (5,6). With improved culture conditions utilizing sequential media the possibility has arisen to prolong culture in vitro for 4–6 days enabling replacement at a more "physiological" stage (7,8).

The morphological evaluation of blastocysts is superior to that of embryos in the four- to eight-cell stage, which means that a single embryo replaced at the blastocyst stage has an increased possibility to implant and develop normally.

Genetic Evaluation of Embryos

A high percentage of the embryos developed in vitro are genetically abnormal, even if they look normal utilizing the blunt morphological criteria. The improvement of the genetic technologies will shortly enable fast and low-cost multiple analyses on embryos cultured in vitro. Preimplantation genetic diagnosis (PGD) will most likely increase dramatically in the future and is probably a prerequisite for more successful elective single embryo transfers.

Freezing of Gametes and Embryos

Improved freezing programs utilizing vitrification in minute amounts of medium will increase the survival of both gametes and embryos of different stages of development. A safe and successful freezing program of gametes and blastocysts is, in fact, a prerequisite for a successful single-embryo replacement program (9,10).

Embryo Reduction

Various techniques for selective embryo reduction have been described. Both from a technical and psychological point of view, early embryo reduction in the eighth to ninth week of pregnancy seems preferable. In the Nordic countries more and more programs apply reduction from three to one performed by embryo aspiration in the eighth week. As mentioned earlier only two embryos are routinely replaced in the Nordic countries, which means that a triplet pregnancy will always be constituted of one pair of monozygotic twins. Because it is known that monocygotic twins run a high risk during pregnancy, the embryo reduction is focused on the twins.

So far, no clinical IVF programs, at least in Europe, run the policy of performing embryo reduction on a "normal" twin pregnancy, even if the survival for the remaining fetus is most likely improved. In many countries law restrictions concerning legal abortions will also make embryo reduction problematic from a legal point of view (11).

Conclusions

Today the multiple pregnancy rate is 8–10 times higher after IVF than after natural conception. This is an unacceptable difference that must be corrected as soon as possible if the society should regard the new developments in ART as acceptable and beneficial. The return to the natural cycle does not seem to be a likely scenario. A better combination and synchronization of the knowledge of COH, culture techniques, genetic analyses, freezing protocols, and embryo reduction will direct us toward the ultimate goal of beating nature in the interest of the infertile couples and their offspring (12) (Fig. 19.2).

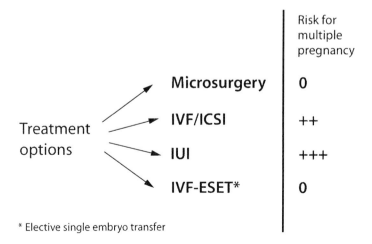

* Elective single embryo transfer

FIGURE 19.2. Infertility treatment options related to risk for multiple pregnancy.

References

1. Edwards RG, Steptoe PC. Current status of human in vitro fertilization and implantation of human embryos. Lancet 1983;2:1265–69.
2. Bergh T, Ericson A, Hillensjo T, Nygren KG, Wennerholm UB. Deliveries and children born after in-vitro fertilisation in Sweden 1982-95: a retrospective cohort study. Lancet 1999;6;354(9190):1579–85.
3. Mikkelsen AL, Smith S, Lindenberg S. Impact of oestradiol and inhibin A concentrations on pregnancies in in-vitro oocyte maturation. Hum Reprod 2000;15(8):1685–90.
4. Mikkelsen AL, Smith SD, Lindenberg S. In-vitro maturation of human oocytes from regularly menstruating women may be successful without follicle stimulating hormone priming. Hum Reprod 1999;14:1847–51.
5. Vilska S, Tiitinen A, Hyden-Granskog C, Hovatto O. Elective transfer of one embryo results in an acceptable p rate and eliminates the risk of multiple birth. Hum Reprod 1999;14(9):2392–95.
6. Gerris J, De Neubourg D, Mangelschots K, Van Royen E, Van de Meerssche, Valkenburg M. Prevention of twin pregnancy after in-vitro fertilization on intracytoplasmic sperm injection based on strict embryo criteria prospective randomized clinical trial. Hum Reprod 1999;14(10):2581–87.
7. Gardner DK, Vella P, Lane M, Wagley L, Schlenker T, Schoolcraft WB. Culture and transfer of human blastocysts increases implantation rates and reduces the need for multiple embryo transfers. Fertil Steril 1998;69:84–88.
8. Schoolcraft WB, Gardner DK, Lane M, Schenkler T, Hamilton F, Meldrum DR. Blastocyst culture and transfer: analysis of results and parameters affecting outcome in two in vitro fertilization programs. Fertil Steril 1999;72:604–9.
9. Kuleshova L, Gianaroli L, Magli C, Ferraretti A, Trounson A. Birth following vitrification of a small number of human oocytes: case report. Hum Reprod 1999;14(12):3077–79.
10. Lane M, Schoolcraft WB, Gardner DK. Vitrification of mouse and human blastocysts using a novel cryoloop container-less technique. Fertil Steril 1999;72:1073–78.
11. Hamberger L, Janson PO. Global importance of infertility and its treatment: role of fertility technologies. Int J Gynaecol Obstet 1997;58(1):149–58.
12. Hazekamp J, Bergh C, Wennerholm U, Hovatta O, Karlstrom PO, Selbing A. Avoiding multiple pregnancies in ART: consideration of new strategies. Hum Reprod 2000;15(6):1217–19.

20

The Niche of the Blastocyst in Human ART

JESSE HADE AND ALAN H. DECHERNEY

As assisted reproductive technology (ART) programs improve their success rate, the number of higher-order multiple pregnancies increases dramatically. Multifetal pregnancy is a concern both of patients undergoing ART as well as to physicians and healthcare insurers alike. High-order multiples increases maternal and neonatal morbidity and mortality. Maternal and fetal health as well as economic considerations are pressing issues of importance when the number of high-order multiples rise.

Aside from the risk associated with carrying multiple fetuses, the risk of hyperstimulation syndrome is likely to occur in women predisposed to having high-order multiples; however, the major problem is with the offspring. Many of these offspring have serious long-term sequelae, with neurologic and gastrointestinal being the primary impairment.

The press frequently clouds readers with schizophrenic jargon. On one hand they create headlines and advertisements marveling at the wonderment of having six or seven offspring at one time, and then simultaneously condemn the medical establishment for being irresponsible in this regard. They also confuse conceptions of higher-order multiple gestations achieved from ovulation induction with that of ART and IVF. In IVF containment of multiples is easier because the number of embryos transferred can be controlled.

IVF initially involved the transfer of Day 2 cleaving embryos into the uterus. Transfers were performed at Day 2 because the culture media used could not support a longer duration of growth. Bolton et al. were the first to describe blastocyst transfer after 5 days of embryo development in culture media (1). This idea was physiologically sound because cleaving embryos normally develop in the fallopian tube and only enter into the uterine cavity and prepares for implantation upon blastocyst formation.

It was not until the use of a co-culture technique that the development of high-quality blastocysts could be performed routinely and with good success (2). This technique, however, is so difficult and labor intensive that only a few labs could offer it routinely. The advent of sequential culture media, in which the culture media is changed to meet the varying metabolic requirements of developing embryos, has revolutionized the ease and accessibility of growing blastocysts. The rate of blastulation is comparable to that of the co-culture technique and is reported to be more than 40% (3–5).

Overall, the embryo implantation rate varies between 10% and 40% among the different ART centers. This variability in implantation is dependent on several factors, including embryo morphology at the time of transfer, maternal age at time of oocyte retrieval, and the quality of clinical treatment during embryo development (6,7). Because there is much variability in the rate of implantation the standard practice in most IVF clinics is to transfer multiple embryos during a single cycle. As a result, there is a high incidence of twins, triplets, and higher-order multiple pregnancies with this process (8).

Most studies to date indicate that the implantation and pregnancy rates for IVF can be improved with the use of an extended culture period. The advantage of this method includes the improved potential for assessing viable from nonviable embryos prior to embryo transfer.

Extended culture periods also allow for a more precise physiologic synchrony between the transferred embryos and the uterine environment. Diagnostic tests (e.g., preimplantation genetic screening) could be achieved with greater ease because more cells would be available for biopsy. This could theoretically reduce the miscarriage rate because chromosomally abnormal embryos tend to develop slower than healthier embryos and could ultimately be selectively removed from those embryos for transfer.

The incidence of multiple and high-order multiple gestation could be reduced because fewer embryos would be required per transfer. Because the implantation rate of each blastocyst can be more than 25% suggests that the transfer of only one embryo should be considered for certain individuals.

The advantage of a Day 5 embryo transfer over a Day 3 embryo transfer is the ability to assess and select the embryos with the best potential for implantation into the uterus. As a result, fewer embryos are transferred and the multiple pregnancy rates are lowered without altering the overall pregnancy rate.

An unfortunate problem to date is the inability to select a Day 3 embryo that is most likely to go on to form a blastocyst. On the other hand others have reported successful correlation with appearance of the blast and subsequent success rates. In August 1999, Dr. David Meldrum wrote an editorial in *Fertility and Sterility* that provided a proper conclusion to the question of the niche of the blastocyst in human ART. His editorial, entitled "Blastocyst Transfer—A Natural Evolution," concluded that high-order multiple gestations will be essentially eliminated when only two blastocysts are transferred back into the patients' uterus.

Studies regarding implantation with 5 days of embryo growth in extended culture appear to be conflicting. Those studies in which a single culture medium formulation was employed for the entire preimplantation period (9,10) observed little benefit from blastocyst transfer. In contrast, when sequential culture media were used, there was a significant increase in implantation rates following blastocyst transfer on Day 5 (55.4%) compared with cleavage-stage embryo transfer on Day 3 (37.0; $p < 0.01$) (4). These data highlight the significance of sequential media and the fact that blastocyst development in culture per se does not relate to subsequent viability.

Other factors that influence implantation include the age of the patient and the number of embryos available for transfer (11). For the most part, patients who have five or more embryos available for transfer will have at least one embryo develop into a blastocyst, resulting in an overall higher implantation rate.

Freezing embryos at the blastocyst stage is associated with a higher birth rate than that from freezing embryos at the early cleavage stage. A study by Gorrill et al. demonstrated that when embryos were frozen at either the 2 PN or cleaving stage Days 1–3 and then thawed and allowed to grow in culture for 5 days to the blastocyst stage, pregnancy rates of more than 66% were achieved. This method of thawing has a statistically significant implantation rate over embryos that are thawed and transferred on either Day 2 or 3 (12).

When embryo development is extended to 5 days of incubation in culture media and fresh blastocysts are transferred, there is significant trend to select male embryos over female embryos (13). This favoring of male embryos occurs as a result of quicker preimplantation development. Because male embryos reach the blastocyst stage sooner than do female embryos, male embryos are preferentially selected over female embryos for fresh transfer. When cryopreserved embryos are transferred, however, this difference in sex bias is eliminated.

It is unclear whether a blastocyst transfer is beneficial for women over 40 years of age or those with a poor prognosis for success with IVF. On average, embryos retrieved from women who are over 40 years of age have a 50% reduction in blastocyst formation than do embryos retrieved from younger women (14). Studies have demonstrated that these embryos from women over 40 have a progressive decline in blastocyst growth and expansion. This decline in blastocyst development is perhaps linked to the decline in fertility associated with advancing age (15). Despite the difficulty in achieving adequate blastocysts for transfer in an older population, favorable results can be achieved in some women (16).

One potential advantage of increased cancellation rates with blastocysts transfers includes a reduction in false expectations for couples with a poor prognosis. Women who are over 40 years old and do not produce any blastocysts during an IVF cycle should be counseled to consider pursuing IVF with donor eggs. Women in this population who attempt a blastocyst transfer have a cancellation rate that is more than twice that of a Day 3 transfer; however, this cancellation is still relatively low and is reported to be about 7% (17).

Containment, although unpopular, must be considered in all ART programs. Multifetal pregnancy is a problem that needs to be resolved. Blastocyst culture and transfer can help to reduce the number of embryos transferred and ultimately reduce and even eliminate the incidence of patients delivering high-order multiples.

Other techniques (e.g., GIFT and ZIFT) do not lend toward selectivity bias and do not offer a solution to reduce the incidence of multiples. Blastocyst transfers will ultimately limit the use of GIFT in ART programs because it can be a selective process that reduces the need to transfer multiple embryos into the uterus (18). A blastocyst transfer, therefore, is the best alternative for patients who seek greater security to prevent the conception and delivering of high-order multiples.

References

1. Bolton VN, Wren ME, Parsons JH. Pregnancies after in vitro fertilization and transfer of human blastocysts. Fertil Steril 1991;55:830–32.
2. Menezo YJR, Guerin JF, Czyba JC. Improvement of human early embryo development in vitro by coculture on monlayers of Vero cells. Biol Reprod 1990;42:301–6.
3. Gardner DK, Lane M. Culture and selection of viable blastocysts: a feasible proposition for human IVF? Hum Reprod Update 1997;3:367–82.
4. Gardner DK, Schoolcraft WB, Wagley L, Schlenker T, Stevens J, Hesla J. A prospective randomized trial of blastocyst culture and transfer in in-vitro fertilization. Hum Reprod 1998;13:3434–40.
5. Milki AA, Fisch JD, Behr B. Two-blastocyst transfer has similar pregnancy rates and a decreased multiple gestation rate compared with three-blastocyst transfer. Fertil Steril 1999;72:225–28.
6. Steer C, Mills C, Tan S, Campbell S, Edwards RG. The cumulative embryo score: a predictive embryo scoring technique to select the optimal number of embryos to transfer in an in-vitro fertilization and embryo transfer program. Hum Reprod 1992;7:117–19.
7. Navot D, Bergh P, Williams MA, Garrisi GJ, Guzman I, Sandler B, et al. Poor oocyte quality rather than implantation failure as a cause of age related decline in female fertility. Lancet 1991;337:1375–77.
8. Staessen C, Camus M, Bollen N, Devroey P, Van Steirteghem AC. The relationship between embryo quality, and the occurrence of multiple pregnancies. Fertil Steril 1992;57:626–30.
9. Scholtes MCW, Zeilmaker GH. A prospective, randomized study of embryo transfer results after 3 or 5 days of embryo culture in in-vitro fertilization. Fertil Steril 1996;65:1245–48.
10. Huisman GJ, Fauser B, Eijkemans M, Pieters M. Implantation rates after in vitro fertilization and transfer of a maximum of two embryos that have undergone three to five days of culture. Fertil Steril 2000;73:117–22.
11. Murdoch AP. How many embryos should be transferred? Hum Reprod 1998;13:2666–69.
12. Gorrill MJ, Kaplan PF, Patton PE, Burry KA. Initial experience with extended culture and blastocyst transfer of cryopreserved embryos. Am J Obstet Gynecol 1999;180:1472–74.
13. Menezo Y, Chouteau J, Torello MJ, Girard A, Veiga A. Birth weight and sex ratio after transfer at the blastocyst stage in humans. Fertil Steril 1999;72:221–24.
14. Pantos K, Athanasiou V, Stefanidis K, Stavrou D, Vaxevanoglou T, Chronopolou M. Influence of advanced age on the blastocyst development rate and pregnancy rate in assisted reproductive technology. Fertil Steril 1999;71:1144–46.

15. Janny L, Menezo YSR. Maternal age effect on early human embryonic development and blastocyst formation. Mol Reprod Dev 1996;45:31–37.
16. Alves da Motta EL, Alegretti JR, Baracat EC, Olive D, Serafini PC. High implantation and pregnancy rates with transfer of human blastocysts developed in preimplantation stage one and blastocyst media. Fertil Steril 1998;70:659–63.
17. Marek D, Langley M, Gardner D, Confer N, Doody KM, Doody KJ. Introduction of blastocyst culture and transfer for all patients in an in vitro fertilization program. Fertil Steril 1999;72:1035–40.
18. Meldrum DR. Blastocyst transfer—a natural evolution. Fertil Steril 1999;72:216–17.

Author Index

B

Bentin-Ley, Ursula, 227–235
Bizzaro, Davide, 38–48

C

Cekleniak, Natalie A., 155–163
Collins, Jane E., 91–102

D

DeCherney, Alan H., 241–245
de Pablo, Jose Louis, 199–209
Destouni, Aspasia, 91–102
Donnay, Isabelle, 61–68
Doody, Kevin, 167–183

E

Eckert, Judith, 91–102

F

Fleming, Tom P., 91–102

G

Galán, Arancha, 199–209

Gardner, David K., 69–90, 118–143
Ghassemifar, M. Reza, 91–102

H

Hade, Jesse, 241–245
Hamberger, Lars, 236–240
Hardy, Kate, 144–154
Houghton, Franchesca D., 61–68

J

Jackson, Katharine V., 155–163
Jones, Howard W. Jr., 3–20

L

Lane, Michelle, 69–90, 118–143
Leese, Henry J., 61–68
Lessey, Bruce A., 210–226

M

Macmillan, Donald A., 61–68
Manicardi, GianCarlo, 38–48
Martin, Julio C., 199–209
Meldrum, David R., 21–28

Menezo, Yves, 188–195
Meseguer, Marcos, 199–209
Moffatt, Odette, 38–48

N

Nikas, George, 227–235

P

Pellicer, Antonio, 199–209
Pierson, Roger A., 29–37
Pool, Thomas B., 105–117

R

Racowsky, Catherine, 155–163

S

Sakkas, Denny, 38–48, 188–195

Schoolcraft, William B., 118–143, 184–187
Schnorr, John A., 3–20
Sheth, Bhavwanti, 91–102
Simón, Carlos, 199–209
Spanos, Sophie, 144–154
Svalander, Peter, 236–240

T

Tasca, Richard J., 51–60
Thomas, Fay, 91–102
Tomlinson, Mathew, 38–48

V

Veiga, Anna, 188–195

W

Wikland, Matts, 236–240

Subject Index

Acquaporins, 57
Adhesion phase, 201–202
Agarose, 110–111
Albumins, and macromolecules, 107–109
American College of Obstetricians and Gynecologists (ACOG), 17
American Society of Reproductive Medicine (ASRM), 16
Amino acid transport (AAT), and preimplantation development, 53–57
   acquaporins, 57
   and mouse PE, 55–56
   Na$^+$ dependent AAT in blastocysts, 54
   NA$^+$/H$^+$ Exchanger 3 (NHE3), 57
   NA$^+$/K$^+$ ATPase (NKA), 56–57
   systems, characterization of, 54–55
Apoptosis, and human preimplantation embryo, 145–151, 200
   cell death genes, 147
   chromatin condensation and nuclear fragmentation, 146
   cytoplasmic fragmentation, 146–147
   DNA fragmentation, 146
   morphological features, 145
   observations of, 145–146
   and protein families, 145
   signals, intra- and extracellular, 145
   and survival factors, 147–151
      growth factors, 147–148
      and IGF-I, 149–151
   timing of, 147
Apposition phase, 201
Artificial ovulation induction, 8
Assisted reproductive technologies (ART), 8–9
   and gonadotropin-releasing hormone (GnRH) agonists, 23–25
      advantages of, 23–24
      future protocols, 24–25
      regimens, 24
   benefits for ART, 21
   and multiple-pregnancy statistics, 12–13
   success rate, improvement of, 241
   See also Blastocyst development; Gonadotropin-releasing hormone (GnRH) agonists
ATP:ADP ratio, 80–81

Biomarkers, 210. *See also* Uterine receptivity
Blastocyst development, 241–244
   as a model system, 67
   morphology of, 160
   protection of in vitro, 114–115
   See also Apoptosis; Blastocyst transfer, patient selection for; Cell junctions and interactions; Cryopreservation of blastocysts; Culture systems, and blastocyst

Blastocyst development (*cont.*)
  development; Human blastocysts; Macromolecules
Blastocyst transfer, patient selection for, 167–182
  general, 174
  good prognosis patients
    determined by cleavage stage parameters, 172
    determined by combination criteria, 171–173
    determined by postinsemination parameters, 171
    determined by preretrieval parameters, 169–170
    determined by retrieval parameters, 170–171
  poor prognosis patients, 173–174
  strategies for, 169
Blastomere homeostasis, 69–85. *See also* Embryo metabolism; Intracellular calcium; Intracellular pH; IVF laboratory and cellular homeostasis

Carbohydrates
  concentration of in human oviduct and uterus, 119
  uptake by embryo, 121
Cavitation, 51
Cell adhesion molecules, 215
Cell biology of preimplantation development, 51–58
Cell death genes, 147
Cell junctions and interactions in blastocyst development, 91–100
  cell-cell interactions, 98–99
  demosomes, 97
  E-cadherin adhesion and compaction, 92–93
  and human embryos, 99–100
  junctions
    gap, 93–94
    tight, 94–96
Chromatin condensation and nuclear fragmentation, 146
Clomiphene citrate, 33
Compaction, 51
Confocal microscopy, 202–203

Controlled ovarian hypterstimulation (COH), 236
Cryopreservation of blastocysts, 75–76, 84–85, 188–194
  background, 188–189
  and birthweights, 192
  cryoprotectants, 190
  freezing protocols, 189–190
    preparation for, 190
    thawing, 190, 191
  implantation rates, comparison of, 192
  results of, 190–193
  and sex ratios, 192
Culture systems, and blastocyst development, 118–138
  cytoplasmic fragmentation, 146–147
  gas phase, 124
  incubation volume:embryo ratio, 120–126
  macromolecules, 126–129
  media, 121–123
  multiple gestation, high-order, elimination of, 115
  success, importance of, 167–169
  transfer, clinical experiences with, 129–133
  and single embryo, 133–138
  See also Nonselective blastocyst culture
Cytokines, 216–217
Cytoplasmic fragmentation, 146–147

Demosomes, 97
Dextrain, 109–110
Developmental plasticity, 105
DNA fragmentation, 146
DNA strand breaks, detection of, 203

E-cadherin adhesion and compaction, 92–93
EEC apoptosis studies, embryonic induction in adhesion phase, 206–207
EEC apoptosis studies, embryonic induction during apposition phase, 206

Subject Index 251

Embryo, interactions with macromolecules in vivo, 111–114
  estrogen-dependent oviduct glycoproteins, 112–113
  mucus glycoproteins, 113–114
Embryo, metabolism of, 61, 78–83
  ATP:ADP ratio, 80–81
  blastocyst, as a model system, 67
  culture, effect of, 79–80
  energy
    production of, 61–62
    utilization of, 62–64
  oxygen consumption, measurements of, 66–67
  protein synthesis, cost of, 64–66
  redox potential, 82–83
  regulation by ionic homeostasis, 81–82
  See also Culture systems, and blastocyst development; Energy metabolism
Embryo, feezing of, 238
Embryo attachment sites
  LM/TEM of, 231–232
  SEM of, 230–231
Embryo-endometrial interactions, 211–212
Embryo implantation, apposition and adhesion phases, 199–208
  methods and materials, 200–202
    adhesion phase, 201–202
    apposition phase, 201
    confocal microscopy, 202–203
    endometrial culture, 200–201
    flow cytometry, 202
  See also Endometrial pinopodes; Northern blot analysis
Embryo implantation, cleavage-stage, 118–120
  concerns, 119–120
  See also Culture systems, and blastocyst development
Embryo-maternal dialogue, 199–208.
  See also Embryo implantation, apposition and adhesion phases
Embryo transfer success, 184–194
  clinical experiences with, 129–133
  and single embryo, 133–138

luteal support for in vitro fertilization, 186–187
ultrasound, use of, 185–186
variables affecting, 184–185
See also Single embryo transfer
Endometrial culture, 200–201
Endometrial/epithelial MUC1 mRNA, embryonic regulation
  during adhesion phase, 206
  at apposition phase, 204–205
  hormonal regulation of, 204
Endometrial pinopodes, 217–218, 227–233
  apical plasma membranes, 232
  detection of, 232
  during in vitro interactions, 230–232
  embryo attachment sites
    LM/TEM of, 231–232
    SEM of, 230–231
  formation of, 228
  scanning electron microscopy, 227–231
Endometrial surface epithelium, 227–230
  animal studies, 227–228
  human studies, 228–230
Energy metabolism, 62–67
  oxygen consumption measurements, 66–67
  protein synthesis, cost of, 64–66
Estrogen-dependent oviduct glycoproteins, 112–113
Exogenous gonadotropins, 33–35

Fertility-enhancing drugs, 8–9
Flow cytometry, 202–203
Follicular development, mathematical modeling of, 35–36
Folliculogenesis, 31–32
Freezing protocols, 189–190
  preparation for, 190
  thawing, 190, 191

Gamete, freezing of, 238
Gamete intrafallopian transfer (GIFT), 8
Gene expression, regulation of, 52–53

Glycolytic activity, as a biochemical marker, 136
Gonadotropin-releasing hormone (GnRH) agonists, 21–23
  and ART, 23–25
    advantages of, 23–24
    future protocols, 24–25
    regimens, 24
  benefits for ART, 21
  hormonal stimulation, 237–238
  oral contraception pretreatment, 22
  ovarian stimulation
    excessive, 23
    and luteinizing hormone (LH), 23
  regimens, 21–22
Growth factors, 216–217

Human blastocysts
  cycle predictors, 156–158
    age of patient, 158
    eight-cell embryo on day 3, 157–158
    ICSI, adverse impact on viability, 158
  embryo predictors of, 159–160
    day 3 morphological characteristics, 159–160
  metabolite production, quantification of, 136
  nutrient consumption, quantification of, 136
  scoring system, 133–136
  viability of, 155–161
Hyaluronan, 110

Incubation volume, and embryo grouping, 120–126, 124–126
Integrins, 214–216
International Federation of Fertility Societies (IFFS), 13–14
Intracellular calcium, 77–78
  channels, 78
  culture, effect of, 77–78
  magnesium, role of, 78
Intracellular pH, 69–78
  buffering capacity
    external, 71
    intrinsic, 70–71
  cumulus cells, 74

  and cryopreserved embryos, 75–76
  embryo metabolism, control of, 75
  and fertilization, 72–74
  HCO_3^-/Cl^- exchanger, 72
  levels of, 69–70
  Na^+/H^+ antiporter, 72
  pHi
    and embryo development, 74–75
    regulation of, 70
  transport proteins, 72
  See also Cryopreservation of blastocysts
Intracytoplasmic sperm injection (ICSI), 39
In vitro fertilization (IVF)
  and sequential culture media, 129–130
  effects on multiple-pregnancy statistics, 13
Ionic homeostasis, regulation of energy by, 81–82
IVG laboratory, and cellular homeostatis, 83–85
  cryopreservation, 84–85
  ICSI, 84

Junctions
  gap, 93–94
  tight, 94–96

Low birth weight infants, 4–5
Luteal phase deficiency (LPD), 212–213
Luteal phase support, and embryo transfer, 184–181, 186–187
Luteinizing hormone (LH), and ovarian stimulation, 23, 34–35

Male germ cells, 38–39
Macromolecules, 105–106
  albumins, use of, 107–109
  blastocysts, protection of in vitro, 114–115
  and embryo, interactions in vivo, 111–114
    estrogen-dependent oviduct glycoproteins, 112–113

mucus glycoproteins, 113–114
and embryo growth, 112–113
plasma proteins, use of, 107–109
protein supplementation, alternatives to, 109–111
  agarose, 110–111
  dextrain, 109–110
  hyaluronan, 110
  polyvinylalcohol, 109
whole serum supplement, 106–107
Mathematical modeling of follicular development, 35–36
Metabolite production, quantification of, 136
  gene expression, regulation of, 52–53
Mitochondria and nucleolus, changes in, 52
Mortality rates, 5, 7
Mucins, 199–200, 216
Mucus glycoproteins, 113–114
Multiple births, cost of, 5–7
  fetus, risks to, 5–6
  mortality, increase in, 7
  mother, risks to, 5
Multiple births, trends in, 3–5
  age of mother, 5
  fertility enhancing therapies, 5
  geographical variations, 4
  low birth weight infants, 4–5
  mortality rate, 5
  statistics, 3–4
Multiple gestation,
  cause of, 8–9
  high-order, elimination of, 115
Multiple pregnancies, high-order, attempted solutions to, 12–14
  American Society of Reproductive Medicine (ASRM), 16
  families, quality of life, 236–237
  International Federation of Fertility Societies (IFFS), 13–14
  surveillance, failure of, 14–16

Na^+ dependent AAT in blastocysts, 54
NA^+/H^+ Exchanger 3 (NHE3), 57
NA^+/K^+ ATPase (NKA), 56–57
Nonselective blastocyst culture, 174-182
  advantages, 175
  disadvantages, 175-176, 182
Northern blot analysis, 203-204
  results of, 204-207
    EEC apoptosis studies, embryonic induction in adhesion phase, 206–207
    EEC apoptosis studies, embryonic induction during apposition phase, 206
    endometrial/epithelial MUC1 mRNA, embryonic regulation during adhesion phase, 206
    endometrial/epithelial MUC1 mRNA, embryonic regulation of at apposition phase, 204–205
    endometrial MUC1 mRNA, hormonal regulation of, 204
    TUNEL studies, 203–204
Nutrient consumption, quantification of, 136

Oocytes
  and DNA-damaged spermatozoa, 43–45
  and donors, 132–133
  high-quality, importance of, 36
Ovaries
  imaging of, 29–32
    folliculogenesis, 31–32
    magnetic resonance imaging, 35
    radioimmunoassay techniques, 29
    three-dimensional, 31
    ultrasonic image analysis, 30–31
  hormonal control of, 32
  oral contraceptives, 32–33
  stimulation of, 23
  See also Superstimulation of ovaries

Paternal influences on embryo development
  male germ cells, effects of radiation on, 38–39
  semen parameters, abnormal, 39–40
  sperm nuclear DNA damage, 42–43
  sperm nucleus, abnormal
    embryo development, effects on, 41–42
    fertilization, effects on, 40–41

Subject Index

Peptide hormones, 214–218
  cytokines, 216–217
  growth factors, 216–217
  integrins, 214–216
  pinopods, 217–218
  secreted proteins, 216–217
  transcription factors, 217
pHi
  and embryo development, 74–75
  regulation of, 70
Plasma protein fractions, 107–109
Polyvinylalcohol, 109
Pregnancy rates, actual versus theoretical, 9–12
Preimplantation development (PD), 51–58
  amino acid transport (AAT), 53–57
  gene expression, regulation of, 52–53
  mitochondria and nucleolus, changes in, 52
  See also Amino acid transport (AAT)
Pronucleate embryos, and number of blastocysts, 130–131
Protein synthesis, cost of, 64–66

Redox potential, 82–83
Replacement policy, 238

Secreted proteins, 216–217
Semen parameters, 39–40
Serum albumin, 126–127
Single embryo transfer
  clinical experiences with, 133–138
  embryo reduction, 239
  freezing of gametes and embryos, 238
  genetic evaluation, 238
  hormonal stimulation, 237–238
  replacement policy, 238

Spermatozoon, role of, 38
Sperm nuclear DNA damage, 42–43
Sperm nucleus, 40–42
Superstimulation of ovaries, 33–35
  clomiphene citrate, 33
  exogenous gonadotropins, 33–35

Transcription factors, 217
TUNEL
  DNA strand breaks, detection of, 203
  and FCM analysis, 203–204
  labeling, 147

Uterine physiology, and cryobiology, 194
Uterine receptivity, and biomarkers, 210–219
  embryo-endometrial interactions, 211–212
  and infertility, 218–219
  occult defects, 218–219
  ovarian steroids, 213–214
  peptide hormones, 214–218
    cytokines, 216–217
    growth factors, 216–217
    integrins, 214–216
    pinopods, 217–218
    secreted proteins, 216–217
    transcription factors, 217
  See also Endometrial pinopods
Voluntary guidelines
  American College of Obstetricians and Gynecologists (ACOG), 17
  failure of in U.S., 16
  Voluntary Licensing Authority (VLA) of Great Britain, 16–17

Whole serum, and macromolecules, 106–107

PROCEEDINGS IN THE SERONO SYMPOSIA USA SERIES

Continued from page ii

BOVINE SPONGIFORM ENCEPHALOPATHY: The BSE Dilemma
 Edited by Clarence J. Gibbs, Jr.

GROWTH HORMONE SECRETAGOGUES
 Edited by Barry B. Bercu and Richard F. Walker

CELLULAR AND MOLECULAR REGULATION OF TESTICULAR CELLS
 Edited by Claude Desjardins

GENETIC MODELS OF IMMUNE AND INFLAMMATORY DISEASES
 Edited by Abul K. Abbas and Richard A. Flavell

MOLECULAR AND CELLULAR ASPECTS OF PERIIMPLANTATION PROCESSES
 Edited by S.K. Dey

THE SOMATOTROPHIC AXIS AND THE REPRODUCTIVE PROCESS IN HEALTH AND DISEASE
 Edited by Eli Y. Adashi and Michael O. Thorner

GHRH, GH, AND IGF-I: Basic and Clinical Advances
 Edited by Marc R. Blackman, S. Mitchell Harman, Jesse Roth, and Jay R. Shapiro

IMMUNOBIOLOGY OF REPRODUCTION
 Edited by Joan S. Hunt

FUNCTION OF SOMATIC CELLS IN THE TESTIS
 Edited by Andrzej Bartke

GLYCOPROTEIN HORMONES: Structure, Function, and Clinical Implications
 Edited by Joyce W. Lustbader, David Puett, and Raymond W. Ruddon

GROWTH HORMONE II: Basic and Clinical Aspects
 Edited by Barry B. Bercu and Richard F. Walker

TROPHOBLAST CELLS: Pathways for Maternal-Embryonic Communication
 Edited by Michael J. Soares, Stuart Handwerger, and Frank Talamantes

IN VITRO FERTILIZATION AND EMBRYO TRANSFER IN PRIMATES
 Edited by Don P. Wolf, Richard L. Stouffer, and Robert M. Brenner

OVARIAN CELL INTERACTIONS: Genes to Physiology
 Edited by Aaron J.W. Hsueh and David W. Schomberg

CELL BIOLOGY AND BIOTECHNOLOGY: Novel Approaches to Increased Cellular Productivity
 Edited by Melvin S. Oka and Randall G. Rupp

PREIMPLANTATION EMBRYO DEVELOPMENT
 Edited by Barry D. Bavister

PROCEEDINGS IN THE SERONO SYMPOSIA USA SERIES

(Continued)

MOLECULAR BASIS OF REPRODUCTIVE ENDOCRINOLOGY
  Edited by Peter C.K. Leung, Aaron J.W. Hsueh, and Henry G. Friesen

MODES OF ACTION OF GnRH AND GnRH ANALOGS
  Edited by William F. Crowley, Jr., and P. Michael Conn

FOLLICLE STIMULATING HORMONE: *Regulation of Secretion and Molecular Mechanisms of Action*
  Edited by Mary Hunzicker-Dunn and Neena B. Schwartz

SIGNALING MECHANISMS AND GENE EXPRESSION IN THE OVARY
  Edited by Geula Gibori

GROWTH FACTORS IN REPRODUCTION
  Edited by David W. Schomberg

UTERINE CONTRACTILITY: *Mechanisms of Control*
  Edited by Robert E. Garfield

NEUROENDOCRINE REGULATION OF REPRODUCTION
  Edited by Samuel S.C. Yen and Wylie W. Vale

FERTILIZATION IN MAMMALS
  Edited by Barry D. Bavister, Jim Cummins, and Eduardo R.S. Roldan

GAMETE PHYSIOLOGY
  Edited by Ricardo H. Asch, Jose P. Balmaceda, and Ian Johnston

GLYCOPROTEIN HORMONES: *Structure, Synthesis, and Biologic Function*
  Edited by William W. Chin and Irving Boime

THE MENOPAUSE: *Biological and Clinical Consequences of Ovarian Failure: Evaluation and Management*
  Edited by Stanley G. Korenman

ISBN 0-387-95245-4